N. Friedel, R. Hetzer, D. Royston (Eds.)

Blood Use in Cardiac Surgery

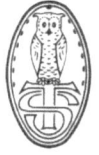 Springer-Verlag Berlin Heidelberg GmbH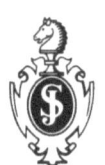

The Editors:
Dr. N. Friedel
Prof. Dr. R. Hetzer
Deutsches Herzzentrum Berlin
Augustenburger Platz 1
1000 Berlin 65, FRG

Dr. D. Royston
Harefield Hospital
Hill End Road
Harefield
Middlesex
UB9 6JH

CIP-Titelaufnahme der Deutschen Bibliothek

Blood use in cardiac surgery / N. Friedel . . . (eds.). — Darmstadt
: Steinkopff; New York: Springer, 1991

NE: Friedel, Norbert [Hrsg.]

ISBN 978-3-662-06121-3   ISBN 978-3-662-06119-0 (eBook)
DOI 10.1007/978-3-662-06119-0

Copyright © 1991 by Springer-Verlag Berlin Heidelberg
Originally published by Dietrich Steinkopff Verlag GmbH & Co. KG, Darmstadt in 1991.
Softcover reprint of the hardcover 1st edition 1991

Medical Editorial: Sabine Müller — English Editor: James C. Willis — Production: Heinz J. Schäfer

Foreword

Cardiac surgery has developed dramatically since the first open-heart operations were performed in the mid 1950s. Although the improvement of surgical technique, extracorporeal circulation, and postoperative management has contributed to a marked reduction of morbidity and mortality, the development of cardiac surgery to its present state would not have been possible without blood substitution by homologous donor blood.

Only 20 years ago, open-heart operations required an average of 8 units of blood preserves. The excessive need of donor blood in those early days was mainly due to premature surgical technique, insecure control of anticoagulation, severe blood trauma by extracorporeal circulation, and the lack of retransfusion technologies that would have allowed the reuse of shed mediastinal blood.

The introduction of new technologies, such as normovolemic hemodilution, intraoperative autotransfusion, postoperative return of shed mediastinal blood, and predonation of autologous blood has greatly reduced donor blood requirements. At present the majority of routine coronary artery surgical procedures can be performed without any blood transfusion. Blood loss, however, may be considerable in patients undergoing complex valve surgery or reoperations, as they often require several units of transfused blood.

Blood conservation has now become an area of major interest for the cardiac surgeon. This increased concern is caused by infectious complications of blood transfusion, in particular hepatitis and, more recently, AIDS.

In the Federal Republic of Germany, posttransfusion hepatitis is reported to develop in approximately 3.8% of patients. Of these, Non A-Non B hepatitis is found in more than 90%. This may be due to the fact that a specific assay for the detection of NANB hepatitis is not available in routine donor screening. In contrast, rigorous donor examination resulted in drastically lowering the risk of contracting hepatitis B. The potential risk of contracting AIDS through blood preserves led to increased public concern. However, since HIV-antibody testing of blood donors began in 1985, the risk of contracting AIDS from blood transfusion is estimated to be only 1 in 250 000. The deleterious effects of blood transfusion have prompted increased efforts to reduce blood loss and the accompanying need for transfusion.

The international conference on "Blood Use In Cardiac Surgery" aimed at reviewing the current state of blood-loss reduction and blood transfusion in open-heart surgery, and at highlighting the problems which remain in this field. Furthermore, it offered discussions of future perspectives and therapies towards "blood-free" cardiac surgery in the 1990s.

The meeting focused on two aspects: The first concern was how to minimize·the risk of transfusion-related infections by improving the quality of blood products, including a better donor selection together with improved methods of blood preservation. Attention was also drawn to predonation programs, which have led to a reduction of blood replacement, but have not yet succeeded in avoiding homologous blood transfusions in the majority of patients.

The second concern was the reduction of blood loss during and after surgery by non-pharmacological and pharmacological intervention. One of the prerequisites for reducing blood loss is the better understanding of pathomechanisms of hematological injury associated with the use of extracorporeal circulation. Other important factors contributing to blood-loss reduction may be the improvement of surgical techniques, the use of fibrin glue, and the retransfusion of shed blood.

Certain pharmacological agents, such as desmopressin and dipyridamole, have been used with some success in reducing postoperative bleeding. However, none of these agents was able to entirely eliminate the need for bank blood.

Since the early 1970s, there has been considerable interest in the antiprotease aprotinin for prevention or reduction of the inflammatory response to tissue injuries of various origins. More recently, aprotinin has also been used to reduce bleeding after open-heart surgery. The high-dose regimen, primarily suggested by Royston and colleagues in 1987, has now been proven to significantly diminish blood loss and postoperative use of blood. As a result of this effect, it could be demonstrated that 70% of treated patients did not require any blood transfusion. Aprotinin was also effective in patients with reoperations or patients under aspirin therapy prior to operation. These data suggest that routine use of aprotinin appears to offer considerable potential for a pharmacological intervention that makes heart surgery less of a risk.

Although it is understood that open-heart surgery cannot be carried out completely without the use of donor blood in the new future, the aim of the symposium and of this volume was to achieve a consensus from an international group of leading clinicians and researchers for improving and further developing present blood-saving measures in order to minimize blood loss and the risk of blood transfusion in the 1990s.

Contents

III: Non-Pharmacological Methods for the Reduction of Blood Use in Cardiac Surgery

IV. Pharmacological Methods for the Reduction of Blood Use in Cardiac Surgery

V. Panel Discussion

I. Pathomechanism of Defective Hemostasis During and After Extracorporeal Circulation

Fibrinolysis

F. Bachmann and P. Parise

Laboratoire Central d'Hématologie, Centre Hospitalier Universitaire Vaudois, Lausanne, Suisse

The activity of the fibrinolytic system is regulated by activators and inhibitors. The inactive zymogen plasminogen, upon activation by the tissue-type plasminogen activator (t-PA) or by the urinary-type plasminogen activator (u-PA or urokinase) is converted to plasmin, a protease which degrades fibrin into soluble fibrin degradation products (Fig. 1). t-PA is synthesized by endothelial cells and is continuously released into the blood stream; its release can be considerably enhanced by many agents, acidosis and hypoxia [1]. In human blood, t-PA exists in two forms: in a free, single-chain form (sct-PA) and in an inactive form bound to the plasminogen activator inhibitor type 1 (PAI-1). Small amounts of plasmin convert sct-PA to two-chain t-PA (tct-PA). The other PA, u-PA, exists in human blood as a true inactive zymogen in single-chain form (scu-PA or pro-urokinase). It can be converted to the active two-chain form (tcu-PA; urokinase) by trace amounts of plasmin or of kallikrein. Beside PAI-1 which inhibits both forms of t-PA and urokinase (but not pro-urokinase) another inhibitor, α_2-antiplasmin, rapidly inactivates free plasmin.

Increased fibrinolytic activity is commonly observed during extracorporeal circulation, as is evidenced by shortening of the euglobulin lysis time, of the dilute whole blood clot lysis time, and of increased levels of fibrin and fibrinogen breakdown products [2, 10, 11, 17]. The generation of these breakdown products is supressed by treatment with high doses of aprotinin [19].

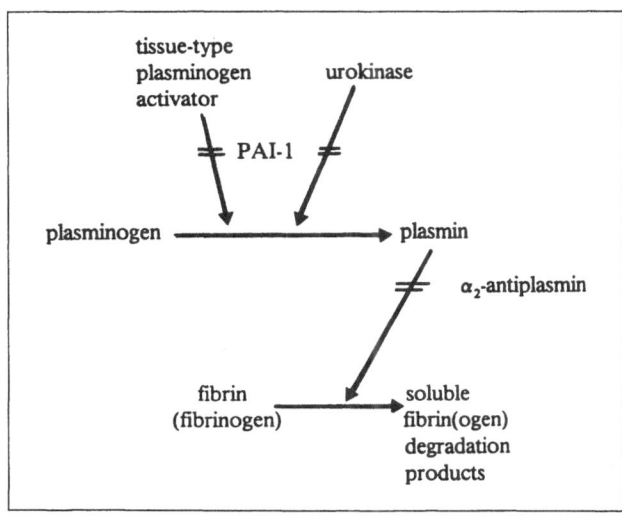

Fig. 1. The fibrinolytic system simplified. PAI-1: plasminogen activator inhibitor type 1.

Table 1 illustrates the pathways that could lead to an increase of fibrinolysis during extracoporeal circulation. Firstly, the contact of blood with a large artificial surface leads to the activation of the contact phase of coagulation and generation of kallikrein. Kallikrein might then convert the inactive zymogen pro-urokinase into urokinase [9]. (This is further discussed in this volume in the contribution of Kluft) Secondly, several hormone enzymes, and other physiological mediators are present in increased concentrations in the blood during extracorporeal circulation. Many of these are capable of stimulating the release of t-PA from endothelial cells [1]. Thirdly, leucocyte proteases, which are released during extracorporeal circulation, are able to degrade fibrin and fibrinogen [7, 23].

What are the consequences when the contact phase system is activated? When the blood coagulation factor XII binds to a negatively charged surface (tubing, membranes) it changes its configuration and becomes autoactivated. The activated form, FXIIa, then triggers a whole series of biochemical events (Fig. 2). It can directly activate the complement system, particularly C1 (8). However, this is probably not a major pathway of the action of FXIIa since the levels of the complement fractions C3a and C4a are hardly elevated in extracorporeal circulation. FXIIa, together with high molecular weight kininogen, brings about the activation of prekallikrein to kallikrein. Kallikrein is an important intermediary product for the activation of the intrinsic coagulation system, t-PA release from endothelium and the conversion of pro-urokinase to urokinase (Fig. 2). There is during extracorporeal circulation, some thrombin formation, as evidenced by the increase of thrombin-antithrombin complexes (TAT) during extracorporeal circulation [5]. This pathway is inhibited to a large extent by heparin which is routinely given during ECC. Kallikrein proteolytically cleaves high molecular weight kininogen which results in the release of the

Table 1. Pathways that could lead to increase of fibrinolysis during ECC.

1) Activation of the contact phase of coagulation;
2) Tissue-type plasminogen activator (t-PA) release;
3) Release of leucocyte proteases.

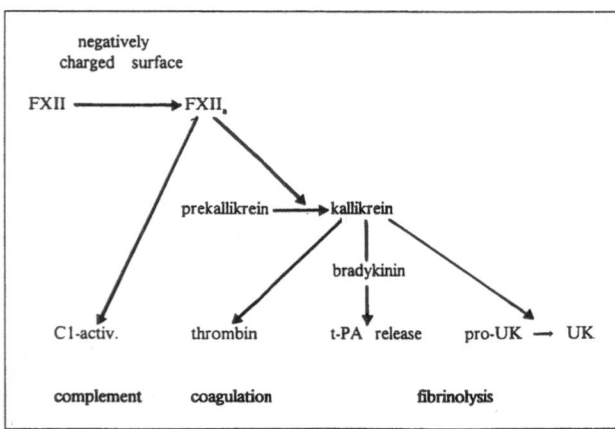

Fig. 2. Consequences of activation of the contact phase of coagulation.

nonapeptide bradykinin. The latter is one of the strongest stimulators of t-PA release. As we have recently shown, kallikrein is also a very efficient enzyme to convert the proenzyme pro-urokinase (scu-PA) into the active enzyme urokinase (tcu-PA) [9]. Trasylol, besides being a kallikrein inhibitor at low doses is also an efficient inhibitor of plasmin [21] and of urokinase [12] at the doses now being used in extracorporeal circulation.

In vivo there is little increase during extracorporeal circulation in the plasma levels of complexes of C1, the first component of the complement system with its inhibitors. This may be due, in part, to the rapid removal of such complexes from the circulation. The group of Colman and collaborators have therefore performed simulated extracorporeal circulation experiments in which blood is circulated in an ECC system not connected to a patient [22]. Under these conditions complexes form between the C1 inhibitor and both activated complement 1 and kallikrein. These experiments then provide evidence that during extracorporeal circulation some complement as well as kallikrein are activated. On the other hand, complexes between plasmin and α_2-antiplasmin were not elevated during simulated extracorporeal circulation [22].

t-PA is released by many different pharmacological agents and physiological stimuli (reviewed in [1]), and during extracorporeal circulation many of these may be operative (Table 2). Thrombin and bradykinin are stimulators of t-PA release: epinephrine and angiotensin levels may be increased. Leukotrienes, generated by activated platelets and leukocytes during extracorporeal circulation, will also release t-PA. Lastly, anoxia should not be completely left out of our consideration.

During extracorporeal circulation a marked shortening of the euglobulin lysis time occurs [11, 17]. If this activity is assayed on fibrin plates in the presence of an inhibitor which does not block the activity of t-PA, about one-third of the fibrinolytic activity is quenched. The remaining activity can be completely blocked with anti-t-PA antibodies [17]. We may thus assume that approximately two-thirds of the fibrinolytic activity generated during extracorporeal circulation is due to t-PA, but that there is some other activity which might well be urokinase. The fibrinolytic activity rapidly disappears at the end of extracorporeal circulation. The disappearance rate approximates that of t-PA, which has a half life of a few minutes.

If there is indeed an increased concentration of plasminogen activators and generation of plasmin during extracorporeal circulation, what are the biological markers of plasmin action? Plasmin converts single- chain t-PA and u-PA to their two-chain forms, releases fibrinopeptide from fibrinogen and forms complexes with its primary inhibitor, α_2-antiplasmin. Free plasmin degrades fibrin, fibrinogen, factor V, factor VIII, von Willebrand factor, and certainly also platelet glycoproteins (Fig. 3).

However, the increase of fibrin(ogen) degradation products and the partial destruction of other coagulation factors and of platelet glycoproteins may not only be

Table 2. Release of t-PA during EEC.

Agents and conditions that are known to release t-PA:	
Bradykinin	Leukotrienes (LTC$_4$, LTD$_4$)
Thrombin	Histamine
Epinephrine	Paf-acether (PAF)
Angiotensin II	Anoxia
Vasopressin	

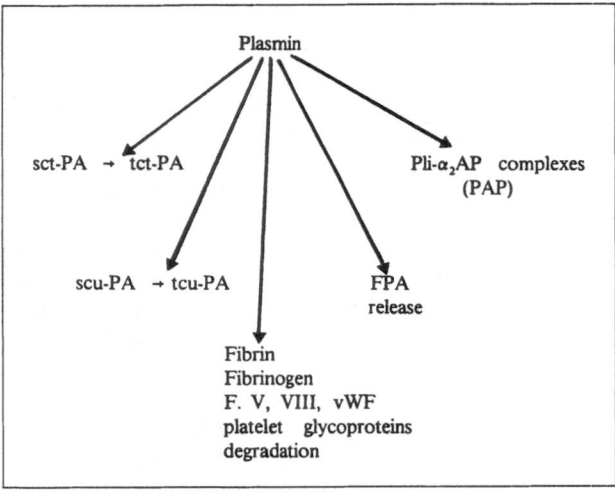

Fig. 3. Biochemical consequences of plasminogen activation.

due to plasmin, it could also be caused by proteases released from leucocytes or monocytes [23]. Von Oeveren et al. found a marked increase of elastase complexes (elastase bound to α_1-proteinase inhibitor) during extracorporeal circulation [19]. This suggests that release of elastase from leukocytes occurs. Trasylol given at high doses does not completely block the release of elastase.

In the initial stages of extracorporeal circulation platelets become activated [7, 24], undergo shape changes [25], and release thromboxane A_2 [19]; at the same time the platelet count drops slightly [7, 19, 25]. Furthermore, there is a decrease of the number of glycoprotein Ib receptors of about 30% within 5 min after starting bypass [18]. This activation is not continuous and the fraction of activated platelets appears to decrease with continuing bypass [25]. However, platelet function gradually and progressively deteriorates during the later stages of bypass. Platelet aggregation in response to the agonists ADP, collagen and epinephrine is impaired, the bleeding time is prolonged [10, 13, 18, 25], and in some studies loss of glycoprotein IIb/IIIa receptors on the surface of platelets has been observed [24]. Several of these changes have been observed during thrombolytic therapy (reviewed in [6]) or after addition of streptokinase or t-PA to human platelet rich plasma [3].

These undesirable abnormalities of platelet functions are partially blocked by the administration of high doses of aprotinin [14, 15]; furthermore, intraoperative and postoperative blood losses are greatly reduced [4, 16, 18, 19].

The question then has to be asked: is the beneficial effect of Trasylol due to the inhibition of fibrinolytic activity? It seems highly unlikely that increased levels of circulating t-PA or plasmin account for the very early degradation of glycoprotein Ib on the platelet surface. Fibrinolytic activity, as measured in the circulating blood, is not very much enhanced in the early phase of bypass [19]. The nearly absent increase of circulating plasmin/α_2-antiplasmin levels further supports the absence of biologically important concentrations of free plasmin [22].

We have studied the changes of platelet receptors in washed platelets exposed to plasmin and to mixtures of plasminogen and t-PA, by fluorescent flow cytometry

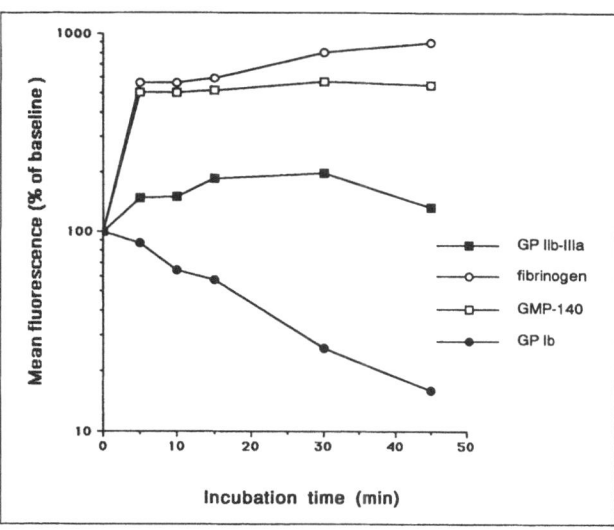

Fig. 4. Platelet surface antigens after in vitro exposure to plasmin (1 IU/ml).

(Fig. 4). When 1 IU/ml of plasmin was incubated with washed platelets at 37 °C there was a five- to sixfold increase of the binding of fluorescent labelled fibrinogen to platelets in the first 5 min. Concomitantly, binding of fluorescent labelled monoclonal antibodies to glycoprotein IIb/IIIa, the main receptor for fibrinogen on platelets increased by approximately 50 %. Furthermore, there was a fivefold increase of GMP-140 epitopes on platelets. GMP-140 is an α-granule-associated glycoprotein which fuses with the platelet membrane upon platelet activation. All these findings are thus consistent with an activation of platelets by plasmin. Glycoprotein Ib, the receptor for von Willebrand factor, showed the opposite behavior. The number of these receptors progressively declined during the 45-min incubation period (Fig. 4).

Figure 5 demonstrates the effect of mixtures of plasminogen and of t-PA on washed platelets. t-PA concentrations of 2—5 µg/ml are commonly observed during thrombolytic therapy of acute myocardial infarction. In our experiments, 1 IU of plasminogen was added to the incubation mixture and after 45 min produced approximately 0.3 U of free plasmin. Comparing Figs. 4 and 5 it is evident that the effect of the plasminogen/t-PA mixtures on glycoproteins was much more marked than that of plasmin.

In the field of fibrinolysis and blood coagulation one should not only consider what happens in the systemic circulation, but also what happens on a local level. Many receptors for coagulation proteins as well as for fibrinolytic components are located on the surface of endothelial cells, of fibrocytes and of other cells. When plasminogen binds to endothelial cells then the efficacy of it being activated to plasmin is severalfold higher than that of free plasminogen in the circulating blood. Also, plasmin and t-PA bound to cell surfaces remain active, whereas in their free forms in the circulation they are immediately blocked by inhibitors.

Such receptors also exist on platelets. Miles et al. have convincingly demonstrated the existence of receptors for plasminogen [14], Vaugham et al. for t-PA [20] and, recently, Park et al. have provided evidence that scu-PA binds to platelets [15]. Thus,

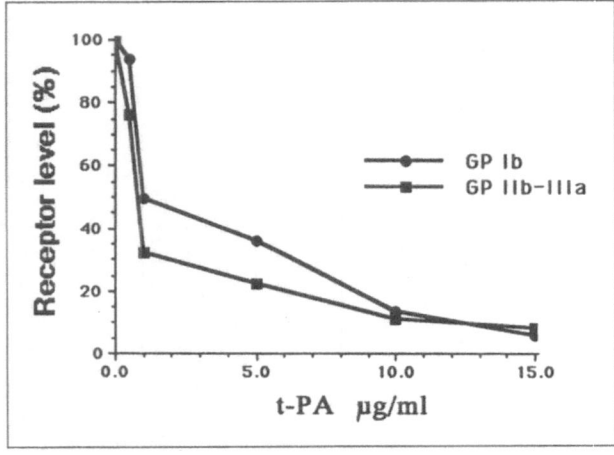

Fig. 5. GP Ib and GPIIb/IIIa levels after in vitro exposure to plasminogen and t-PA at low Ca+ concentration for 45'.

it is entirely possible that the measurements of fibrinolytic activity in the whole blood reported previously are not a good reflection of what happens on the platelet surface and that sct-PA and scu-PA bound to the platelet surface undergo activation to their two-chain forms and thus convert platelet-bound plasminogen locally and with great efficacy. Further studies will be necessary to determine whether this hypothesis can be validated.

References

1. Bachmann F (1987) Fibrinolysis. In: Verstraete M, Vermylen J, Lijnen R, Arnout J (eds) Thrombosis and Haemostasis. Leuven University Press, pp 227—265
2. Bachmann F, McKenna R, Cole ER, Najafi H (1975) The hemostatic mechanism after open-heart surgery. I. Studies on plasma coagulation factors and fibrinolysis in 512 patients after extracorporeal circulation. J Thorac Cardiovasc Surg 70: 76—85
3. Berridge DC, Burgess-Wilson ME, Westby JC, Hopkinson BR, Makin GS (1989) Differential effects of low-dose tissue plasminogen activator and streptokinase on platelet aggregation. Br J Surg 76: 1026—1030
4. Bidstrup BP, Royston D, Sapsford RN, Taylor KM (1989) Reduction in blood loss and blood use after cardiopulmonary bypass with high dose aprotinin (Trasylol). J Thorac Cardiovasc Surg 97: 364—372
5. Bleyl H, Roka L (1988) Serpincomplexes as indicators of thrombophilic states. Haemostasis 18 (Suppl S2): 54
6. Coller BS (1990) Platelets and thrombolytic therapy. N Engl J Med 322: 33—42
7. Edmunds LH (1989) Blood platelets and bypass [invited letter]. J Thorac Cardiovasc Surg 97: 470—471
8. Ghebrehiwet B, Randazzo BP, Dunn JT, Silverberg M, Kaplan AP (1983) Mechanism of activation of the classical pathway of complement by Hageman factor fragment. J Clin Invest 71: 1450—1457
9. Hauert J, Nicoloso G, Schleuning WD, Bachmann F, Schapira M (1989) Plasminogen activators in Dextran sulfate-activated euglobulin fractions: A molecular analysis of factor XII- and pre-kallikrein-dependent fibrinolysis. Blood 73: 994—999
10. Holloway DS, Summaria L, Sandesara J, Vagher JP, Alexander JC, Caprini JA (1988) Decreased platelet number and function and increased fibrinolysis contribute to postoperative bleeding in cardiopulmonary bypass patients. Thromb Haemost 59: 62—67

11. Kucuk O, Kwaan HC, Frederickson J, Wade L, Green D (1986) Increased fibrinolytic activity in patients undergoing cardiopulmonary bypass operation. Am J Hematol 23: 223—229
12. Lottenberg R, Sjak-Shie N, Fazleabas AT, Roberts RM (1988) Aprotinin inhibits urokinase but not tissue-type plasminogen activator. Thromb Res 49: 549—556
13. McKenna R, Bachmann F, Whittaker B, Gilson JR, Weinberg M (1975) The hemostatic mechanism after open-heart surgery. II. Frequency of abnormal platelet functions during and after extracorporeal circulation. J Thorac Cardiovas Surg 70: 298—308
14. Miles LA, Ginsberg MH, White JG, Plow EF (1986) Plasminogen interacts with human platelets with two distinct mechanisms. J Clin Invest 77: 2001—2009
15. Park S, Harker LA, Marzec UM, Levin EG (1989) Demonstration of single chain urokinase-type plasminogen activator on human platelet membrane. Blood 73: 1421—1426
16. Royston D, Bidstrup BP, Taylor KM, Sapsford RN (1987) Effect of aprotinin on need for blood transfusion after repeat open-heart surgery. Lancet ii: 1289—1291
17. Stibbe J, Kluft C, Brommer EJP, Gomes M, De Jong DS, Nauta J (1984) Enhanced fibrinolytic activity during cardiopulmonary bypass in open-heart surgery in man is caused by extrinsic (tissue-type) plasminogen activator. Eur J Clin Invest 14: 375—382
18. Van Oeveren W, Harder MP, Roozendaal KJ, Eijsman L, Wildevuur CRH (1990) Aprotinin protects platelets against the initial effect of cardiopulmonary bypass. J Thorac Cardiovas Surg 99: 788—797
19. Van Oeveren W, Jansen NJG, Bidstrup BP, Royston D, Westaby S, Neuhof H, Wildevuur CRH (1987) Effects of aprotinin on hemostatic mechanisms during cardiopulmonary bypass. Ann Thorac Surg 44: 640—645
20. Vaughan DE, Mendelsohn ME, Declerck PJ, Van Houtte E, Collen D, Loscalzo J (1989) Characterization of the binding of human tissue-type plasminogen activator to platelets. J Biol Chem 264: 15869—15874
21. Verstraete M (1985) Clinical application of inhibitors of fibrinolysis. Drugs 29: 236—261
22. Wachtfogel YT, Harpel PC, Edmunds LH, Colman RW (1989) Formation of $C\bar{1}_s$—$C\bar{1}$-inhibitor, kallikrein-C1-inhibitor, and plasmin-α_2-plasmin-inhibitor complexes during cardiopulmonary bypass. Blood 73: 468—471
23. Wachtfogel YT, Kucich U, Greenplate J, Gluszko P, Abrams W, Weinbaum G, Wenger RK, Rucinski B, Niewiarowski S, Edmunds LH, Colman RW (1987) Human neutrophil degranulation during extracorporeal circulation. Blood 69: 324—330
24. Wenger RK, Lukasiewicz H, Mikuta BS, Niewiarowski S, Edmunds LH (1989) Loss of platelet fibrinogen receptors during clinical cardiopulmonary bypass. J Thorac Cardiovasc Surg 97: 235—239
25. Zilla P, Fasol R, Groscurth P, Klepetko W, Reichenspurner H, Wolner E (1989) Blood platelets in cardiopulmonary bypass operations. Recovery occurs after initial stimulation, rather than continual activation. J Thorac Cardiovasc Surg 97: 379—388

Authors' address:
Prof. Fedor Bachmann
Laboratoire central d'hematologie
CHUV
CH-1011 Lausanne

Pathomechanisms of Defective Hemostasis During and After Extracorporeal Circulation: Contact Phase Activation

C. Kluft

Gaubius Institute TNO, Leiden, The Netherlands

Introduction

Contact of blood with so-called foreign surfaces or macromolecular structures results in activation of both coagulation and fibrinolysis. This activation is mediated by the contact phase system. This system was originally discovered in vitro in relation to coagulation [13] and also fibrinolysis [12], but has since been implicated in several other processes and reactions, such as vasodilatation, activation of complement, of neutrophils, and of the renin/angiotensin system.

The scope of this paper is restricted to the effects on coagulation and fibrinolysis. It aims at summarizing the situation that exists during extracorporeal circulation, with respect to activation and inhibition of the contact system. The present paper considers which effects on the hemostatic system might be exerted and might contribute to bleeding problems and how such an effect might be controlled by exogenous inhibition.

Contact activation mechanisms

The biochemical nature of the components involved in contact phase activation and their molecular interactions has been largely unravelled for reviews see (8, 11, 14, 17).

The results of a contact of the three components, factor XII (or Hageman factor), and the high-molecular-weight (HMW) kininogen in complex with prekallikrein is depicted in Fig. 1. This contact is invited by the activating surface or macromolec-

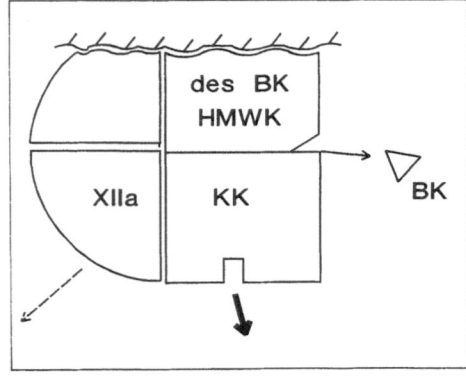

Fig. 1. Schematic summary of the results of the early contact activation process. HMWK = high molecular weight kininogen, BK = bradykinin, KK = kallikrein, XIIa = factor XIIa.

ular structure. During this contact, mutual activation that involves conformational changes and hydrolysis of peptide bonds occurs, and several activation products are formed. The activation products include the peptide hormone bradykinin, the serine proteases kallikrein (bound to des-BK HMW kininogen) and factor XIIa. Depending upon the extent of proteolysis of factor XII (by kallikrein), either the active site containing part of factor XIIa remains attached to the heavy chain that contains the surface binding domain, or is separated from the heavy chain and called factor XIIf (f for fragment) or β-factor XIIa.

Contribution of contact phase activation to coagulation and fibrinolysis

From the activation products of the contact activation, factor XIIa contributes to coagulation activation while kallikrein and bradykinin contribute to fibrinolysis activation [10] (see scheme in Fig. 3).

The effects on coagulation concern activation of factor XI by the surface bound factor XIIa, a mainly local phenomenon; and "activation" of factor VII to a more readily activatable form. Only the exhaustion of coagulation factors could contribute to an acquired bleeding tendency, but activation is usually only limited [1].

The effects on fibrinolysis concern all three routes of plasminogen activation (cf. [10]). Bradykinin is capable of releasing t-PA from endothelial sources, and kallikrein (also shown to be able to recruit t-PA [2]) is capable of activating both plasma pro-urokinase and the factor XII-dependent plasminogen proactivator. Theoretically, these contributions to activation of fibrinolysis add to a bleeding tendency.

Contact activation acting at distance

As illustrated in Fig. 2, the activation of the contact system by the foreign surface of the extracorporeal tubing is distant from the sites in the body with active hemostatic processes from the surgery.

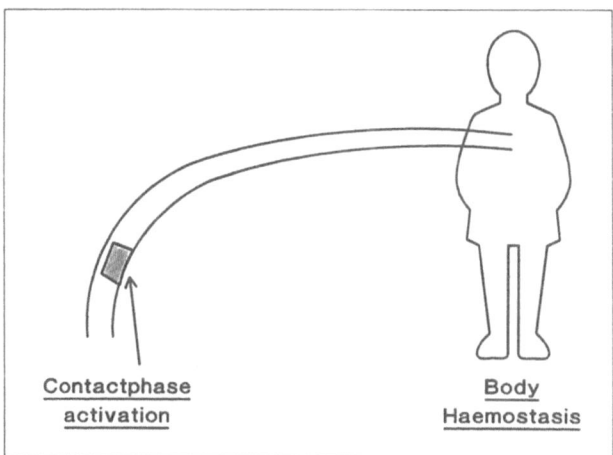

Contactphase activation

Body Haemostasis

Fig. 2. Situation of extracorporeal circulation where contact activation takes place at a site other than where hemostasis is required.

11

The question is thus one of identifying which active factors, generated at the site of contact activation, enter the circulation and can survive to contribute to hemostasis at a distance.

It has previously been suggested that the contact system contributes in a balanced way to both coagulation and fibrinolysis [12, 9]. This mainly applies to localized hemostasis. In the case of extracorporeal circulation, it can be suggested that the balance "at distance" is shifted in favor of fibrinolysis, due to the fact that the mainly local activation of coagulation via factor XI significantly loses momentum.

For fibrinolysis, infusions of bradykinin and kallikrein have shown their capacity to act at a distance in releasing t-PA [2]. The amounts infused in such experiments amount to a few percent activation of prekallikrein and few percent conversion of HMW kininogen to bradykinin. It is unknown whether pro-urokinase and the factor XII-dependent plasminogen proactivator become activated and enter the circulation at the site of contact activation.

Contact activation during extracorporeal circulation

During extracorporeal circulation, the exposure to foreign surfaces is obvious. Thusfar, no artificial materials are known [19] that are completely devoid of contact activation, but materials can vary significantly in the degree of induction of contact activation. Also, the balance between activation of fibrinolysis and coagulation can be different depending upon the material (cf [10]).

In simulated extracorporeal circulation it has been shown that a low degree of contact activation (few percent prekallikrein conversion) takes place, as is evident

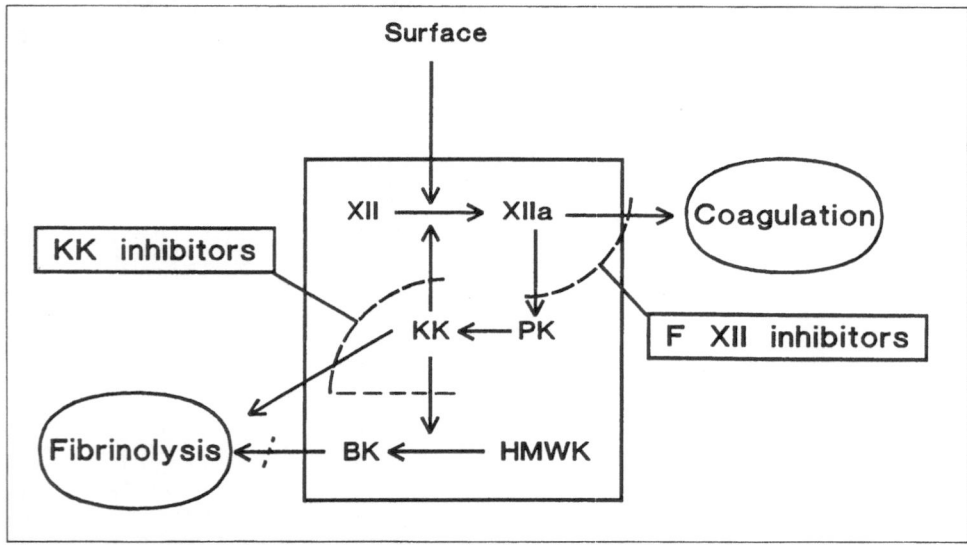

Fig. 3. Scheme of early contact activation (in box) and subsequent effects on coagulation and fibrinolysis (For abbreviations see legend to Fig. 1).

12

from the generation of complexes between kallikrein and its main inhibitor Cl-inactivator [20]. The main activation appears to occur in the early period of circulation. This pattern in simulated extracorporeal circulation resembles that in patients exhibiting appearance of activity on synthetic substrates for kallikrein, presumed to represent the complex of kallikrein with its secondary inhibitor α_2-macroglobulin [5]. The pattern of appearance of kallikrein-Cl-inactivator complexes is not confirmed in patients [20]. It is possible that the complexes between kallikrein and Cl-inactivator are not very well formed during hypothermia. It is known that α_2-macroglobulin increases its share in inhibition of kallikrein at lower temperatures, because Cl-inactivator loses its activity [7]. The simulated extracorporeal circulation mentioned above was performed at 37 °C.

Reduced inhibition during extracorporeal circulation

Usually, the survival of components is reduced by inactivation or inhibition. Bradykinin is normally inactivated in the circulation and to a large extent on first passage through the lung [4]. During extracorporeal circulation this inactivation, however, is minimal and circulating inactivating enzymes are reduced in concentration (hemodilution) and gradually decrease further, due to reduced synthesis in the lung.

Factor XIIf and kallikrein are mainly inactivated by Cl-inactivator (half-life about 2 and 5 min, respectively) [14, 18]. However, during extracorporeal circulation this inactivation will be reduced due to the lowering of temperature, which strongly affects the inactivation rate.

Urokinase is mainly inactivated by PAI-1. During extracorporeal circulation, however, the increased t-PA [16] will neutralize circulating PAI-1 readily and generated urokinase will have an increased survival.

It can be concluded that factors generated at the site of contact activation have, during extracorporeal circulation, an increased possibility to act on distance, due to the reduced inhibition in circulation of these factors. Thus, supply of activated contact factors and, subsequently, generated factors (e.g., t-PA) to the sites of fibrin formation will result in incorporation into forming fibrin and enhancement of the lysis of the fibrin. In such fibrin clots the reduced inhibition of contact factors and generated factors continues to exist. A further significant aspect of reduced fibrinolysis inhibition concerns PAI-1 released from platelets during coagulation [15]. It should be noted that platelets are strongly affected by extracorporeal circulation and that this possibly also involves a reduced PAI-1 supply to fibrin clots by platelets [6]. Consequently, fibrin clots formed during extracorporeal circulation might lyse prematurely, either during or after the extracorporeal circulation due to a built-in program of both enhanced lysis and reduced inhibition.

Intervention with inhibitors

If the above discussed contact phase mechanisms contribute to bleeding problems associated with extracorporeal circulation, intervention in the mechanism is indicated. Such intervention can aim at preventing the occurrence of contact activation or can involve the administration of inhibitors to reinforce the reduced inhibition of the contact activation process.

Figure 3 shows the early activation process schematically within a box. To prevent any contribution of the contact system to hemostasis (outside the box) it can be attempted to inhibit the effect of the surface with "for example" hexadimethrine [3].

Inhibition of the activities of one of the generated proteases, factor XIIa and kallikrein, theoretically have different effects, depending upon which protease is inhibited and depending upon the degree of inhibition.

Complete inhibition of factor XIIa results in a complete block of the activation process for fibrinolysis and coagulation. Partial or slow inhibition of factor XIIa results in a stronger inhibition of coagulation relative to fibrinolysis, shifting the balance in the case of extracorporeal circulation in the wrong direction. The use of factor XIIa inhibitors in extracorporeal circulation therefore seems only justified when a very effective inhibition can be instituted.

Complete inhibition of kallikrein also results, in view of the reciprocal activation mechanism (see Fig. 3), in a complete block of the activation process for fibrinolysis, but it leaves a slow contact activation process between factor XII and XI (not indicated in Fig. 3) [11]. Also partial (though increased) inhibition of kallikrein is theoretically favorable. In that case, the effects are stronger on fibrinolysis than on coagulation (cf. Fig. 3).

Reinforcement of the inactivation of bradykinin would be inhibitory for fibrinolysis; but opposite measures of reduction of inactivation (ACE-inhibitors), rather than those of reinforcement are available. It seems undesirable to perform extracorporeal circulation on patients using ACE-inhibitors.

All interventions aimed at reducing contact activation effects on fibrinolysis should be effective *during* extracorporeal circulation. At that moment the contact-activation-mediated effects operate and program of inhibition and lysis built into fibrin clots formed at that moment should be modulated.

It is, at present, unknown whether or not one or more of the reviewed profibrinolytic effects derived from contact activation do contribute to the bleeding problems associated with extracorporeal circulation. To investigate the significance of such contributions might become possible, especially with the use of very specific kallikrein inhibitors. The present successes in reduction of blood losses with aprotinin at high dosages, which are effective against kallikrein, are in agreement with a possible role of the contact activation process. However, aprotinin has broader specificity, leaving possibilities for other target enzymes.

References

1. Bick RL (1985) Hemostasis defects associated with cardiac surgery, prosthetic devices, and other extracorporeal circuits. Semin Thromb Haemostas 11: 249—280
2. Egberg N, Gallimore M, Green K, Jakobsson J, Vesterqvist O, Wiman B, (1988) Effects of plasma kallikrein and bradykinin infusions into pigs on plasma fibrinolytic variables and urinary excretion of thromboxane and prostacyclin metabolites. Fibrinolysis 2: 101—106
3. Eisen V (1964) Effect of hexadimethrine bromide on plasma kinin formation, hydrolysis of p-tosyl-L-arginine methyl ester and fibrinolysis. Brit J Pharmacol 22: 87—103
4. Erdös EG (1979) Inhibitors of kininases. Federation Proc 38: 2774—2777
5. Fuhrer G, Heller W, Hoffmeister H-E (1985) Das Verhalten von Plasma-Präkallikrein/-Kalli-

krein bei Patienten mit aorto-koronarer Bypass-Operation unter Anwendung zweier verschiedener Aprotinin-Dosierungsschemata. In: Dudziak R, Kirchhoff PG, Reuter HD, Schumann F (eds) Proteolyse und Proteinaseninhibition in der Herz- und Gefäßchirurgie. Schattauer, Stuttgart, New York, pp 255—261

6. Gomez MJ, Carroll RC, Hansard MR, Kidd M, Goldman MH (1988) Regulation of fibrinolysis in aortic surgery. J Vasc Surg 8: 384—388
7. Harpel PC, Lewin MF, Kaplan AP (1985) Distribution of plasma kallikrein between Cl inactivator and α_2-macroglobulin in plasma utilizing a new assay for α_2-macroglobulin-kallikrein complexes. J Biol Chem 260: 4257—4263
8. Iwaarden van F, Bouma BN (1987) Role of high molecular weight kininogen in contact activation. Semin Thromb Haemostas 13: 15—24
9. Kluft C, Dooijewaard G, Emeis JJ (1985) Contact product formation: balanced activation of coagulation and fibrinolysis. In: Schmid-Schönbein H, Wurzinger LJ, Zimmerman RE (eds) Enzyme Activation in Blood-perfused Artificial Organs. Martinus Nijhoff Publishers, Boston Dordrecht, pp 9—31
10. Kluft C, Dooijewaard G, Emeis JJ (1987) Role of the contact system in fibrinolysis. Semin Thromb Haemostas 13: 50—68
11. Mannhalter CH (1987) Biochemical and functional properties of factor XI and prekallikrein. Semin Thromb Haemostas 13: 25—35
12. Niewiarowski S, Prou-Wartelle O (1959) Rôle du facteur contact (facteur Hageman) dans la fibrinolyse. Thromb Diath Haemorrh 3: 593—603
13. Ratnoff OD (1980) A quarter century with Mr Hageman. Thromb Haemostas 43: 95—98
14. Schapira M (1987) Major inhibitors of the contact phase coagulation factors. Semin Thromb Haemostas 13: 69—78
15. Sprengers ED, Kluft C (1987) Plasminogen activator inhibitors. Blood 69: 381—387
16. Stibbe J, Kluft C, Brommer EJP, Gomes M, de Jong DS, Nauta J (1984) Enhanced fibrinolytic activity during cardiopulmonary bypass in openheart surgery in man is caused by extrinsic (tissue-type) plasminogen activator. Eur J Clin Invest 14: 375—382
17. Tans G, Rosing J (1987) Structural and functional characterization of factor XII. Semin Thromb Haemostas 13: 1—14
18. Trumpi-Kalshoven MM, Kluft C (1979) Cl inhibitor: the main inhibitor of human plasma kallikrein. In: Haberland GL, Hamberg U (eds) Current concepts in kinin research. Pergamon Press, Oxford, New York, pp 93—101
19. Vroman L (1987) The importance of surfaces in contact phase reactions. Semin Thromb Haemostas 13: 79—85
20. Wachtfogel YT, Harpel PC, Edmunds LH Jr, Colman RW (1989) Formation of Cls-Cl-inhibitor, kallikrein-Cl-inhibitor, and plasmin-α_2-plasmin-inhibitor complexes during cardiopulmonary bypass. Blood 73: 468—471

Author's address:
C. Kluft
Gaubius Institute TNO
P.O. Box 612
2300 AP Leiden
The Netherlands

Pathomechanism of Defective Hemostasis During and After Extracorporeal Circulation: The Role of Platelets

A. D. Michelson*)

Department of Pediatrics, University of Massachusetts Medical School, Worcester, Massachusetts, USA

Introduction

The pathomechanism of defective hemostasis during and after cardiopulmonary bypass surgery may be related to multiple factors, including: surgical damage to blood vessels, thrombocytopenia, defects in platelet function, a fibrinolytic state, unneutralized heparin, and excessive protamine [1, 2]. The most important factor in post-bypass hemorrhage is considered to be an acquired defect in the formation of the platelet plug [3]. In this chapter, the role of platelets in the hemostatic defect associated with extracorporeal circulation will be reviewed.

Normal platelet physiology (Fig. 1)

Platelets are essential for normal hemostasis. The main functions of platelets are adhesion to damaged blood vessel walls, aggregation to form a platelet plug, and promotion of fibrin clot formation. Platelet adhesion is primarily mediated by the adhesive molecule von Willebrand factor, which binds both to a specific receptor on the platelet surface glycoprotein (GP) Ib-IX complex and to exposed subendothelial components [4, 5]. Platelet-to-platelet aggregation is primarily mediated by fibrinogen binding to its receptor on the platelet surface GPIIb-IIIa complex [4, 6]. Normal circulating platelets are in a resting state and, despite the presence of platelet surface GPIb-IX and GPIIb-IIIa complexes, they bind neither plasma von Willebrand factor nor plasma fibrinogen. In vitro, the cationic antibiotic ristocetin induces binding of von Willebrand factor to its receptor on GPIb [4], but the in vivo analogue of ristocetin remains uncertain. Thrombin and other physiological platelet agonists (e.g., adenosine diphosphate (ADP), epinephrine) induce exposure of the fibrinogen receptor on the platelet surface GPIIb-IIIa complex [6]. These agonists also stimulate platelets to change shape, secrete the contents of their granules (e.g., β-thromboglobulin, platelet factor 4, thrombospondin), and aggregate. Secreted thrombospondin binds to a receptor on the platelet surface membrane, as well as to fibrinogen, thereby stabilizing platelet-to-platelet aggregates [7]. GMP-140, also referred to as PADGEM protein [8], is a component of the α-granule membrane of resting platelets that is only expressed on the platelet plasma membrane after platelet activation and secretion [9]. Platelet surface expression of GMP-140 is therefore a

---

*) Dr. Michelson was supported by FIRST Award HL38138 from the National Heart, Lung, and Blood Institute.

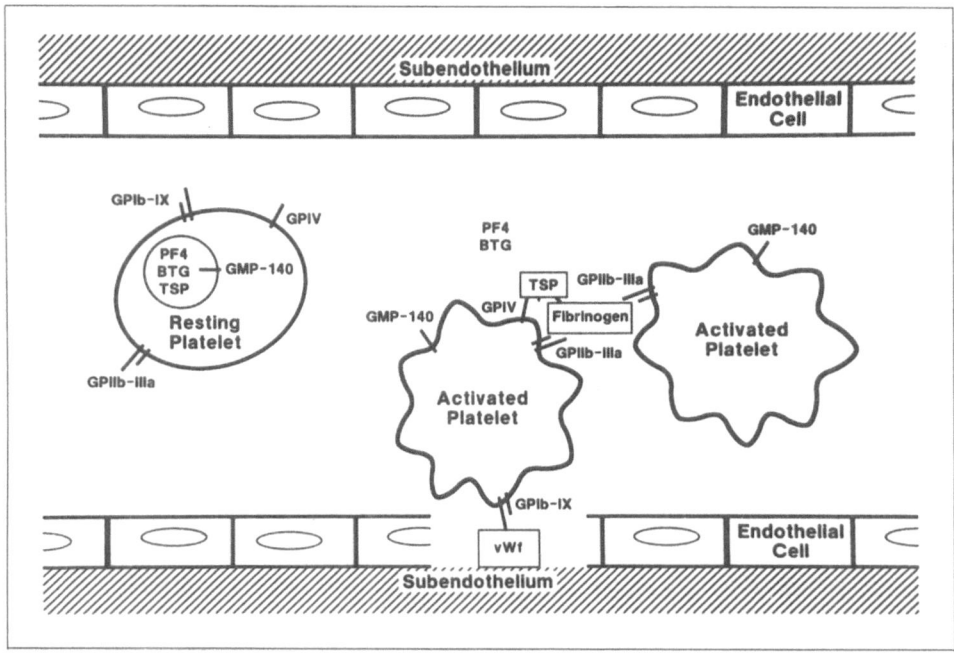

Fig. 1. Normal platelet physiology (see text). Abbreviations: βTG = β-thromboglobulin; GMP-140 = granule membrane protein 140; GP = glycoprotein; PF4 = platelet factor 4; TSP = thrombospondin; vWf = von Willebrand factor.

very precise marker of platelet secretion. Although its physiologic role remains speculative, GMP-140 mediates in vitro adhesion of activated platelets to monocytes and neutrophils [10]. In contrast to its effect on GMP-140 and the fibrinogen receptor on GPIIb-IIIa complex, thrombin downregulates the platelet surface expression of the von Willebrand factor receptor on the GPIb-IX complex [11—13].

The role of platelets in defective hemostasis during and after extracorporeal circulation

An anticoagulant, usually heparin, is required during extracorporeal circulation to prevent clotting due to contact of blood with synthetic, non-endothelial surfaces. Heparin, however, prevents neither adsorption nor activation of platelets [1]. Thus, both thrombocytopenia and platelet function defects occur during extracorporeal circulation and are generally considered to be the major contributors to the hemostatic defect associated with cardiopulmonary bypass [1—3].

17

Thrombocytopenia

Thrombocytopenia has been widely reported in association with cardiopulmonary bypass surgery [1, 14, 15] and generally persists for several days after the bypass procedure [15, 16]. However, not all investigators have found significant thrombocytopenia during cardiopulmonary bypass [2]. The wide variability in the reported degree of thrombocytopenia in different series most likely reflects differences in equipment and techniques, for example: synthetic materials in the extracorporeal perfusion apparatus, oxygenation system, pumping system, normothermic or hypothermic perfusion, type and volume of the priming solution, flow rate, time on bypass, and effects of pharmacologic agents administered during or after bypass.

The predominant causes of the thrombocytopenia associated with cardiopulmonary bypass surgery are considered to be hemodilution and removal of activated platelets from the circulation, especially by platelet adherence to synthetic surfaces. Less common causes include disseminated intravascular coagulation, heparin, and cyanotic congenital heart disease.

Hemodilution: During extracorporeal circulation for cardiac surgery, blood is diluted by priming of the extracorporeal perfusion system with either crystalloids (5 % dextrose, saline, Ringer's lactate) or colloids (albumin, dextran, starch solutions, plasma). This hemodilution is generally considered to be the major cause of thrombocytopenia during cardiopulmonary bypass [1, 14]. However, some investigators have failed to demonstrate a correlation between hematocrit and platelet count, suggesting that hemodilution may not be the major cause of the thrombocytopenia [17].

Removal of activated platelets from the circulation: Platelets have been demonstrated by scanning electron microscopy to adhere to extracorporeal synthetic surfaces [18]. Fibrinogen appears to be the most important cofactor in platelet adhesion to synthetic surfaces [19], as it is for platelet-to-platelet aggregation [4]. Plasma fibrinogen is preferentially adsorbed onto synthetic surfaces [20, 21] and platelet reactivity with these surfaces has been reported to be directly proportional to the adsorbed fibrinogen concentration [22], although this is controversial [23]. The mechanism(s) by which platelets are initially activated within extracorporeal perfusion systems is not completely clear, but possible causes include: direct surface contact, thrombin, and ADP. Thrombin, which is generated in small amounts despite the presence of heparin, is adsorbed onto synthetic surfaces [24]. ADP is stored in platelet dense granules and is therefore released both by platelet lysis and platelet activation. Hemolysis of red cells also releases ADP. In any event, platelet activation results in exposure of fibrinogen receptors on the GPIIb-IIIa complex [6] and thereby permits binding to fibrinogen molecules previously adsorbed onto the surface [25]. Gluszko et al. [23] provided evidence that exposure of fibrinogen receptors associated with the GPIIb-IIIa complex contributes to platelet consumption during cardiopulmonary bypass. These investigators [23] demonstrated that blood from patients with Glanzmann's thrombasthenia (an inherited deficiency of the GPIIb-IIIa complex) had reduced cardiopulmonary bypass-induced thrombocytopenia, whereas patients with Bernard-Soulier syndrome (an inherited deficiency of GPIb, GPIX, and GPV) did not.

In addition to adherence to the synthetic surfaces of the cardiopulmonary bypass tubing, activated platelets are more likely to adhere to injured endothelial surfaces, to deposit in the heart after cardioplegic arrest [26], and to be removed by the reticuloendothelial system. Support for the concept that platelet activation, adherence, and/or clearance is important in the etiology of thrombocytopenia during cardiopulmonary bypass comes from the effects of infusion of drugs (PGE_1, PGI_2, iloprost, and dipyridamole) that inhibit platelet activation. Infusion of any of these drugs during cardiopulmonary bypass can result in inhibition of platelet activation, a marked reduction in platelet adherence to the synthetic surfaces, maintenance of platelet counts at near normal levels, and reduction in postoperative blood loss [23, 27—33].

An adsorbed protein layer that reduces the affinity of synthetic surfaces for platelets may eventually form [34, 35]. Although the exact physiological basis for this process, termed passivation [1], remains unclear, support for the concept derives from studies with PGI_2 [29]. When PGI_2 is used to inhibit platelets during 2 h of recirculation in a membrane oxygenator system, platelet activation is inhibited only during the first hour [29]. PGI_2 is extremely unstable in plasma, and after 1 h the recirculated platelets regain their ability to aggregate in the presence of ADP and epinephrine, yet do not react with the synthetic surface [29].

Oxygenators, and to a lesser extent filters, contain the largest surface areas in contact with blood and therefore, are the most prominent sites of platelet deposition [1]. Thrombocytopenia is of a greater degree with bubble oxygenators than with membrane oxygenators [2], apparently as a result of the greater platelet damage caused by the direct blood-gas interface created in bubble oxygenators [36]. Cardiotomy sucker systems further decrease platelet counts [37]. Turbulence and high flow ratios also increase platelet adhesion [38].

The reported occurrence of platelet aggregates during cardiopulmonary bypass [39] is a further potential activation-dependent contributor to thrombocytopenia.

Disseminated intravascular coagulation: Although probably uncommon (as distinct from primary fibrinolysis [2]), disseminated intravascular coagulation is a cause of thrombocytopenia following cardiopulmonary bypass [40, 41]. Disseminated intravascular coagulation can occasionally be a cause of bleeding soon after cardiopulmonary bypass [40], but this complication more often occurs later, in association with septicaemia or low cardiac output [1].

Heparin-induced thrombocytopenia: Heparin-induced thrombocytopenia is of two types [42]. Type I is a transient thrombocytopenia of immediate onset and mild degree that accompanies heparin therapy in approximately 5 % of patients [42]. The mechanism is probably non-immune and related to a direct proaggregatory effect of heparin [43]. Type II occurs in approximately 0.6 % of patients receiving heparin and is a delayed, severe, and probably immune-mediated thrombocytopenia that may occur in association with platelet activation, aggregation, and, on occasion, massive arterial thrombosis [42].

Cyanotic congenital heart disease: The mechanism of the association between cyanotic congenital heart disease and thrombocytopenia [44, 45] is unclear.

Platelet function defects

Cardiopulmonary bypass surgery is clearly associated with a platelet function defect [2]. The standardized template bleeding time is prolonged during cardiopulmonary bypass [15]. The bleeding time is unaffected by heparinization, but increases abruptly following the initiation of bypass, and lengthens progressively during the first 2 h of bypass [15]. Bleeding time measurements decrease rapidly after the end of bypass [15]. That the prolongation of the bleeding time reflects a platelet function defect is established by the normal [46] or increased [47, 48] plasma levels of von Willebrand factor and by the increasing divergence during bypass of the normal relationship between platelet count and bleeding time [15].

What causes the platelet function defect? The cause(s) of the platelet function defect during cardiopulmonary bypass is not entirely clear. Possible causes of the platelet function defect include: contact with synthetic surfaces [1], shear force [38], oxygenation [2], hypothermia [15], plasmin generated by a fibrinolytic state [2], fibrin(ogen) degradation products [2], denatured plasma proteins [1], thrombin (which is generated in small amounts despite the presence of heparin [24]), ADP (released from platelet dense bodies or by lysis of platelets or red cells), drugs (e.g., aspirin [49], heparin [42], protamine [50], sodium nitroprusside [51], penicillins [52]), and underlying diseases (e.g. cyanotic congenital heart disease [53, 54]). Many of these factors are discussed elsewhere in this chapter. The presence of a circulating platelet inhibitor is mitigated against by the finding that plasma from patients undergoing cardiopulmonary bypass does not inhibit the function of normal platelets [1]. Circulating fibrin(ogen) degradation products can interfere with platelet function [55] and these are present in the majority of patients undergoing cardiopulmonary bypass surgery [2]. However, there is a poor correlation between levels of circulating fibrin(ogen) degradation products and the degree of abnormal platelet function during bypass surgery [17]. Plasma proteins are denatured during cardiopulmonary bypass, particularly in bubble oxygenator perfusion systems [56, 57], and high concentrations of denatured plasma proteins reduce platelet function [58]. Patients with cyanotic congenital heart disease have been reported to have preoperative decreases in platelet aggregation in response to ADP, epinephrine, and collagen, as well as platelet release abnormalities [53, 54].

Why has it been difficult to characterize the platelet-function defect? The precise nature of the platelet function defect(s) during and after cardiopulmonary bypass remains contentious. The variability in reported defects in platelet function during and after bypass reflects, in part, the same differences in equipment and techniques referred to above with regard to thrombocytopenia: synthetic materials in the extracorporeal perfusion apparatus, oxygenation system, pumping system, normothermic or hypothermic perfusion, type and volume of the priming solution, flow rate, time on bypass, and effects of pharmacologic agents administered during or after bypass. In addition, however, methodological problems have bedeviled attempts to characterize in vivo platelet function defects in clinical settings. During their separation from whole blood for functional assays, platelets are susceptible to membrane alterations [59] and in vitro activation. Plasma assays of the secretion products of platelet α-granules (platelet factor 4 and β-thromboglobulin) have been widely used to study the platelet defect in cardiopulmonary bypass. However, the

20

potential problem of in vitro secretion is of particular concern, because 1 % platelet secretion may cause as much as a 30-fold increase in the plasma level of platelet factor 4 [60]. In addition, plasma assays of platelet factor 4 and β-thromboglobulin reflect, not only the number of circulating activated platelets, but also lysed platelets and non-circulating activated platelets adherent to synthetic surfaces or vessel walls.

Do platelet microparticles, and/or platelets with partial α-granule release, circulate? In an attempt to circumvent these problems with regard to platelet function testing, whole blood assays that do not involve any separation or manipulation of platelets have been developed [11, 61]. George et al. [11] directly measured platelet surface glycoproteins in immediately fixed whole blood samples with ^{125}I-labeled monoclonal antibodies. These investigators [11] were able to define two prototypic types of acquired abnormalities of platelet surface glycoproteins. Patients with adult respiratory distress syndrome had an increased concentration of GMP-140 and thrombospondin on the surface of their platelets, demonstrating in vivo platelet secretion, but had no increase in platelet microparticles in their plasma. In contrast, patients after cardiac surgery with cardiopulmonary bypass demonstrated changes consistent with membrane fragmentation without secretion: a decreased platelet surface concentration of GPIb and GPIIb, no increase in platelet surface GMP-140 or thrombospondin, and an increased plasma concentration of platelet membrane microparticles. The production of platelet microparticles was assumed to be the result of turbulence and shear stress [11]. Using an electron-microscopic analysis of fixed, separated platelets and plasma assays of platelet factor 4 and β-thromboglobulin, Harker et al. [15] did find evidence of platelet α-granule secretion during cardiopulmonary bypass. However, the findings of George et al. [11] are supported by a report by Abrams et al. [62]. These authors [62], utilizing a whole-blood-flow cytometric assay [61], also found that cardiopulmonary bypass results in platelet fragmentation with the production of microparticles, but not platelet secretion, as determined by a GMP-140-specific monoclonal antibody. In further agreement with George et al. [11], Dechavanne et al. [63] demonstrated reduction in the binding of a monoclonal antibody directed against the platelet GPIIb-IIIa complex, with no evidence of degranulation, as evidenced by electron microscopy and lack of binding of monoclonal antibodies directed against an α-granule membrane glycoprotein and thrombospondin.

What is the mechanism of the platelet aggregation defect? During cardiopulmonary bypass, circulating platelets become less responsive to agonists such as ADP, collagen, and epinephrine [14, 15, 64, 65]. The mechanism may be loss of platelet membrane fibrinogen [25, 66] and epinephrine [65] receptors. Loss of these receptors in circulating platelets may be caused by platelet microparticle formation [11] or by detachment of adherent platelets, with some fibrinogen receptors remaining on still-adherent fragments of platelet membrane [66]. After protamine sulfate administration, there is a further decrease in ADP-induced platelet aggregation [14, 67]. Mammen et al. [14] reported that ristocetin-induced platelet agglutination is relatively unchanged during cardiopulmonary bypass, but decreases after administration of protamine sulfate, remaining abnormal for 24 h postoperatively. Although protamine effects on platelets are well-documented [50, 68], the mechanisms by which it induces these effects are uncertain. In vitro experiments have suggested the possibility that the effects are mediated by a protamine-heparin complex rather than by protamine alone [50]. Given that an increase in circulating plasmin has been reported in association with infusion of protamine [69, 70], one possible explanation for the protamine-induced decreases in ristocetin- and ADP-induced platelet aggregation is plasmin-induced cleavage of platelet surface GPIb [71—73] and the GPIIb-IIIa complex [73].

What is the role of plasmin-induced cleavage of platelet surface GPIb? The majority of patients undergoing cardiopulmonary bypass surgery have a primary fibrino(geno)lytic state, resulting in the generation of plasmin [2]. We have demonstrated that plasmin cleaves platelet surface GPIb in vitro [71, 72]. This could be important in the hemostatic defect of cardiopulmonary bypass, because GPIb is essential for normal platelet adhesion (via its von Willebrand factor receptor [4, 5]) and activation (via its thrombin receptor [74—76]). Mohr et al. [46] reported that, in all 20 patients studied, after cardiopulmonary bypass surgery there was impaired platelet aggregation to ADP, collagen, and ristocetin. In this study [46], the only aggregation response that correlated with clinical bleeding was the response to ristocetin. Assays for von Willebrand factor were normal, strongly suggesting that the abnormality in ristocetin-induced platelet agglutination was the result of a defect in platelet surface GPIb [46]. Redistribution of intraplatelet stores of GPIb to the platelet surface [77] could account for the rapid decrease in the bleeding time that occurs after the end of bypass [15]. Aprotinin has been demonstrated in vitro to inhibit the plasmin-mediated cleavage of platelet surface GPIb [71]. Furthermore, it has been suggested [78] that the in vivo effectiveness of aprotinin in decreasing bleeding during and after cardiopulmonary bypass surgery [79, 80] may relate to inhibition of plasmin-induced cleavage of platelet surface GPIb.

Summary

During cardiopulmonary bypass surgery, the thrombocytopenia is mainly the result of hemodilution and removal of activated platelets from the circulation. The nature of the platelet function defect has not been completely characterized, but there are decreases in platelet surface GPIb (the von Willebrand factor receptor) and the GPIIb-IIIa complex (the fibrinogen receptor). The pathophysiological significance of the increased platelet membrane microparticles remains to be determined. Previously reported evidence of selective platelet α-granule release [15] is not supported by recent studies in whole blood [11, 62].

References

1. Edmunds LH and Addonizio VP (1987) Extracorporeal circulation. In: Hemostasis and thrombosis Basic principles and clinical practice. Colman RW, Hirsh J, Marder VJ and Salzman EW (ed.) Lippincott, Philadelphia: 901—912
2. Bick RL (1985) Hemostasis defects associated with cardiac surgery, prosthetic devices, and other extracorporeal circuits. Semin Thromb Hemost 11: 249—280
3. Harker LA (1986) Bleeding after cardiopulmonary bypass. N Engl J Med 314: 1446—1448
4. George JN, Nurden AT and Phillips DR (1984) Molecular defects in interactions of platelets with the vessel wall. N Engl J Med 311: 1084—1098

5. Michelson AD, Loscalzo J, Melnick B, Coller BS and Handin RI (1986) Partial characterization of a binding site for von Willebrand factor on glycocalicin. Blood 67: 19—26
6. Shattil SJ, Hoxie JA, Cunningham M and Brass LF (1985) Changes in the platelet membrane glycoprotein IIb-IIIa complex during platelet activation. J Biol. Chem 260: 11107—11114
7. Leung LLK (1984) Role of thrombospondin in platelet aggregation. J. Clin Invest 74: 1764—1772
8. Hsu-Lin S-C. Berman CL, Furie BC, August D and Furie B (1984) A platelet membrane protein expressed during platelet activation and secretion. Studies using a monoclonal antibody specific for thrombin-activated platelets. J Biol. Chem 259: 9121—9126
9. Stenberg PE, McEver RP, Shuman MA, Jacques YV and Bainton DF (1985) A platelet alpha-granule membrane protein (GMP-140) is expressed on the plasma membrane after activation. J Cell Biol 101: 880—886
10. Larsen E, Celi A, Gilbert GE, Furie BC, Erban JK, Bonfanti R, Wagner DD and Furie B (1989) PADGEM protein: A receptor that mediates the interaction of activated platelets with neutrophils and monocytes. Cell 59: 305—312
11. George JN, Pickett EB, Saucerman S, McEver RP, Kunicki TJ, Kieffer N and Newman PJ (1986) Platelet surface glycoproteins. Studies on resting and activated platelets and platelet membrane microparticles in normal subjects, and observations in patients during adult respiratory distress syndrome and cardiac surgery. J Clin. Invest 78: 340—348
12. Michelson AD and Barnard MR (1987) Thrombin-induced changes in platelet membrane glycoproteins Ib, IX, and IIb-IIIa complex. Blood 70: 1673—1678
13. George JN and Torres MM (1988) Thrombin decreases von Willebrand factor binding to platelet glycoprotein Ib. Blood 71: 1253—1259
14. Mammen EF, Koets MH, Washington BC, Wolk LW, Brown JM, Burdick M, Selik NR and Wilson RF (1985) Hemostasis changes during cardiopulmonary bypass surgery. Semin Thromb Hemost 281: 292
15. Harker LA, Malpass TW, Branson HE, Hessel EA and Slichter SJ (1980) Mechanism of abnormal bleeding in patients undergoing cardiopulmonary bypass: Acquired transient platelet dysfunction associated with selective α-granule release. Blood 56: 824—834
16. Martin JF, Daniel TD and Trowbridge EA (1987) Acute and chronic changes in platelet volume and count after cardiopulmonary bypass induced thrombocytopenia in man. Thromb Haemostas 57: 55—58
17. Bick RL, Schmalhorst SW and Arbegast NR (1976) Alterations of hemostasis associated with cardiopulmonary bypass. Thromb Res 8: 285—291
18. Salzman EW, Linden J, Brier D and Merrill EW (1977) Surface-induced platelet adhesion, aggregation and release. Ann NY Acad Sci 283: 114—127
19. George JN (1982) Direct assessment of platelet adhesion to glass: A study of the forces of interaction and the effects of plasma and serum factors, platelet function and modification of the glass surface. Blood 40: 862—874
20. Uniyal S and Brash JL (1982) Patterns of adsorption of proteins from human plasma onto foreign surfaces. Thromb Haemostas 47: 285—290
21. Lindon JN, McNamara G, Kushner L, Merrill EW and Salzman EW (1986) Does the conformation of adsorbed fibrinogen dictate platelet interactions with artifical surfces? Blood 68: 355—362
22. Lindon J, McNamara G, Pekala R and et al (1984) Fibrinogen platelet interactions on hydrophilic and hydrophobic surfaces. Circulation 70: II358—II364
23. Gluszko R, Rucinski B, Musial J, Wenger RK, Schmaier AH, Colman RW, Edmunds LH and Niewiarowski S (1987) Fibrinogen receptors in platelet adhesion to surfaces of extracorporeal circuit. Am J Physiol. 21: H615—H621
24. Chuang HYK, Sharma NC, Mohammed SF and Mason RG (1979) Adsorption of thrombin onto artificial surfaces and its detection by an immunoradiometric assay. Artif Organs 3: 226—231
25. Musial J, Niewiarowski S, Hershock D, Morinelli TA, Colman RW and Edmunds LH (1985) Loss of fibrinogen receptors from the platelet surface during simulated extracorporeal circulation. J Lab Clin Med 105: 514—522
26. Teoh KH, Christakis GT, Weisel RD, Mullen JC and et al (1986) Prevention of myocardial platelet deposition and thromboxane release with dipyridamole. Circulation 74: III145—III152

23

27. Addonizio VP, Macarak EJ, Colman RW, Niewiarowski S and Edmunds LH (1979) Preservation of human platelets with prostaglandin E₁ during in vitro simulation of cardiopulmonary bypass. Circ Res 44: 350—355

28. Walker ID, Davidson JF, Faichney A, and et al. (1981) A double-blind study of prostacyclin in cardiopulmonary bypass surgery. Br J Haematol 49: 415—423

29. Addonizio VP, Macarak EJ, Nicolaou KC, Edmunds LH and Colman RW (1979) Effects of prostacyclin and albumin on platelet loss during in vitro simulation of extracorporeal circulation. Blood 53: 1033—1039

30. Addonizio VP, Strauss JF, Colman RW and Edmunds LH (1979) Effects of prostaglandin E₁ on platelet loss during in vitro cardiopulmonary bypass. Circ Res 44: 350—359

31. Aren C, Feddersen K and Radegran K (1983) Effects of prostacyclin infusion on platelet activation and postoperative blood loss in coronary bypass. Ann Thorac Surg 36: 49—54

32. Addonizio VP, Fisher CA, Jenkin BK and et al. (1985) Iloprost (ZK36374), a stable analogue of prostacyclin, preserves platelets during simulated extracorporeal circulation. J Thorac Cardiovasc Surg 89: 926—933

33. Teoh KH, Christakis GT, Weisel RD, Wong P, Mee AV, Ivanov J, Madonik M, Levitt DS, Reilly PA, Rosenfeld JM and Glynn MFX (1988) Dipyridamole preserved platelets and reduced blood loss after cardiopulmonary bypass. J Thorac Cardiovasc Surg 96: 332—341

34. Packham MA, Evans G, Glynn MF and Mustard JF (1969) The effect of plasma proteins on the interaction of platelets with glass surfaces. J Lab Clin Med 73: 686—673

35. Salzman EW, Merrill EW, Binder A and et al. (1969) Protein-platelet interaction on heparinized surfaces. J Biomed Mater Res 3: 69—75

36. Van den Dungen JJ, Karliczek GF, Brenken U, Homan van der Heide J N and Wildevuur CR (1982) Clinical study of blood trauma during perfusion with membrane and bubble oxygenators. J Thorac Cardiovasc Surg 83: 108—116

37. Edmunds LH, Saxena NC, Hillyer P and Wilson TJ (1978) Relationship between platelet count and cardiotomy suction return. Ann Thorac Surg 25: 306—310

38. Addonizio VP, Colman RW and Edmunds LH (1978) Effect of blood flow and surface area on platelets during extracorporeal circulation. Trans Am Soc Artif Intern Organs 24: 650—655

39. Dutton RC, Edmunds LH, Hutchinson JC and Roe BB (1974) Platelet aggregate emboli produced in patients during cardiopulmonary bypass with membrane and bubble oxygenators and blood filters. J Thorac Cardiovasc Surg 67: 258—263

40. Bachmann F, McKenna R, Cole ER and Najafi H (1975). The haemostatic mechanism after open-heart surgery. J Thorac Cardiovasc Surg 70: 76—85

41. Young JA (1982) Coagulation abnormalities with cardiopulmonary bypass. In Pathophysiology and techniques of cardiopulmonary bypass. JR Utley, editor. Williams and Wilkins Baltimore. 88—105

42. Berndt MC, Chong BH and Andrews RK (1989) Biochemistry of drug-dependent platelet autoantigens. In Platelet immunobiology. Molecular and clinical aspects. TJ Kunicki and JN George, editors. JB Lippincott, Philadelphia. 132—147

43. Salzman EW, Rosenberg RD, Smith MH, Lindon JN and Favreau L (1980) Effect of heparin and heparin fractions on platelet aggregation. J Clin Invest 65: 64—70

44. Ekert H, Gilchrist GS, Stanton R and Hammond D (1970) Hemostasis in cyanotic congenital heart disease. J Pediatr. 76: 221—230

45. Gross S, Keefer V and Liebman J (1968) The platelets in cyanotic congenital heart disease. Pediatrics 42:, 651—655

46. Mohr R, Golan M, Martinowitz U, Rosner E, Goor DA and Ramot B (1986) Effect of cardiac operation on platelets. J Thorac Cardiovasc Surg 92: 434—441

47. Jones DK, Luddington R, Higenbottam TW, Scott J, Cavarocchi N, Reardon D, Calvin J and Wallwork J (1988) Changes in factor VIII proteins after cardiopulmonary bypass in man suggest endothelial damage. Thromb Haemostas 60: 199—204

48. Hackmann T, Gascoyne RD, Naiman SC, Growe GH, Burchill LD, Jamieson WRE, Sheps SB, Schechter MT and Townsend GE (1989) A trial of desmopressin (1-desamino-8-D-arginine vasopressin) to reduce blood loss in uncomplicated cardiac surgery. N Engl J Med 321: 1437—1443

49. Salzman EW (1987) Hemostatic problems in surgical patients. In Hemostasis and thrombosis. Basic principles and clinical practice. RW Colman, J Hirsh, VJ Marder and EW Salzman, editors. JB Lippincott, Philadelphia. 920—925

24

50. Ellison N, Edmunds LH and Colman RW (1978) Platelet aggregation following heparin and protamine administration. Anesthesiology 48: 65—68

51. Hines, R and Barash PG (1989) Infusion of sodium nitroprusside induces platelet dysfunction in vitro. Anesthesiology 70: 611—615

52. Carvalho ACA and Rao AK (1987) Acquired qualitative platelet defects. In Hemostasis and thrombosis. Basic principles and clinical practice. RW Colman, J Hirsh, VJ Marder and EW Salzman, editors. JB Lippincott, Philadelphia, pp 750—771

53. Ekert H and Dowling SV (1977) Platelet release abnormality and reduced prothrombin levels in children with cyanotic congenital heart disease. Aust Paediatr J 13: 17—21

54. Maurer HM, McCue CM, Caul J and Still WJS (1972) Impairment in platelet aggregation in congenital heart disease. Blood 40: 207—211

55. Kowalski E, Kopec M and Wegrzynowicz Z (1963) Influence of fibrinogen degradation products (FDP) on platelet aggregation, adhesiveness, and viscous metamorphosis. Thromb Diath Haemorrh 10: 406—413

56. Lee WH, Krumhaar D, Fonkalsrud E and et al. (1961) Denaturation of plasma proteins as the cause of morbidity and death after intracardiac operation. Surgery 50: 29—39

57. Pruitt KM, Stroud RM and Scott JW (1971) Blood damage in the heart-lung machine. Proc Soc Exp Biol Med 137: 714—718

58. Wallace HW, Liquoir EM, Stein TP and Brooks H (1975) Denatured plasma and platelet function. Trans Am Soc Artif Intern Organs 21: 450—455

59. George JN, Thoi LL and Morgan RK (1981) Quantitative analysis of platelet membrane glycoproteins: Effect of platelet washing procedures and isolation of platelet density subpopulations. Thromb Res 23: 69—77

60. Levine SP and Krentz LS (1977) Development of a radioimmuncassay for human platelet factor 4. Thromb. Res. 11: 673—686

61. Shattil SJ, Cunningham M and Hoxie JA (1987) Detection of activated platelets in whole blood using activation-dependent monoclonal antibodies and flow cytometry. Blood 70: 307—315

62. Abrams CS, Ellison N, Budzynski A and Shattil SJ (1990) Direct defection of actrated platelets and platelet — derived microparticles in humans. Blood 75: 128—138

63. Dechavanne M, Ffrench M, Pages J, Ffrench P, Boukerche H, Bryon PA and McGregor JL (1987) Significant reduction in the binding of a monoclonal antibody (LYP 18) directed against the IIb-IIIa glycoprotein complex to platelets of patients having undergone extracorporeal circulation. Thromb Haemostas 57: 106—109

64. Edmunds LH, Ellison N, Colman RW and et al (1982) Platelet function during open heart surgery: Comparison to the membrane and bubble oxygenators. J Thorac Cardiovasc Surg 83: 805—812

65. Wachtfogel YT, Musial J, Jenkin B, Niewiarowski S, Edmunds LH and Colman RW (1985) Loss of platelet α2-adrenergic receptors during simulated extracorporeal circulation: Prevention with prostaglandin E_1 J Lab Clin Med 105: 601—607

66. Wenger RK, Lukasiewicz H, Mikuta BS, Niewiarowski S and Edmunds LH (1989) Loss of platelet fibrinogen receptors during clinical cardiopulmonary bypass. J Thorac Cardiovasc Surg 97: 235—239

67. Holloway DS, Summaria L, Sandesara J, Vagher JP, Alexander JC and Caprini JA (1988) Decreased platelet number and function and increased fibrinolysis contribute to postoperative bleeding in cardiopulmonary bypass patients. Thromb Haemostas 59: 62—67

68. Velders AJ and Wildevuur CRH (1986) Platelet damage by protamine and the protective effect of prostacyclin: an experimental study in dogs: Ann Thorac Surg 42: 168—171

69. Bick RL, Arbegast N, Crawford L, Holterman M, Adams T and Schmalhorst W (1975) Hemostatic defects induced by cardiopulmonary bypass. Vasc. Surg 9: 228—243

70. Ekert H, Montgomery D and Aberdeen E (1971) Fibrinolysis during extracorporeal circulation: Comparison of the effects of disc and membrane oxygenators. Circ Res 28: 512—517

71. Adelman B, Michelson AD, Loscalzo J, Greenberg J and Handin RI (1985) Plasmin effect on platelet glycoprotein Ib-von Willebrand factor interactions. Blood 65 32—40

72. Adelman B, Michelson AD, Greenberg J and Handin RI (1986) Proteolysis of platelet glycoprotein Ib by plasmin is facilitated by plasmin lysine-binding regions. Blood 68: 1280—1284

25

73. Stricker RB, Wong D, Shiu DT, Reyes PT and Shuman MA (1986) Activation of plasminogen by tissue plasminogen activator on normal and thrombasthenic platelets: Effects on surface proteins and platelet aggregation. Blood 68: 275—280
74. Takamatsu J, Horne MK and Gralnick HK (1986) Identification of the thrombin receptor on human platelets by chemical crosslinking. J Clin Invest 77: 362—368
75. Harmon JT and Jamieson GA (1986) The glycocalicin portion of platelet glycoprotein Ib expresses both high and moderate affinity receptor sites for thrombin. J Biol Chem 261: 13224—13229
76. Michelson AD and Barnard MR (1989) The role of glycoprotein Ib in thrombin-induced modulation of platelet surface receptor expression. Blood 74: 172a—172a (Abstr.)
77. Michelson AD, Adelman B, Barnard MR, Carroll E and Handin RI (1988) Platelet storage results in a redistribution of glycoprotein ib molecules. Evidence for a large intraplatelet pool of glycoprotein Ib. J Clin Invest 81: 1734—1740
78. van Oeveren W, Eijsman L, Roozendaal KJ and Wildevuur CRH (1988) Platelet preservation by aprotinin during cardiopulmonary bypass. Lancet i: 644—644
79. Royston, D, Bidstrup BP, Taylor KM and Sapsford RN (1987) Effect of aprotinin on need for blood transfusion after repeat open-heart surgery. Lancet ii: 1289—1291
80. Bidstrup BP, Royston D, Sapsford RN and Taylor KM (1989) Reduction in blood loss and blood use after cardiopulmonary bypass with high dose aprotinin (Trasylol). J Thorac Cardiovasc Surg 97: 364—372

Author's address:
Dr. Alan D. Michelson,
Department of Pediatrics,
University of Massachusetts,
Medical School,
55 Lake Avenue North,
Worcester,
MA 01655, U.S.A.

Blood-Surface Interactions During Cardiopulmonary Bypass

L. H. Edmunds, Jr., R. W. Colman and S. Niewiarowski

Division of Cardiothoracic Surgery, Harrison Department of Surgery, University of Pennsylvania, Philadelphia and the Thrombosis Research Center and the Hematology-Oncology Sections and Department of Physiology, Temple University School of Medicine, Philadelphia, Pennsylvania, USA

Approximately 15 years ago, we began to investigate what happens to blood during extracorporeal circulation. We were discouraged by attempts to develop a non-thrombogenic synthetic surface and observed that only the endothelial cell possesses this attribute [50]. Endothelial cells have a vast surface area in contact with blood [51] and achieve the property of nonthrombogenicity by active metabolic processes. We concluded that short-term development of a synthetic, nonthrombogenic surface was unlikely, and decided to look at the other side of the blood-surface relationship. Over the next 10 years, we presented evidence supporting our hypothesis that complete inhibition of the initial reactions of blood constituents that are activated directly by surface contact will prevent all subsequent reactions of blood elements during cardiopulmonary bypass [31]. This strategy offers the possibility of controlling both the bleeding problems and the "whole body inflammatory response" associated with clinical cardiopulmonary bypass. This "overview" will summarize some of the data relevant to this hypothesis and present our current concept of what is happening during clinical cardiopulmonary bypass.

As soon as heparinized blood contacts a synthetic surface, plasma proteins are adsorbed onto that surface [11]. The concentrations of adsorbed proteins are not related to bulk concentrations in plasma [12], but are influenced by the chemical composition and physical properties of the surface. Factor XII, von Willebrand factor, fibronectin, and thrombospondin are immediately adsorbed [7, 57, 78, 89]. Fibrinogen is selectively adsorbed, but soon thereafter, surface fibrinogen undergoes conformational changes that alter its reactivity with platelets. Lindon, Salzman and colleagues have recently shown that fibrinogen adsorbed onto hydrophilic surfaces causes less platelet adhesion than fibrinogen adsorbed onto hydrophobic surfaces. In vitro preadsorption of albumin attenuates adhesion of platelets [65]; in vivo this strategy fails [13], probably because albumin is desorbed rapidly from the surface or is replaced by proteins with greater affinity to platelets. Platelets adhere to surface-adsorbed fibrinogen at binding sites located in both the alpha chain [55] and at the C terminal domain of the gamma chain [36] within 1 to 2 min of surface contact. Thereafter, platelets do not appear to adhere to the surface [76], probably because of conformational changes in adsorbed fibrinogen which no longer recognizes antifibrinogen antibody [91]. Alternatively, fibrinogen is displaced by high-molecular-weight kininogen [79]. Thus the synthetic surface becomes "passivated" (i.e., unreactive to platelets) [76] shortly after cardiopulmonary bypass with membrane oxygenator systems. With bubble oxygenators, each bubble represents a new

Supported by National Heart, Lung & Blood Institute Grant HL 19055.

surface and, therefore, platelet loss in these systems follows a more exponential curve [3].

During clinical cardiopulmonary bypass, platelets are directly activated by surface contact [77] and undergo shape change [100]. Other coagulation factors are not diluted or depleted sufficiently to cause postoperative coagulation deficits in patients who do not have preexisting abnormalities [44]. Activated platelets form circulating aggregates as detected on filters [30] and adhere to surface-adsorbed fibrinogen via the platelet GPIIb/IIIa membrane receptor complex [20, 39]. The mechanism by which platelets are initially activated is not known; adenine diphosphate (ADP) may be involved since the plasma concentration from lysed red cells is elevated. Some of the activated platelets release alpha and dense granular contents [43] and synthesize thromboxane A_2; others do not release [100]. The mean number of platelet membrane "fibrinogen receptors" (GPIIb/IIIa complex) receptors decreases [97]. Platelet membrane fragments, presumably from platelets that detach from the surface, appear in plasma [37]. Morphologic studies show a mixture of unactivated, activated, degranulated, and lysed platelets [100]. Platelet sensitivity to soluble agonists such as ADP, epinephrine, and thrombin decreases [32, 100]. Both platelet loss, which primarily occurs in the oxygenator [47, 68], and dilution decrease the platelet count. The decrease in platelet count contributes to the prolonged bleeding time after bypass [9, 32], but it is not the only cause. The functional deficit of platelets also contributes to an increase in bleeding time [9, 32].

Recirculation of fresh heparinized human blood in a simple membrane oxygenator-roller pump extracorporeal circuit is a useful model for study of the interaction of blood with the synthetic surfaces of the heart-lung machine [45]. Although the system does not include a cardiotomy sucker system which clearly contributes to platelet activation and destruction [33], the use of human blood permits sophisticated assays of blood constituents that are not available in animal models. Moreover, large sample volumes that are necessary for some assays are available, and drugs and chemicals which are not available for human use can be tested. The absence of an animal prevents in vivo clearance of released products and metabolites and also prevents the addition of new platelets from the bone marrow and other blood constituents from hepatic cells. The system can be rinsed with a detergent after recirculation for analysis of adsorbed proteins and blood elements [39]. In vitro recirculation provides a severe test of the ability of heparin to maintain the fluidity of blood, and it is a sensitive system for assessing activated and/or altered blood constituents.

During in vitro recirculation of fresh heparinized human blood in a membrane oxygenator circuit, platelet count decreases immediately to approximately 20% of control values [45]. Plasma low-affinity platelet factor 4 increases [45], thromboxane B_2 appears in plasma [3, 4], and none of the remaining circulating platelets react to ADP or epinephrine. After 2 h of recirculation, approximately 20% of previously adherent platelets detach from the surface; after 6 h, 40% have returned to the circulation [45, 5]. Surface adhesion of platelets requires the presence of the GPIIb/IIIa complex; platelets from patients with Glanzmann's thrombasthenia, which lack this complex, do not adhere, whereas platelets from patients with Bernard-Soulier's disease, which lack von Willebrand receptor, GPI/IX complex, do attach [39]. Recirculation reduces the mean number of circulating platelet alpha adrenergic [92] and fibrinogen receptors [64]. Transmission electron microscopy shows a mixture of partially degranulated and totally degranulated, destroyed platelets [5]. Analysis of Triton X 100 washings of the rinsed circuit after 2 h of recirculation shows a disproportionate amount of platelet GPIIIa on the surface as compared to beta thromboglobulin, which indicates that the amount of membrane material still attached to the surface far exceeds that contained in attached intact platelets [39].

At the end of cardiopulmonary bypass with either a membrane or bubble oxygenator, the platelet population is heterogeneous [97]. It is composed of platelet membrane fragments [37], totally degranulated platelets [15], detached platelets with resealed membranes [97], intact platelets [100] and newly arrived platelets from the bone marrow [58, 61]. Platelet aggregates have broken up or been removed in arterioles, capillaries, and filters. The ability of this heterogeneous mixture to aggregate and form platelet plugs is reduced; the qualitative defect in platelet function is probably the major reason that post-bypass bleeding times are increased [9, 32].

Platelet activation and loss during cardiopulmonary bypass can be altered in several ways. The chemical composition and physical characteristics of the synthetic surfaces of the bypass system affect both the adsorption and conformation of fibrinogen [59]. Theoretically, selective blockade of exposed fibrinogen platelet receptors with specific Fab fragments should prevent platelet adhesion and "passivate" the surface [60]. This strategy raises the concern that digestion, desorption or reconformation of the surface fibrinogen may expose platelet-binding sites later.

An alternative strategy involves temporary inhibition of platelets during the period of bypass with reversible inhibitors such as the prostanoids [1, 2, 5, 71], dipyridamole [86] or a new class of peptides derived from the venom of snakes (e.g., the Trimeresurus gramineus). Prostanoids reversibly inhibit platelets and prevent platelet activation, aggregation, adhesion, and release during in vitro recirculation [5]. Prostaglandin E_1 preserves platelet numbers and function during cardiopulmonary bypass in rhesus monkeys and prevents the expected increase in postoperative bleeding times [2]. In patients with heparin-induced antibodies to platelets iloprost, a stable analog of prostacyclin prevents platelet activation and loss during open-heart surgery [53]. Unfortunately, the prostanoids are potent vasodilators; clinical use requires simultaneous administration of potent vasoconstrictors or large fluid volumes to maintain acceptable blood pressures.

Dipyridamole is a vasodilator and a weak platelet inhibitor. The drug inhibits platelet cyclic AMP phosphodiesterase [67] and platelet adenosine uptake, and can attenuate platelet loss during cardiopulmonary bypass [71]. The half-life in plasma is approximately 100 min [67].

Huang and coworkers recently developed a potent inhibitor of the platelet GPIIb/IIIa complex which, in the presence of fibrinogen, is responsible for both aggregation and adhesion to synthetic surfaces [49]. This inhibitor, trigramin, was isolated from the venom of the Trimeresurus gramineus snake. A number of similar inhibitors from other viper venoms have been isolated, including echistatin, bitistatin [82], albolabrin and elegantin [99], and applogin [17]. This group of inhibitors contains an RGD sequence; however, they are 500 to 2000 times more potent than RGDs and block platelet GPIIb/IIIa, as well as other integrins (i.e., adhesive receptors). For this reason, the name "disintegrins" was proposed for this group of peptides [40]. Trigramin also blocks the binding of von Willebrand factor to the GPIIb/IIIa complex [48].

During in vitro recirculation of fresh heparinized human blood, disintegrins block adhesion of platelets to synthetic surfaces and release of beta thromboglobulin (BTG) [63]. Echistatin at a concentration of 200 nM completely prevents platelet loss and BTG release during in vitro recirculation. These peptides alone or in combination with prostanoids may produce normal bleeding times after clinical cardiopulmonary bypass by temporarily inhibiting platelets and preventing activation during the period of bypass.

Temporary inhibition of platelets during the initial moments of blood-synthetic surface contact may also create "passivated" synthetic surfaces that do not react to platelets [67, 91]. Early observations by Salzman, Vroman, and others showed that surface-adsorbed fibrinogen undergoes conformational changes that inhibit platelet adhesion. During recirculation of fresh heparinized human blood, Addonizio observed that prostacyclin inhibited platelet adhesion, aggregation, and release, and that inhibition of adhesion and release outlasted the presence of the drug in plasma and the restoration of platelet sensitivity to soluble agonists [1]. Addonizio extended these studies in dogs and showed that temporary inhibition of platelets during initial blood-surface contact with iloprost preserves platelet numbers and function during partial cardiopulmonary bypass long after the drug is metabolized [27]. Thus, reversible inhibition of platelets during initial blood-surface contact can create "passivated" synthetic surfaces in vivo, as well as in vitro.

Blood contact with synthetic surfaces also directly activates the contact activation system and specifically Factor XII, Hageman Factor. Rapid adsorption of plasma proteins produces a mosaic of positive and negative surface charges [41]; Factor XII is activated [85], bound by contact with negatively charged surfaces, and cleaved to form Factors XIIa and XIIf [29, 80]. Factor XIIa cleaves the procofactor high-molecular-weight kininogen (HK) which binds prekallikrein and Factor XI to the surface near XIIa [80, 81, 85]. Surface-bound XIIa cleaves bound prekallikrein to kallikrein, and Factor XI to XIa. Factor XIa is tightly bound to activated HK and slowly dissociates to catalyze Factor IX to IXa [87]. Kallikrein readily dissociates from the surface [87] to accelerate and amplify the contact pathway. Kallikrein reciprocally activates Factor XII, but also cleaves and activates HK, plasminogen [22], prorenin, C_1 [26], and it stimulates neutrophils [24, 94]. Activation of the contact system initiates coagulation, activates neutrophils, and produces kallikrein, bradykinin, renin and plasmin [25].

Both cardiopulmonary bypass and hemodialysis [8, 28] activate the contact pathway. Coagulation is blocked by heparin; however, uninhibited reactions contribute to the whole body reponse associated with clinical cardiopulmonary bypass. Cardiopulmonary bypass with either bubble or membrane oxygenators sharply increases plasma C3a (activated C3) and causes sequestration of leukocytes within the lungs. C5a does not increase in plasma, probably because it is rapidly bound and internalized by leukocytes [19]; however, an increase in C5a has been demonstrated indirectly [34]. Most studies fail to show a decrease in plasma C4 [18, 34, 54]; therefore, most investigators conclude that complement is activated to the anaphylatoxins C3a and C5a by the alternative (properdin) pathway [16, 18, 34, 42, 54, 98]. Collett has found direct evidence of alternative pathway activation. Jones, however, found small, inconstant reductions of C4 during clinical cardiopulmonary bypass and concluded that complement was activated via the classical pathway, possibly due to aggregation (and denaturation of IgM) [52]. Recently, we proved that cardiopulmonary bypass activates complement by the classical pathway by demonstrating increases in C1-C1 inhibitor complex and kallikrein-C1 inhibitor complex [93]. The increase in C-C1 inhibitor complex is direct evidence of C1 activation and probably occurs via Factor XIIf [38]. Thus, there is evidence that complement is activated by both classical (though non-immune) and alternative pathways during cardiopulmonary bypass.

Complement activation is not the only means by which neutrophils are activated during cardiopulmonary bypass. Both kallikrein [94] and Factor XIIa [45] directly activate neutrophils and both are produced by initial reactions of the contact pathway. Activation of neutrophils causes release of powerful proteolytic enzymes [23, 69, 83, 94, 95, 96], including elastase [69, 94, 95, 96], collagenase, cathepsin G and D [83, 96], and acid hydrolases [6]. Other biologically active components secreted include neutrophil thromboxane, myleoperoxidase, lactoferrin, superoxide [10, 75], hydrogen peroxide, and procoagulants [62, 70, 73]. Activation of neutrophils and monocytes causes sequestration of these cells within the lung[18, 28, 54]. Release of leukocyte proteases and oxygen radicals [10, 56, 75] from sequestered cells are likely responsible for pulmonary endothelial cell injury [46, 74], extravasation of blood and fluid into the lung [66, 72, 88], loss of pulmonary compliance and much of the morbidity associated with cardiopulmonary bypass [54, 98], and hemodialysis [8, 28].

From what we now know, only platelets and Factor XII are directly activated by blood contact with synthetic surfaces. All other reactions — including coagulation — are consequences of activated platelets and activated Factor XII. Theoretically, inhibition of these two initial reactions should prevent both the bleeding diathesis and the whole-body inflammatory response associated with extracorporeal perfusion, and should obviate the need for heparin. Some platelet inhibitors are already available and a new group of platelet membrane receptor inhibitors has recently been discovered. The means to control platelets does not appear far off. Effective inhibitors of various steps in the contact activation system are also known. Aprotinin, an inhibitor of plasma kallikrein, is one of these, but paradoxically, aprotinin appears to have a greater salutary effect on the bleeding diathesis than on the whole-body inflammatory response. As the mysteries of the contact activation system unfold and as new specific inhibitors are discovered, the goal of controlling the blood-surface interface comes closer. Complete control not only pre-empts much of the morbidity of cardiopulmonary bypass, but also conquers the thromboembolic complications associated with prosthetic heart valves, small-vessel prostheses, artificial hearts, and the development of other artificial internal organs.

References

1. Addonizio VP Jr, Macarak EJ, Nicolaou, KC, et al (1979c) Effects of prostacyclin and albumin on platelet loss during in vitro simulation of extracorporeal circulation. Blood 53: 1033
2. Addonizio VP Jr, Strauss JF III, Macarak EJ, Colman RW, Edmunds LH Jr (1978) Preservation of platelet number and function with prostaglandin E_1 during total cardiopulmonary bypass in rhesus monkeys. Surgery 83: 619—625
3. Addonizio VP Jr, Smith JB, Strauss JF III, Colman RW, Edmunds LH Jr (1980) Thromboxane synthesis and platelet secretion during cardiopulmonary bypass with bubble oxygenator. J Thorac Cardiovasc Surg 79: 91—96
4. Addonizio VP Jr, Smith JB, Guiod LR, Strauss JF III, Colman RW, Edmunds LH Jr (1979s) The relationship between thromboxane synthesis and blood protein release during simulated extracorporeal circulation. Blood 54: 371
5. Addonizio VP Jr, Strauss JF III, Colman RW, Edmunds LH Jr (1979) Effects of prostaglandin E_1 on platelet loss during in vitro cardiopulmonary bypass. Circ Res 44: 350

6. Addonizio VP Jr, Chang LK, Strauss JR III, Colman RW, Edmunds LH Jr (1982) Release of lysosomal hydrolases during extracorporeal circulation. J Thorac Cardiovasc Surg 84: 28—34
7. Andrade JD, Nagaoka S, Cooper S, Okano T, Kim SW (1987) Surfaces and blood compatibility: Current hypotheses. Trans Am Soc Artif Intern Organs 33: 75—84
8. Arnaout MA, Hakim RM, Todd RF III, Dana N, Colten HR (1985) Increased expression of an adhesion-promoting surface glycoprotein in the granulocytopenia of hemodialysis. N Engl J Med 312: 457—462
9. Bachmann F, McKenna R, Cole ER, Najafi H (1975) The hemostatic mechanism after open-heart surgery. J Thorac Cardiovasc Surg 70: 76—85
10. Badway JA, Karnovsky ML (1980) Active oxygen species in the functions of fagocytic leukocytes. Ann Rev Biochem 49: 695—726
11. Baier RC, Dutton RC (1969) Initial events in interactions of blood with a foreign surface. J Biomed Mater Res 3: 191
12. Brash JL, Uniyal S (1979) Dependence of albumin-fibrinogen simple and competitive adsorption on surface properties of biomaterials. J Polymer Sci 166: 377
13. Brash JL, ten Hove P (1984) Effect of plasma dilution on adsorption of fibrinogen to solid surfaces. Thromb Haemost 51: 326—330
14. Brach JL, Scott CF, Move P, Wojciechowski P, Colman RW (1988) Mechanism of transient adsorption of fibrinogen from plasma to solid surfaces: Role of the contact and fibrinolytic system. Blood 71: 932—939
15. Brueling-Harbury C, Galvan CA (1978) Acquired decrease in platelet secretory ADP associated with increased postoperative bleeding in post-cardiopulmonary bypass patients and in patients with severe valvular heart disease. Blood 52: 13
16. Cavarocchi NC, Pluth JR, Schaff HV, et al (1986) Complement activation during cardiopulmonary bypass. J Thorac Cardiovasc Surg 91: 252—258
17. Chao BH, Jakubowski JA, Savage B, Ping Chow E, Marzec UM, Harker LA, Maraganore JM (1989) Agkistrodon piscivorus piscivorus platelet aggregation inhibitor: A potent inhibitor of platelet activation. Proc Natl Acad Sci 86: 8050—8054
18. Chenoweth DE, Cooper SW, Hugli TE, Stewart RW, Blackstone EH, Kirklin JW (1981). Complement activation during cardiopulmonary bypass. N Engl J Med 304: 497—503
19. Chenoweth DE, Hugli TE (1980) Binding internalization and degradation of C5a by neutrophils. Fed Proc 39: 1049
20. Coller BS, Peerschke EI, Scudder LE, Sullivan CA (1983) A murine monoclonal antibody that completely blocks the binding of fibrinogen to platelets produces a thromboasthenic-like state in normal platelets and binds to glycoproteins IIb and/or IIIa. J Clin Invest 72: 325
21. Collett B, Alhaq A, Abdullah NB, et al (1984) Pathways to complement activation during cardiopulmonary bypass. Brit Med J 289: 1251—1254
22. Colman RW (1969) Activation of plasminogen by human plasmin kallikrein. Biochem Biophys Res Commun 35: 273
23. Colman RW, Scott CF, Schmaier AH, Wachtfogel YT, Pixley RA, Edmunds LH Jr (1987) Initiation of blood coagulation at artificial surfaces. In press, NY Acad Sci
24. Colman RW, Wachtfogel YT, Kucich U, et al (1985) Effect of cleavage of the heavy chain of human plasma kallikrein on its functional properties. Blood 65: 311—318
25. Colman RW (1984) Surface-mediated defense reactions. J Clin Invest 73: 1249
26. Cooper NR, Miles LA, Griffin JH (1980) Effects of plasma kallikrein and plasmin of the first component of complement. J Immunol 124: 1517
27. Cottrell ED, Kappa JR, Stenach N, Fisher CA, Tuszynski GP, Switalska HI, Addonizio VP (1988) Temporary inhibition of platelet function with iloprost (ZK36374) preserves canine platelets during extracorporeal membrane oxygenation. J Thorac Cardiovasc Surg 96: 535—541
28. Craddock PR, Fehr J, Brigham KL, Kronenberg RS, Jacob HS (1977) Complement and leukocyte-mediated pulmonary function in hemodialysis. N Engl J Med 296: 769—774
29. Dunn JT, Silberberg M, Kaplan AP (1982) The cleavage and formation of activated human Hageman factor by autodigestion and by kallikrein. J Biol Chem 257: 1779
30. Dutton RC, Edmunds LH Jr (1973) Measurement of emboli in extracorporeal perfusion systems. J Thorac Cardiovasc Surg 65: 523—530
31. Edmunds LH Jr (1985) The sangreal. J Thorac Cardiovasc Surg 90: 1

32. Edmunds LH Jr, Ellison N, Colman RW, Niewiarowski S, Rao AK, Addonizio VP Jr, Stephenson LW, Edie RN (1982) Platelet function during open heart surgery: Comparison of membrane and bubble oxygenators. Thorac Cardiovasc Surg 83: 805—812

33. Edmunds LH Jr, Saxena NC, Hillyer P, Wilson TJ (1978) Relationship between platelet count and cardiotomy suction return. Ann Thorac Surg 25: 306—310

34. Fosse E, Mollnes TE, Ingvaldsen B (1987) Complement activation during major operations with or without cardiopulmonary bypass. J Thorac Cardiovasc Surg 93: 860—866

35. Gan ZR, Gould RJ, Jacobs JW, Friedman PA, Polokoff MA (1988) Echistatin; A potent platelet aggregation inhibitor from the venom of the viper. Echis carinatus. J Biol Chem 263: 19827—19832

36. Gartner TK, Bennett JS (1985) The tetrapeptide analogue of cell attachment site of fibronectin inhibits platelet aggregation and fibrinogen binding to activated platelets. J Biol Chem 260: 3931—3936

37. George JN, Picket EB, Saucerman S, et al (1986) Platelet surface glycoproteins: Studies on resting and activated platelets and platelet microparticles in normal subjects and observations in patients during adult respiratory distress syndrome and cardiac surgery. J Clin Invest 78: 40—48

38. Ghebrehiwet B, Silverberg M, Kaplan AP (1981) Activation of the classical pathway of complement by Hageman factor fragment. J Exper Med 153: 665

39. Gluszko P, Rucinski B, Musial J, Wenger RK, Schmaier AH, Colman RW, Edmunds LH Jr, Niewiarowski S (1987) Fibrinogen receptors in platelet adhesion to surface of extracorporeal circuit. Amer J Physiol 252: H615—H621

40. Gould RJ, Gan Z-R, Polokoff MA, Carsky VM, Shebuski RJ, Friedman PA, Niewiarowski S, Rucinski B, Williams JA, Cook JJ, Holt JC, Huang T-F (1990) Disintegrins: A family of integrin inhibitory proteins from viper venoms. In press, Faseb J

41. Griffin JH, Cochrane CG (1979) Recent advances in the understanding of contact activation reactions. Semin Thromb Hemost 5: 254

42. Hammerschmidt DE, Stroncek DF, Bowers TK, Lammi-Keefe CJ, Kurth DM, Ozalins A, Nicoloff DM, Lillehei RC, Craddock PR (1981) Complement activation and neutropenia occuring during cardiopulmonary bypass. J Thorac Cardiovasc Surg 81: 370—377

43. Harker LA, Marzec UM, Ginsberg MH (1983) Thrombospondin levels in plasma, platelets and urine in normal subjects, subjects receiving heparin, thoracotomy patients and patients undergoing cardiopulmonary bypass. Thromb Haemost 50: 0040

44. Harker LA, Malpass TW, Branson HE, Hessel EA II, Slichter SJ (1980) Mechanisms of abnormal bleeding in patients undergoing cardiopulmonary bypass: Acquired transient platelet dysfunction associated with seletive alpha granule release. Blood 55: 824

45. Hennessey VL Jr, Hicks RE, Niewiarowski S, Edmunds LH Jr, Colman RW (1977) Effects of surface area and composition on the function of human platelets during extracorporeal circulation. Amer J Physiol 232: H622—H628

46. Henson PM, Larsen GL, Webster O, Mitchell BC, Goins AJ, Henson JE (1981) Pulmonary microvascular alterations and injury induced by complement fragments: synergistic effect of complement activation, neutrophil sequestration and prostaglandins. Ann NY Acad Sci 384: 287—300

47. Hope AF, Heyns A duP, Lotter MG, van Reenen OR, deKock F, Badenhorst PN, Pieters H, Kotze H, Meyer JM, Minnaar PC (1981) Kinetics and sites of sequestration of indium III-labeled human platelets during cardiopulmonary bypass. J Thorac Cardiovasc Surg 81: 880—886

48. Huang TF, Holt JC, Kirby EP, Niewiarowski S (1989) Trigramin: Primary structure and its inhibition of von Willebrand Factor binding to glycoprotein IIb/IIIa complex on human platelets. Biochemistry 28: 551—666

49. Huang TF, Holt JC, Lukasiewicz H, Niewiarowski S (1987) Trigramin: A low molecular weight peptide inhibiting fibrinogen interaction with platelet receptors expressed on glycoprotein IIb/IIIa complex. J Biol Chem 262: 16157—16163

50. Jaffe EA, Weksler VP (1979) Recovery of endothelial cell prostacyclin production after inhibition of low doses of aspirin. J Clin Invest 63: 532

51. Jaffe EA (1984) Biology of Endothelial Cells. Nijhoff, Boston

52. Jones HM, Matthews N, Vaughan RS, Stark JM (1982) Cardiopulmonary bypass and complement activation: Involvement of classical and alternative pathways. Anaesthesia 37: 629—633

33

53. Kappa JR, Fisher CA, Bell P, Campbell F, Ellison N (1990) Intraoperative management of patients with heparin-induced thrombocytopenia: The University of Pennsylvania experience. In press, Ann Thorac Surg

54. Kirklin JK, Westaby S, Blackstone EH, Kirklin JW, Chenoweth DE, Pacifico AD (1983) Complement and the damaging effects of cardiopulmonary bypass. J Thorac Cardiovasc Surg 86: 845—857

55. Kloczewiak M, Timmons S, Lukas TJ, Hawiger J (1984) Platelet recognition of human fibrinogen: Synthesis and structure-function relationship of peptides corresponding to the carboxy-terminal segment of the gamma chain. Biochem

56. Korchak HM, Vienne K, Rutherford LE, Weissman G (1984) Neutrophil stimulation: Receptor membrane and metabolic events. Fed Proc 43: 2749—2754

57. Lambrecht LK, Young DR, Stafford RE, Albrecht RM, Mosher DF, Cooper SL (1986) The influence of preabsorbed canine von Willebrand factor, fibronectin and fibrinogen on in vivo artificial surface-induced thrombosis. Thromb Res 41: 99—117

58. Laufer N, Merin G, Grover NB, Pessachowicz B, Borman JB (1975) The influence of cardiopulmonary bypass on the size of human platelets. J Thorac Cardiovasc Surg 70: 727—731

59. Lindon JN, McManama G, Kushner L, et al (1986) Does the conformation of adsorbed fibrinogen dictate platelet-surface interactions? Blood 68: 355

60. McManama G, Lindon JN, Kloczewiak M et al (1986) Platelet aggregation by fibrinogen polymers cross-linked over the E domain. Blood 68: 363

61. Mohr R, Golan M, Martinowitz U, Rosner E, Goor DA, Ramot B (1986) Effect of cardiac operation on platelets. J Thorac Cardiovasc Surg 92: 434—441

62. Muhlfelder TW, Niemetz J, Kreutzer D, Beebe D, Ward PA, Rosenfeld SI (1979) C5 chemotactic fragment induces leukocyte production of tissue factor activity. J Clin Invest 63: 147—150

63. Musial J, Rucinski B, Williams JA, Stewart GJ, Edmunds LH Jr, Niewiarowski S (1990) Inhibition of platelet adhesion to surfaces of the extracorporeal circuit by disintegrins: RGD-containing peptides from viper venoms. In press, Circulation

64. Musial J, Niewiaroski S, Hershock D, Morinelli TA, Colman RW, Edmunds LH Jr (1985) Loss of fibrinogen receptors from the platelet surface during stimulated extracorporeal circulation. J Lab Clin Med 105: 513—522

65. Packham MA, Evans G, Glynn MF, Mustard JF (1969) The effect of plasma proteins on the interaction of platelets on glass surfaces. J Lab 6 Clin Med 73: 686

66. Parker DJ, Karp RB, Kirklin JW, Bedard P (1972) Lung water and alveolar and capillary volumes after intracardiac surgery. Circulation 45 (Suppl 1): 139

67. Pedersen AK, Fitzgerald GA (1985) The human pharmacology of platelet inhibition: Pharmacokinetics relevant to drug action. Circulation 72: 1164—1176

68. Peterson KA, Dewanjee MK, Kaye MP (1982) Fate of indium II-labeled platelets during cardiopulmonary bypass performed with membrane and bubble oxygenators. J Thorac Cardiovasc Surg 84: 39—43

69. Plow EP (1982) Leukocyte elastase release during blood coagulation. J Clin Invest 69: 564—572

70. Pyrdz H, Allison AC, Schorlemmer HU (1977) Further link between complement activation and blood coagulation. Nature 270: 173—174

71. Radegran K, Papaconstantinou C (1980) Prostacyclin infusion during cardiopulmonary bypass in man. Thromb Res 19: 267—270

72. Ratliff NB, Young WG Jr, Hackel DB, Mikat E, Wilson JW (1973) Pulmonary injury secondary to extracorporeal circulation. J Thorac Cardiovasc Surg 65: 425—432

73. Rothberger H, Zimmerman TS, Spiegelberg HL, Vaughan JH (1977) Leukocyte procoagulant activity. J Clin Invest 59: 549—557

74. Ryan US, Schultz DR, Ryan JW (1981) Fc and C3b receptors on pulmonary endothelial cells: Induction by injury. Science 214: 557—558

75. Sacks T, Moldow CF, Craddock PR, Bowers TK, Jacob HS (1978) Oxygen radicals mediate endothelial cell damage by complement-stimulated granulocytes. J Clin Invest 61: 1161—1167

76. Salzman EW, Landon J, Brier D (1977) Surface-induced platelet adhesion, aggregation and release. In: Vroman L, Leonard EF (eds) The Behavior of Blood and Its Components at Interfaces. N.Y. Academy of Sciences, N.Y., p. 114

34

77. Salzman EW (1963) Measurement of platelet adhesiveness. J Lab Clin Med 62: 724
78. Salzman EW, Merrill EW (1987) Interaction of blood with artifical surfaces. In: Colman RW, Hirsh J, Marder VJ, Salzman EW (eds) Hemostasis and Thrombosis. Lippincott, Philadelphia, pp 1335—1347
79. Schmaier AH, Silver L, Adams AL, Fischer GC, Munoz PC, Vroman L, Colman RW (1984) The effect of high molecular weight kininogen on surface-adsorbed fibrinogen. Thromb Res 33: 51—57
80. Schmaier AH, Silberberg M, Kaplan AP, Colman RW (1987) Contact activation and its abnormalities. In: Colman RW, Hirsh J, Marder VJ, Salzman EW (eds) Hemostasis and Thrombosis. Lippincott, Philadelphia, p. 18—38
81. Scott CF, Silver LD, Schapira M, Colman RW (1984) Cleavage of human high molecular weight kininogen markedly enhances its coagulant activity: Evidence that this molecule exists as a procofactor. J Clin Invest 73: 954—962
82. Shebuski RJ, Ramjit DR, Bencen GH, Polokoff MA (1989) Characterization of platelet inhibitory activity of bitistatin, a potent RGD containing peptide from the venom of the viper, bitis arietans. In press, J Biol Chem
83. Silber R, Moldaw CF (1983) Biochemistry and function of neutrophils. In: Williams WJ, Beutler E, Erslev AJ, Lichtman MA (eds) Hematology. McGraw Hill, N.Y., pp 726—734
84. Silberberg M, Nicoll JE, Kaplan AP (1980) The mechanism by which the light chain of cleaved HMW-kininogen augments the activation of prekallikrein, Factor XII and Hageman factor. Thromb Res 20: 173
85. Silverberg M, Dunn JT, Garen L, Kaplan AP (1980) Autoactivation of human Hageman factor; Demonstration utilizing a synthetic substrate. J Biol Chem 255: 7281—7296
86. Teoh KH, Christakis GT, Weisel RD, Wong PY, Mee AU, Ivanov J, Madonik M, Levitt DS, Reilly PA, Rosenfeld JM, Glynn MFX (1988) Dipyridamole preserved platelets and reduced blood loss after cardiopulmonary bypass. J Thorac Cardiovasc Surg 96: 332—341
87. Thompson RE, Mandle R Jr, Kaplan AP (1979) Studies of the binding of prekallikrein and Factor XII to high molecular weight kininogen and its light chain. Proc Natl Acad Sci USA 79: 4862
88. Toren M, Goffinet JA, Kaplow LS (1970) Pulmonary bed sequestration of neutrophils during hemodialysis. Blood 36: 337—340
89. Uniyal S, Brash JL (1982) Patterns of adsorption of proteins from human plasma onto foreign surfaces. Thromb Haemost 47: 285—290
90. Vroman L, Adams AL (1969) Findings with the recording ellipsometer suggesting rapid exchange of specific plasma proteins at liquid/solid interfaces. Surface Science 16: 438
91. Vroman L, Adams AL, Fischer GC, Munoz PC (1980) Interaction of high molecular weight kininogen, Factor XII and fibrinogen in plasma at interfaces. Blood 55: 156
92. Wachtfogel YT, Musial J, Jenkin B, Niewiarowski S, Edmunds LH Jr, Colman RW (1985) Loss of platelet alpha 2-adrenergic receptors during simulated extracorporeal circulation: Prevention with prostaglandin E₁. J Lab Clin Med 105: 601—607
93. Wachtfogel YT, Harpel PC, Edmunds LH Jr (1989) Formation of Cls-Cl-inhibitor, kallikrein-Cl-inhibitor and plasmin-alpha 2-plasmin-inhibitor complexes during cardiopulmonary bypass. Blood 73: 468—471
94. Wachtfogel YT, Kucich U, James HL, Scott CF, et al (1983) Human plasma kallikrein releases neutrophil elastase during blood coagulation. J Clin Invest 72: 1672—1677
95. Wachtfogel YT, Pixley RA, Kucich U, et al (1986) Purified plasma Factor XIIa aggregates human neutrophils and causes degranulation. Blood 67: 1731—1737
96. Weitz JI, Landman SL, Crowley KA, Birken S, Morgan FJ (1986) Development of an assay for in vivo human neutrophil elastase activity. J Clin Invest 78: 155—162
97. Wenger RK, Lukasiewicz H, Mikuta BS, Niewiarowski S, Edmunds LH Jr (1989) Loss of platelet fibrinogen receptors during clinical cardiopulmonary bypass. J Thorac Cardiovasc Surg 97: 235—239
98. Westaby S (1983) Complement and the damaging effects of cardiopulmonary bypass. Thorax 38: 321—325
99. Williams JA, Rucinski B, Holt JC, Niewiarowski S (1989) Purification and amino acid sequence of two RGD-containing peptides from the venoms of Trimeresurus elegans and T. albolabris. FASEB J 3: 487 (abstract). Submitted Bioch Bioph Acta

100. Zilla P, Fasol R, Groscurth P, Klepetko W, Keichenspurner H, Wolner E (1989) Blood platelets in cardiopulmonary bypass operations: Recovery occurs after initial stimulation rather than continual activation. J Thorac Cardiovasc Surg 97: 379—388

Author's address:
L. Henry Edmunds, JR., MD.
W. M. Measey Professor
Chief, Cardiothoracic Surgery
Hospital of the University of Pennsylvania
3400 Spruce Street
Philadelphia
PA 19104

A Clinical Study on Platelet Preservation in Coronary Artery Bypass Surgery During Cardiopulmonary Bypass Without Oxygenator

A. Bochenek, Z. Religa, J. Wojnar, A. Wnuk-Wojnar, M. Zembala, J. Hołłowiecki, A. Bochenek

1st Clinic of Cardiac Surgery, Department of Cardiac Surgery, Clinic of Haematology, and 1st Clinic of Cardiology, Institute of Cardiology, Silesian Medical Academy, Katowice-Zabrze, Poland

Introduction

The direct blood gas interface in bubble oxygenators is thought to be the main causative factor in the production of platelet (Plt) damage and bleeding unrelated to technical problems. To diminish the unphysiological surface area, the elimination of membrane or bubble oxygenator by the technique of extracorporeal circulation (ECC) with patient's lungs used for oxygenation (autooxygenation technique [2]) was introduced.

The aim of this study was to evaluate the hemocompatibility of ECC using the lungs in comparison to the extracorporeal bubble oxygenator in coronary artery bypass (CAB) surgery.

Material and methods

Thirty male patients undergoing elective CAB surgery were divided into two equal groups. In group-A (autooxygenation) patients (mean age 53 ± 6.7 years), a double reservoir system (Polystan Reservoir catalog no 892910) was used, utilizing, patients' lungs in ECC [2]. In group-B (bubble oxygenator) patients (mean age 59 ± 2.1 years) a conventional technique of CPB with a bubble oxygenator (Polystan Venotherm 5000) was used. No patient from any group had abnormal coagulation parameters.

Whole blood samples were drawn before, during, and after CPB to evaluate: 1) platelets (Plt) count, measured by an electronic Platelet Counter MK 4HC, Baker; 2) β-thromboglobulin (BTG) concentrations measured by means of commercial radio-immunoassay (Radio Chemical Centre); 3) Plt aggregation measured using a modified Born method (1) in an agregometer (Chronolog Corp.) at 37 °C after stimulation by epinephrine and adenosine diphosphate (ADP) (Sigma Medical Co.); 4) Blood loss through the chest-tube drainage and requirements of blood transfusions up to 18 h after protamine administration. The Plt count, plasma Hb and BTG values were corrected for hemodilution. Statistical analysis included paired and unpaired Student's t-test.

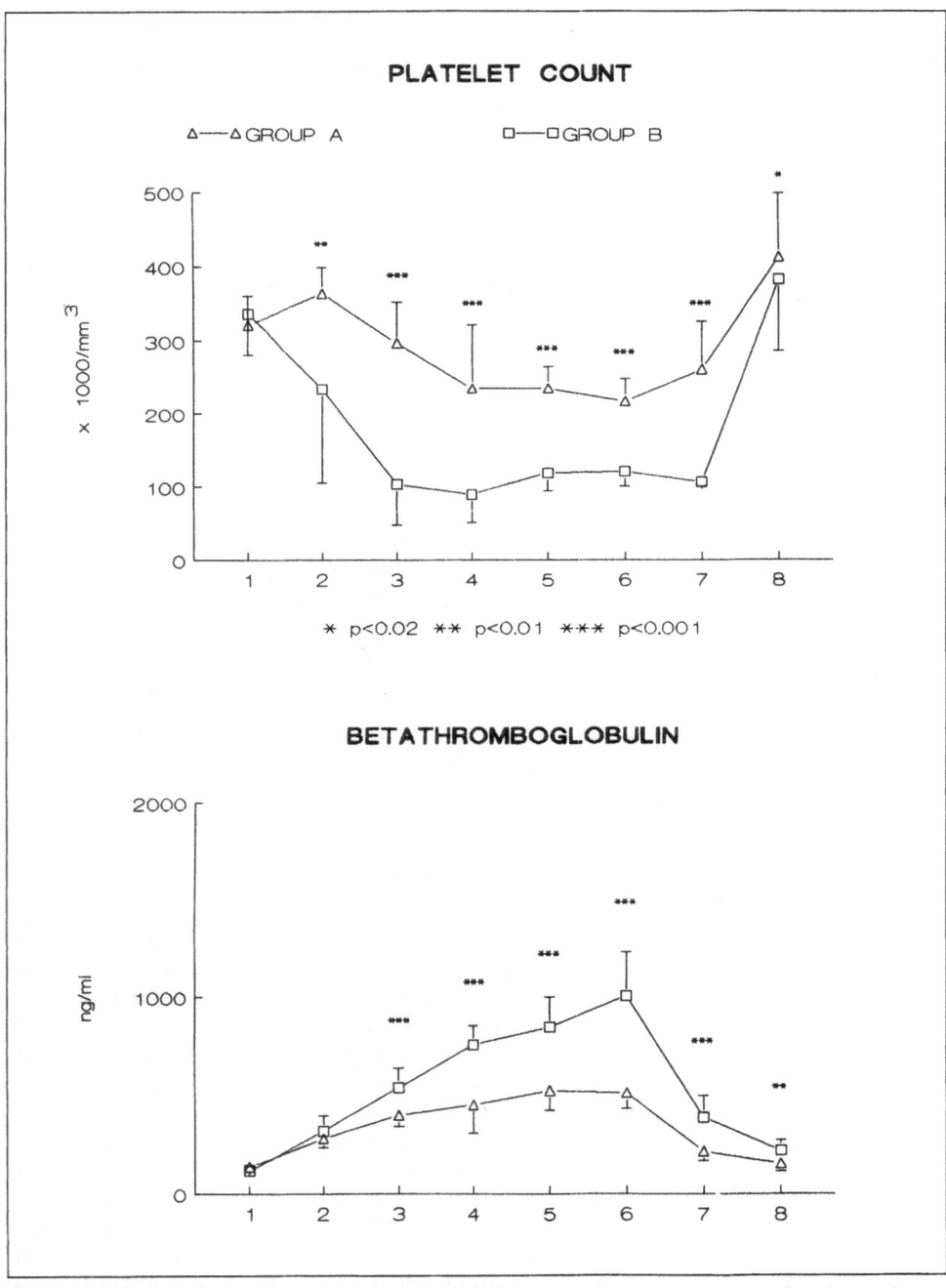

Fig. 1. Platelet count and β-thromboglobulin release during CPB in two groups of patients. Group A: autooxygenation with patient's lungs; Group B: bubble oxygenator in ECC. Sample 1: Pre-CPB (before heparin); Sample 2: 5 min after institution of CPB; Sample 3: 30 min after sample 2; Sample 4: following removal of aortic clamp; Sample 5: end of CPB; Sample 6: 30 min after protamine sulfate administration; Sample 7: 4 h after end of CPB; Sample 8: 18 h after end of CPB.

Results

There were no significant differences between groups in anthropometric and bypass data. The most enhanced changes during and after ECC (Fig. 1) were observed in group B in Plt count and function; the significant decrease in Plt count was observed starting from sample 1 ($p < 0.01$) until sample 7 ($p < 0.001$), and the lowest Plt count was observed at sample 4: -73% of initial value in group B vs only -27% in group A.

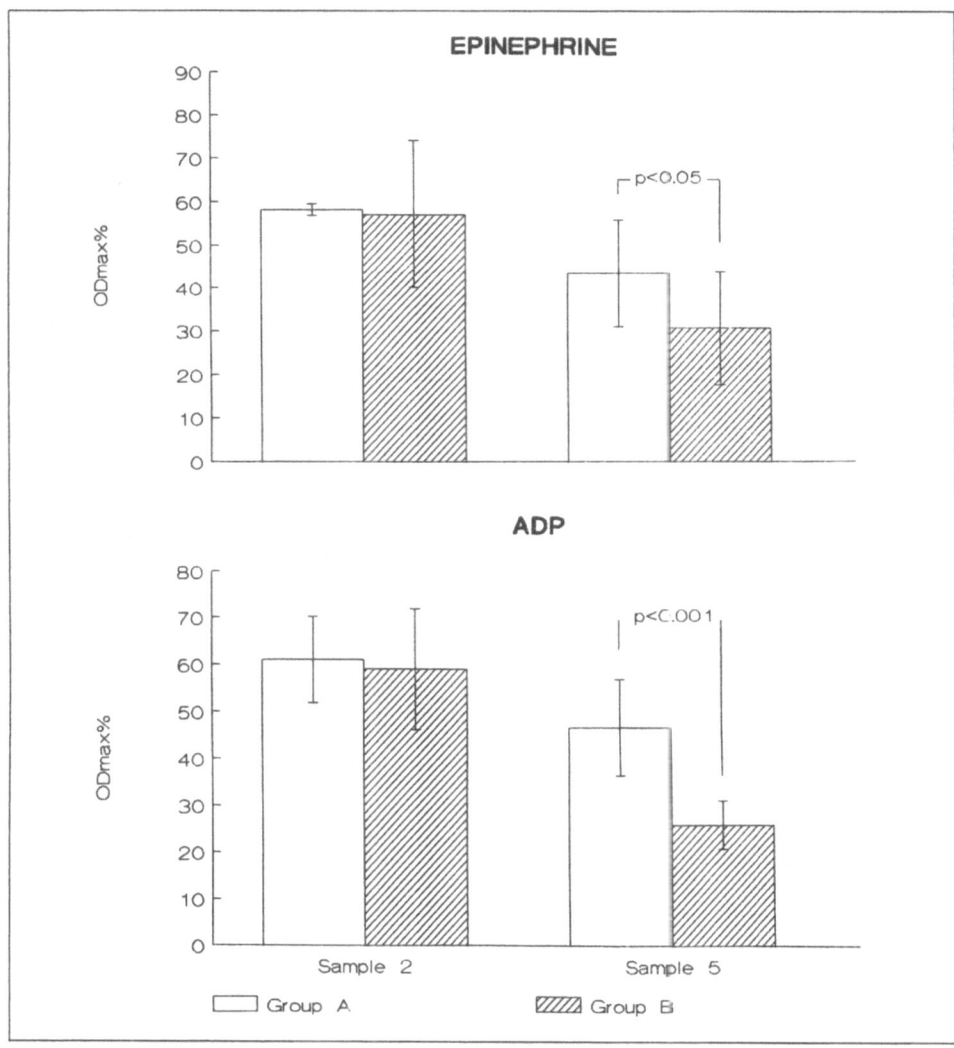

Fig. 2. Platelet aggregation to epinephrine and ADP during CPB in two groups of patients. Group A: autooxygenation with patient's lungs; Group B: bubble oxygenator in ECC. Sample 2: 5 min after institution of CPB; Sample 5: end of CPB.

In both groups a rise in BTG was shown with a significant inverse correlation to the degree of Plt depletion, but starting from the sample 3 a higher BTG release was observed in group B, $p < 0.001$, with the maximum increase being $+ 286\%$ in group A (sample 4) and $+ 769\%$ in group B (sample 5).

No significant difference in initial Plt aggregation (Fig. 2) as assessed using epinephrine and ADP was observed between groups: 56 ± 4 $OD_{max\%}$ and 60 ± 7 $OD_{max\%}$ in group A, and 56 ± 19 $OD_{max\%}$ and 58 ± 11 $OD_{max}\%$ in group B, respectively, but at the end of CPB in group A aggregation decreased only slightly to 41 ± 11 $OD_{max\%}$ after epinephrine and 48 ± 8 $OD_{max\%}$ after ADP, and barely decreased in group B to 29 ± 9 $OD_{max\%}$ and 25 ± 4 $OD_{max\%}$, respectively. The differences between Plt aggregation induced by both agents were significant between two groups, $p < 0.2$ and $p < 0.001$, respectively.

In group A the mean blood loss was 287 ± 35 ml/m^2 and 476 ± 58 ml/m^2 in group B, $p < 0.001$. The mean homologous blood transfusion in group A and B was 189 ± 79 ml/m^2 and 417 ± 81 ml/m^2, respectively ($p < 0.001$).

Discussion

Bubble oxygenators have been recognized as a main source of Plt damage [3, 4]: Plt are activated, adhere to synthetic surfaces, form circulating aggregates, release granule contents or are refractory to activating stimuli. Mechanical Plt damage, dilution and aggregation by ADP released from hemolyzed red cells may contribute to bleeding diathesis after CPB.

Our results demonstrate clearly that the elimination of artificial oxygenator from the ECC and installation of double reservoir system with autooxygenation diminished markedly the decline in Plt count and Plt activation during CPB.

References

1. Born G, Cross M (1963) The aggregation of blood platelets. J Physiol 168: 178—80
2. Glenville B (1987) Cardiac surgery using the patient's lungs as the oxygenator. Perfusion 2: 161—166
3. Harker L, Malpass T, Branson H, Hessel E, Slichter S (1980) Mechanism of abnormal bleeding in patients undergoing cardiopulmonary bypass: acquired transient platelet dysfunction associated with selective α-granule release. Blood 56: 824—834
4. Pearson D, McArdle B (1989) Haemocompatibility of membrane and bubble oxygenators. Perfusion 4: 9—24

Authors' address:
Andrzej Bochenek, MD
I Klinika Kardiochirurgii
Slaskiej Akademii Medycznej
Ślaski Ośrodek Kardiologii
Ul. Ziołlowa 47,
PL-40 635 Katowice, Poland

The Effect of Aprotinin on Platelet Function and Coagulation In Vitro

C. P. Ratnatunga*, P. Gorog, I. B. Kovacs, G. M. Ress

* Department of Cardiothoracic Surgery and Thrombosis Unit,
  St. Bartholomew's Hospital, London, UK

Introduction

Aprotinin is associated with an impressive reduction in postoperative blood loss after cardiac surgery [1]. The risk of transmission of infection with homologous blood transfusion has led to the call for the use of haemostatic agents, such as aprotinin, routinely during cardiopulmonary bypass [2]. There is concern however, that the haemostatic effect of the drug may reflect its thrombogenic potential and therefore, preclude its routine use.

The aim of this study was to investigate the possible thrombogenecity of aprotinin, by using a new technique (the Haemostatometer) to measure the effect of aprotinin on platelet function under physiologically relevant conditions.

Methods

Non-anticoagulated blood (2 ml) was studied alone or following mixing with aprotinin (Trasylol, Bayer) (0.5 ml) or 0.9 % saline (0.5 ml). Haemostatic-plug formation and the coagulation process were studied in 14 subjects, and occlusive platelet thrombus formation on collagen fibre was studied in 11 subjects.

Platelet formation and coagulation measurements

The Haemostatometer technique has been described in detail elsewhere [3, 4]. Non-anticoagulated blood was perfused through polyethylene tubing. The pressure changes monitored continuously were due to 1) the punching of holes in the tube and the subsequent haemostatic-plug formation (haemostatogram), 2) the formation of an occlusive thrombus on a collagen fibre mounted in the lumen of the tube (thrombogram), and 3) the coagulation process subsequent to haemostasis (coagulogram). The analysis of the recordings has been described elsewhere [3, 4] (for definitions see Table 1).

Statistical Analysis

All the data are represented as the mean ± SEM. Comparisons within groups were made using the paired t-test.

Table 1. The in vitro effect of aprotinin on haemostasis, coagulation and thrombus formation on a collagen fibre. 1 = Initial platelet reactivity due to activation by haemodynamic forces; 2 = Complete haemostasis due to thrombin generation and platelet-plug stabilization; and 3 = The integrated area under the thrombogram expressed as a percentage of a maximum possible area over 7 min (0 % = no thrombosis; 100 % total occlusion). p-values are differences from the respective control data: * p < 0.01, ** p < 0.005, *** p < 0.001.

	Subjects	native blood alone	native blood and saline	native blood and aprotinin
Haemostasis phase I [1]	14	581±101	561±75	3379±1064*
Haemostasis phase II [2]	14	4137±665	3387±467	16484±3170***
Coagulation (seconds)	14	776±40	644±60	1244±57***
Thrombus formation [3] on collagen fibre (%)	11	57.3±6.4	54.0±6.7	12.2±1.9**

Results

Aprotinin mixed with blood had a significantly prolonged first phase of haemostasis (3379 ± 1046), completion of haemostasis (16484 ± 3170) and coagulation (1244 ± 51), when compared with blood alone or blood mixed with saline (p < 0.01, p < 0.001 and p < 0.001, respectively). Aprotinin, furthermore, had a significant inhibitory effect on thrombus formation on a collagen fibre (12.2 ± 1.9) when compared as above (p < 0.005).

Discussion

The reduction of postoperative blood loss with the use of aprotinin has led to the call for its more widespread use. It has, for instance, been advocated for use in patients undergoing coronary artery bypass grafting (CABG), who give a history of chronic aspirin ingestion or who have a bleeding tendency identified on conventional preoperative coagulation screens [2].

Enhanced haemostasis can be achieved either by stimulation of platelet activity, of the coagulation process, or both. Aprotinin prolonged the coagulation of whole native blood in a dynamic (flowing) system, which proved to be sensitive in detecting coagulation abnormalities [4]. As far as the effect on platelet reactivity is concerned, emphasis of the differences between haemostasis and thrombosis is mandatory. Although the two processes appear different only in definition (thrombosis has been defined as haemostasis in the wrong place), there are significant differences between them in the conditions affecting platelet function. While the skin-bleeding time is a relevant test for overall haemostasis (the arrest of blood from small vessels), it lacks those haemodynamic conditions (shear-stress and turbulence) that are determinants of thrombus formation at arterial stenoses or at ruptured atherosclerotic plaques. The Haemostatometer, a true model of arterial thrombogenesis, simulates such conditions as shear-stress, platelet-collagen interaction and thrombin generation [3]. The fact that aprotinin inhibits shear- and collagen-induced thrombus (platelet plug) formation makes thrombogenecity with its use in vivo unlikely.

By inhibiting platelet reactivity to stimuli such as high shear-stress, exposure to deep layers of the vessel wall (collagen) and artificial surfaces (extracorporeal circuits and oxygenators), aprotinin may preserve haemostatically competent platelets during bypass and thus later enable them to fulfil their function. The fact that aprotinin does not induce a significant prolongation of skin-bleeding time after bypass [1] shows that the basic haemostatic mechanism is undisturbed by this therapy.

In conclusion, our present findings exclude the possibility of risk of thrombosis, as a consequence of aprotinin therapy when used for the reduction of blood loss after CABG.

References

1. Bildstrup BP, Royston D, Sapsford RN, Taylor KM (1989) Reduction in blood loss and blood use after cardiopulmonary bypass with high dose aprotinin (Trasylol). J Thorac Cardiovasc Surg 97: 364—373
2. Ferraris VA, Gildengorin V (1989) Predictors of excessive blood use after coronary artery bypass grafting. J Throac Cardiovasc 98: 492—497
3. Gorog P, Kovacs IB (1990) Modelling coronary thrombosis from non-anticoagulated human blood in-vitro. Haematologic Pathology 4(1): 43—52.
4. Kovacs IB, Hutton RA, Kernoff PBA (1989) Haemostatic evaluation in bleeding disorders from native blood. Clinical experience with the Haemostatometer. Am J Clin Pathol 91: 271—179

Authors' address:
C. P. Ratnatunga, M.D.
Department of Cardiothoracic Surgery
and Thrombosis Unit
St. Bartholomew's Hospital
London, EC 1 A 7 BE UK

Clinical Impact of Reduced Blood Cell Deformability During Cardiopulmonary Bypass

N. Al-Khaja, A. Belboul, B. Liu, D. Roberts

Department of Thoracic and Cardiovascular Surgery, Sahlgrenska Hospital, Göteborg, Sweden

Introduction

During cardiopulmonary bypass (CPB), red cells are traumatized [1—3], resulting in hemolysis, reduced rheological properties, and a shortened lifespan that leads to postoperative anemia [4]. Following surgery there is a further deterioration of red cell deformability for several days [2]. The effects of this rheological disturbance on postoperative morbidity has been suspected recently. In this study, red cell filtrability was studied in order to note if it could predict postoperative bleeding following heart operations. Such a test would help in selecting or anticipating high-risk bleeders on the basis of red cell rheological function.

Patients and methods

Eighty-two patients in NYHA classification III undergoing open heart surgery were investigated prospectively. Patient data are given in Tab. 1. The same standard technique for anesthesia and CPB was used in all patients. The same type of bubble oxygenator was used and the perfusion circuit was primed with Ringerdex (Pharmacia, Uppsala, Sweden), and CPB was performed at moderate hypothermia (28—30 °C). A cold crystalloid cardioplegia (Pharmacia, Uppsala, Sweden) was used for myocardial protection. A previously described filtration method [5] was used to assess red cell deformability. Deformability was expressed as red cell filtration rate (RFR) in microliters per s (μl/s). Samples for RFR were collected preoperatively 1 day before surgery, at the start and the end of CPB, and 12 h and 24 h after starting CPB. The amount of postoperative bleeding was defined as all fluid from the mediastinal drains starting from the end of the operation until they were removed, or a maximum of 24 h.

Table 1. Patient data (n = 82).

Sex	
Male	58
Female	24
Mean age (years)	59
Perfusion time (min)	123 ± 33
Aortic occlusion (min)	62 ± 18

Statistical Methods

Intergroup comparisons were done using the appropriate Student's t-test [6]. All means were expressed with one standard deviation. Correlations were done using the linear regression test [6].

Results

Red cell deformability

There were no significant differences in the mean RFR and bleeding values between males and females. The mean preoperative RFR in all patients was 42.6 ± 6.5 µl/s. At the end of CPB this fell significantly by 43 % to 23.6 ± 5.0 µl/s (p < 0.01), by 64 % at 12 h to 15.3 ± 4.8 µl/s (p < 0.01), and by 54 % at 24 h to 19.2 ± 5.9 (p < 0.01) postoperatively (Fig. 1).

RFR and postoperative bleeding

The mean postoperative blood loss at 24 h was 870 ± 280 ml. The mean preoperative RFR in high bleeders (> 870 ml, n = 33) was 46.6 ± 5.0 µl/s and this was significantly higher than the low bleeders (< 870 ml, n = 49) who had a mean preoperative RFR of 36.6 ± 5.1 µl/s (p < 0.05). Table 2. There were significant differences in the mean RFR values between these two groups of bleeders at the end of CPB, and 12 h and 24 h postoperatively (Table 2). The preoperative RFR values

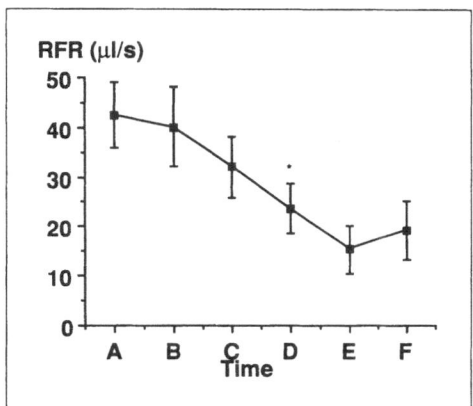

Fig. 1. Reduction in red cell filtrability (RFR) in cardiac surgery. Note that the RFR is significant 30 min, after starting cardiopulmonary bypass (CPB). RFR was measured preoperatively (A), at the start of CPB (B), 60 min during CPB (C), end of CPB (D), 12 h (E) and 24 hours (F) after starting CPB.

Table 2. Mean RFR values (µl/s) in patients bleeding less than or more than 870 ml.

Bleeding (ml)	RFR			
	Pre CPB	End CPB	12 h post op	24 h post op
< 870 ml (n = 49)	42.9 ± 11	26.0 ± 5	19.3 ± 4	23.0 ± 6
> 870 ml (n = 33)	36.6 ± 5	19.4 ± 3	10.8 ± 5	13.8 ± 4
p	< 0.05	< 0.02	< 0.01	< 0.01

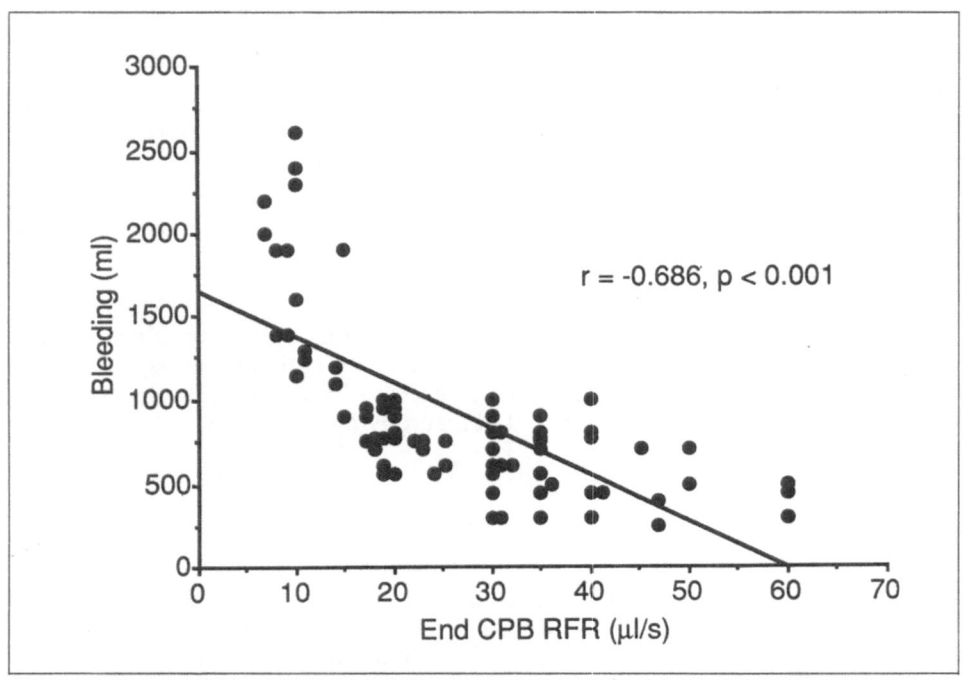

Fig. 2. Correlation between preoperative red cell filtrability (RFR) and postoperative blood loss.

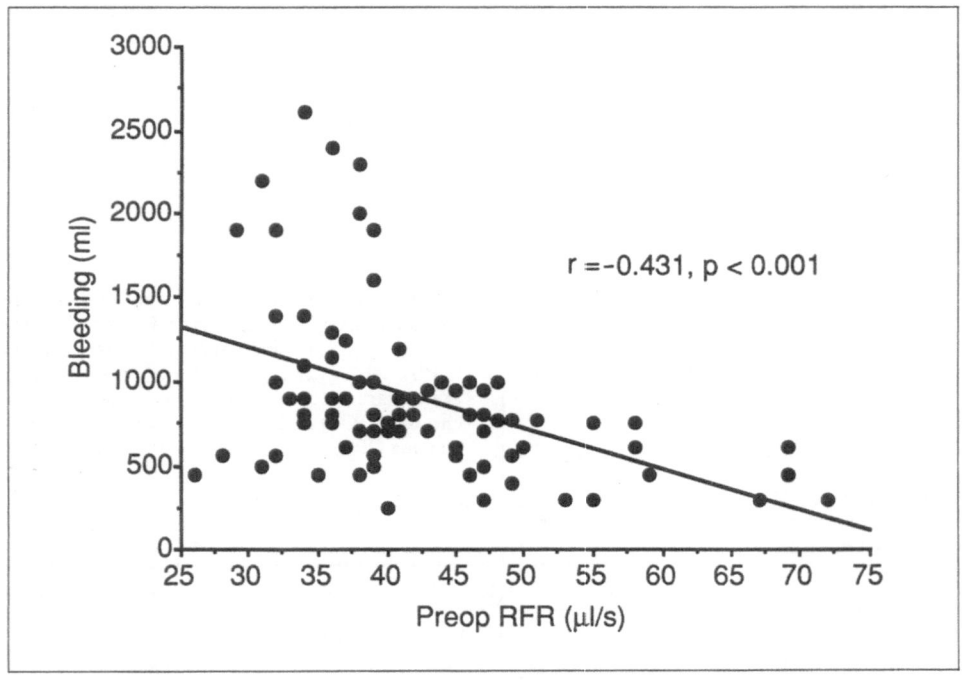

Fig. 3. Correlation between red cell filtrability (RFR) at the end of CPB and postoperative blood loss.

were significantly correlated with the postoperative blood loss ($r = -0.43 \pm 0.084$ SE, $p < 0.001$) (Fig. 2). The RFR values at end of CPB were significantly correlated with the postoperative blood loss also ($r = -0.68 \pm 0.038$ SE, $p < 0.001$) (Fig. 3).

Discussion

This study shows that RFR is reduced during CPB. Similar results have been seen in previous studies [5]. The reduction is attributed to continuous mechanical trauma caused by artificial surfaces of the extra-corporeal circulation [2, 7], the effect of anesthesia, and direct surgical trauma [8]. Following surgery, RFR continued to be reduced up to 24 h. This could be due to the response to blood trauma and surgery which is known to take several weeks to recover. This response involves immuno-logical, inflammatory, endocrinological, and humoral changes following surgery. Bleeding is a well known postoperative complication in cardiac surgery. It is inter-esting that red cell filtrability reflected the bleeding in a nonspecific way, which makes it an interesting parameter to study postoperative morbidity in open heart surgery. However, red cell rheology is sensitive, but not specific to trauma. The significant correlations between RFR and postoperative bleeding could be used as a prognostic indicator of this complication. However, the correlation for bleeding is somewhat stronger at the end of CPB, probably due to the mechnical trauma and the operative factors. One can tentatively suggest that RFR values below approxi-mately 30 µl/s preoperatively and 20 µl/s at end of CPB would be expected to predict increasing blood losses. Perhaps such patients should be assisted pharmacologically (Aprotinin, etc.) to improve hemostatic function in order to reduce bleeding. Rhe-ological improvement could also be attempted, preferably before surgery. These possibilities need further study.

References

1. deLeval MR, Hill, Mielke CH (1976) Heamatological aspects of extracorporeal circulation. In: Ionescu MI, Wooler GH, eds. Techniques in extracorporeal circulation. London: Butterworths, p. 369—390
2. Ekström S, Koul BL, Sonnenfeld T (1983) Decreased red cell deformability following open heart surgery. Scand J Thor Cardiovasc Surg 17: 41—44
3. Hill DJ, Gerbode F (1976) Prolonged extracorporeal circulation. In: Sabiston D, Spencer F, (eds.) Gibbons surgery of the chest. Philadelphia: WB Saunders p. 867—877
4. Kreel I, Zaroff LI, Canter JW, Krasna I, Baronofsky ID, A syndrome following total body per-fusion. Surg Gynecol Obstet 1960: 111: 317—321
5. Yamaguchi H, Allers M, Roberts D. The effects of urea on red cell deformability during cardio-pulmonary bypass. Scand J Thor Cardiovasc Surg 1984; 18: 119—122
6. Swinscow TDV. Statistics at square one. London: British Medical Association, 1983
7. Belboul A, Al-Khaja N, Hirayama T, Dahlin A, Karlsson H and Roberts D. Comparision of Terumo hollow fibre membrane and Harvey 1500 bubble oxygenators using red cell microrheo-logy analysis during cardiopulmonary bypass. JECT 1987; 19: 209—215.
8. Hirayama T, Yamaguchi H, Allers M, Roberts DG and William-Olsson G. Changes in red cell deformability associated with anaesthesia and cardiopulmonary bypass in open-heart surgery. Scand J Thor Cardiovasc Surg 1985; 19: 257—262

Author's address:
Najib Al-Khaja, MD
Department of Thoracic and
Cardiovascular surgery
Sahlgreuska Hospital
S-41345 Göteborg, Sweden

Diagnostic Value of Hemostatic Parameters for Prediction of Complications in Patients Undergoing Aorto-Coronary Bypass Grafting

H. Teufelsbauer[2,3], M. Havel[3], P. Knöbl[2], S. Andert[3], P. Jaksch[1], M. Müller[3], T. Vukovich[1,2]

Dept. Med. Physiology[1], Dept. Medicine II[2], Dept. Surgery II[3], University of Vienna, Vienna, Austria

Introduction

Though there has been rapid progress in coronary bypass surgery, postoperative hemostatic disorders due to extracorporeal circulation (ECC) are one of the remaining obstacles of this technique. Thrombocytopenia and platelet dysfunction [5], hyperfibrinolysis [3, 7] or activation of the anticoagulant system [4] going along with consumption of pro- and anticoagulant proteins [3—5] can cause extensive postoperative bleeding. Furthermore, the activation of intravasal coagulation might be the pathophysiological base for complex postoperative complications [4]. Thus, the aim of this study was to investigate whether a reduction in the preoperative thromboresistant potential quantified by various hemostatic parameters is linked to intra- or postoperative complications.

Patients and methods

Forty-seven of 50 consecutive patients who underwent coronary bypass surgery were included in this study. Patients with a prolonged stay in the intensive care unit (3 days or more) and/or a blood loss exceeding 1000 ml during the first 24 h postoperatively were allocated to a complication subgroup. Three patients who died (of the 47 patients) were added to this subgroup. All operations were carried out by conventional ECC with moderate hypothermia. For myocardial revascularization saphenous vein grafts and/or the left mammarian artery were used. At the end of the procedure thoracic drains were inserted, enabling measurements of the postoperative blood loss.

Immediately before and after surgery, blood was sampled from all patients through a central venous line. Then hematocrit and platelet count were determined from EDTA-blood. After the preparation of plasma by addition of Na_3-citrate and centrifugation plasma levels of α_1-protease inhibitor (α_1-pi), α_2-antiplasmin (α_2-ap), α_2-macroglobulin (α_2-mg), and C1-inhibitor (C1-inh) were measured by electroimmunodiffusion with specific antisera (Behring, Marburg, Germany). Plasma concentrations of protein C, protein S, von Willebrand factor (vWf) (Boehringer Mannheim, Germany), respectively), thrombin-antithrombin III complexes (tat) (Behring) and cross-linked fibrin degradation products (d-dimer) (Mabco, Australia) were quantified by commercially available enzyme-linked immunosorbent assays.

Plasma levels of fibrinogen, plasminogen (Boehringer Mannheim, respectively) and antithrombin III (at-III) (Kabi-Vitrum Diagnostica) were measured by automatic kinetic tests using a Hitachi 705 analyzer.

For raw statistical analysis medians and interquartile ranges of all described parameters stratified for patients with and without complications were calculated first. Significance ($p < 0.1$) of group differences was tested by non-parametric variance analysis.

Logistic regression [2] was used to provide preoperative predictions of intra- or postoperative complications. Maximum likelihood parameter and intercept estimates were computed by the modified Gauss-Newton method. Logistic probabilities as decision criterion were obtained by the formula shown in Table 1. Furthermore, the significance of the whole logistic model and the influence of the actual parameters were tested. For avoiding statistical errors regression models with a maximum of two or three parameters showing the highest multiple correlation coefficient regarding complications after rank transformation were selected for this logistic analysis.

Table 1. Formula and parameter value estimates for the calculation of logistic probabilities.

Test combination	Parameter estimate		Joint association of parameters p-value
	values $\pm$ SD	p-value	
fibrinogen	-0.01391 ± 0.00502	0.006	
α_1-pi	$+4.97031 \pm 2.18167$	0.02	0.0009
vWf	$+1.96329 \pm 0.93903$	0.04	
intercept	-4.78396 ± 2.76422		
fibrinogen	-0.01076 ± 0.00439	0.01	
vWf	$+2.11474 \pm 0.91677$	0.02	0.005
intercept	-0.13099 ± 1.45668		

$$\text{logistic probability} = \frac{\exp (\text{intercept} + \Sigma \text{ parameter estimate} \times \text{parameter raw value})}{1 + \exp (\text{intercept} + \Sigma \text{ parameter estimate} \times \text{parameter raw value})}$$

Table 2. Preoperative values of hemostatic parameters significantly different in patients with and without complication.

	Complications:		p-value
	n = 19 YES (median; Q1—Q3)	n = 28 NO (median; Q1—Q3)	
α_1-pi (U/ml)	1.22; 1.15—1.37	1.16; 0.99—1.22	< 0.05
α_2-ap (U/ml)	1.00; 0.92—1.06	1.06; 0.99—1.12	< 0.10
vWf (U/ml)	154; 1.42—1.82	1.44; 1.21—165	< 0.10
fibrinogen (mg/dl)	306; 257—345	364; 260—423	< 0.10
tat (ng/ml)	5; 4—11	4; 2—6	< 0.10

49

Results

Medians and interquartile ranges of the preoperatively measured hemostatic parameters revealing significant group differences between patients with (n = 19) and without (n = 28) complications are illustrated in Table 2. Concerning protein C, protein S, at III, α_2-mg, C1-inh, plasminogen, platelets, and d-dimer, no significant group differences were found. Furthermore, the patients in both groups were comparable in age, sex, duration of ECC, and aortic cross-clamping time.

In all patients the hemostatic system was activated during ECC. Comparing patients with complications to those without complications significant higher plasma levels of tat (median: 59 ng/ml vs 20; p < 0.01) and d-dimer (median: 317 ng/ml vs 226; p < 0.05) were measured.

The combinations of two and three parameters showing the best multiple correlation coefficients and, thus, the best predictive power for complications consisted of fibrinogen + α_1-pi + vWf ($R^2 = 0.3$) and fibrinogen + vWf ($R^2 = 0.2$). Parameter estimates of logistic regression are presented in Table 1. Defining a logistic probability of 0.3 or more as complication-predicting equivalent the parameter triplet (duplet) had a sensitivity of 95% (84%) with a specificity of 68% (54%). The three patients who died intra- or postoperatively showed logistic probabilities of 0.95, 0.78, 0.31 and 0.91, 0.46, 0.42, respectively.

Discussion

The results presented confirm the assumption of a linkage between activation of hemostasis and the onset of complications in patients undergoing coronary bypass surgery. Clearly, tat and d-dimer levels were more increased in patients with subsequent complications without showing any dependence on surgical parameters. Furthermore, the preoperatively increased tat and decreased fibrinogen and α_2-ap suggest moderate activation of coagulation and fibrinolysis even prior to the start of surgery. Elevated vWf concentrations also represent a finding consistent with such an activation [6, 8]. The increase in serine protease inhibitors and there mainly in α_1-pi may indicate an acute phase reaction in response to tissue damage [1], indicating a preoperatively compromised physical status of patients with subsequent complications.

The results of the logistic regression analysis provide an adequate preoperative screening of high-risk patients. The main limitation of this prognostic feature lies in measuring comparable values of the necessary parameters, independent of the

Table 3. Classification schema for simplified prediction of complications after coronary bypass surgery.

	Sensitivity	Specificity
fibrinogen < specific median	32 %	68 %
fibrinogen < specific median and vWf > specific median	47 %	82 %
fibrinogen < specific median or fibrinogen < specific median and vWf > specific median	79 %	50 %

50

respective laboratory. Thus, for the application of the described method in other hospitals it would be necessary to repeat the whole logistic analysis [2] on a sufficient large population of patients with and without complications. To avoid such extensive statistical computations a simplified procedure would be to calculate first labor-specific median values of fibrinogen and vWf in patients without complications and then to classify the actual values according to the scheme shown in Table 3.

In conclusion, the results of this study suggest that a preoperative hemostatic inbalance induces severe alterations of the hemostatic system during ECC, leading to severe subsequent complications. Further studies will show whether the high predictive power of hemostatic parameters can be successfully transformed into a significant reduction of complications by enabling specific prophylaxis.

References

1. Dinarello CD (1984) Interleukin-1 and the pathogenesis of acute phase response. New Engl J Med 311: 1413—1417
2. Harrel FE (1986) The logist procedure. In: Sugi Supplemental library user's guide 5th edition. Sas Institute 2: 269—293
3. Kalter RD, Saul CM, Wetstein L, Soriano C, Reiss RF (1979) Cardiopulmonary bypass: associated hemostatic abnormalities. J Thorac Cardiovasc Surg 77: 427—435
4. Knöbl PN, Zilla P, Fasol R, Müller MM, Vukovich TC (1987) The protein C system in patients undergoing cardiopulmonary bypass. J Thorac Cardiovasc Surg 94: 600—605
5. Mammen EF, Koets MH, Wolk LW, et al. (1985) Hemostasis changes during cardiopulmonary bypass surgery. Semin Thromb Hemost 11: 281—291
6. Rowland FN, Donovan FJ, Picciano PT, Wilner GD, Kreutzer DL (1984) Fibrin mediated vascular injury. Am J Pathol 117: 418—428
7. Stibbe J, Kluft C, Brommer EJP, Gomes M, deJong D, Nauta J (1984) Enhanced fibrinolytic activity during cardiopulmonary bypass in open-heart surgery in man is caused by extrinsic (tissue-type) plasminogen activator. Eur J Clin Invest 14: 375—382
8. Vukovich TC, Schernthaner G, Knöbl PN, Hay U (1989) The effect of near-normoglycemic control on plasma factor VIII/von Willebrand factor and fibrin degradation products in insulin-dependent diabetic patients. J Clin Endocrin Meatabol 60: 84—89

Authors' address:
Dr. H. Teufelsbauer
Dept. of Medicine II
Garisongasse 13
A-1090 Vienna

Summary of Lectures, Posters and Discussions: Pathomechanism

C. Prentice, Leeds, England

It is very difficult to summarise all the information from a two-day meeting. I will therefore concentrate solely on the uresolved questions about mechanisms of proteolytic inhibition. As always, any scientific subject is filled with good news and bad news. The good news is that all of the speakers who discussed the haemostatic mechanisms are probably correct. There is no one single mechanism that causes bleeding after surgery and aprotinin is likely to work through a number of mechanisms; so each speaker has focussed on one aspect of the problem and all are, in general, correct. Now, for the bad news, we still do not know the fundamental haemostatic mechanism which causes bleeding after bypass surgery and there remain many questions to be answered.

The first question is, how does aprotinin work in reducing postoperative blood loss? The three main mechanisms for the inhibitory action of aprotinin are shown in Table 1.

Contact system inhibition

The inhibition of the contact system is the main site of aprotinin action, via blocking of XIIa and the XIIa-XI complex. This causes an anticoagulant effect, a reduction in the coagulation potential, and a reduction in complement activation. These actions are important, but I am not sure how important they are; remember that the alternative name for factor XII is Hageman factor, and Mr. Hageman was a very healthy person; despite having no factor XII, he had a perfectly normal coagulation system, and a normal immune system. Clearly, the body has bypass mechanisms for getting round these pathways, so another question is, how important is the contact activation process during extracorporeal circulation? It is potentially important because the artificial surface activates the contact system. However, even in the congenital absence of the contact mechanism there are other mechanisms which can stimulate the coagulation and the immune mechanisms.

Inhibition of fibrinolysis

Possibly the most important action of aprotinin, a serum protease inhibitor, is to inhibit plasmin. In the presence of aprotinin the secondary fibrinolytic response is inhibited; again, we do not know the importance of this in extracorporeal surgery. Hyperplasminaemia is a rare phenomenon. The presence of free plasmin in the circulation during or after surgery is most unusual and is normally only seen with the disseminated intravascular coagulation syndromes. The body has an effective system of plasmin and activator inhibitors, so-called PAI-1 (plasminogen activator

52

Table 1. Inhibitory actions of aprotinin.

1) Contact Activation System Inhibits Factor XIIa	Normal Actions of Factor XIIa — activates intrinsic coagulation system (factor XI); — converts prekallikrein to kallikrein; — complement activation (CI); — activates fibrinolytic system; (converts pro-UK to uPA).
2) Fibrinolysis Inhibits Plasmin	Normal Actions of Plasmin — proteolysis of fibrin to fibrin-degradation products; — activates tPA and uPA; — proteolysis of factor V and factor VIII; — proteolysis of platelet membrane glycoprotein Ib — activates complement (CI).
3) Kallikrein-Kinin System inhibits Kallikrein	Normal actions of Kallikrein — activates fibrinolysis (tPA und uPA) — releases kinins from kininogens — activates complement (CI) — activates factor XII — activates factor IX

Abbreviations

tPA — tissue-type plasminogen activator
uPA — urokinase-type plasminogen activator

inhibitor 1) and also α_2-antiplasmin to neutralise plasmin. Also, in the kallikrein-kinin system, surface contact leads to kallikrein formation and that in itself has a positive feedback mechanism which can stimulate fibrinolysis and also contact activation.

If I was asked to guess the most important mechanism by which aprotinin reduced operative and post-operative blood loss, I would choose its antifibrinolytic action. Even in the absence of overt hyperplasminaemia it seems plausible that local plasmin action at the site of forming fibrin could cause sufficient disruption of the haemostatic thrombus to initiate sustained haemorrhage.

Consideration of fibrinolysis before surgery, or fibrinolysis during surgery, shows that about two-thirds of the fibrinolytic mechanism is contributed by the tissue plasminogen activator (t-PA), and probably about one-third from the endogenous pro-urokinase to urokinase mechanism. t-PA release does not seem to be affected by aprotinin, but, of course, if any free plasmin is produced, either by t-PA or urokinase, it will be inhibited by aprotinin. Hyperplasminaemia can lead to a fall in factor V and VIII, but that is very rare in major extracorporeal surgery and I would agree with Prof. Edmunds, who said that loss of coagulation factors during extracorporeal surgery is not very important.

Antiplatelet action

A third possible mechanism of the protective action of aprotinin is on the platelets. Whether there is a clinically significant fall of glycoprotein Ib (the von Willebrand

53

receptor) is not certain; there appears to be a fall of about 50% or so in glycoprotein Ib, but, as has been pointed out in the Bernard Soulier syndrome, there are patients with less than 50% of glycoprotein Ib receptors and they do not have a bleeding problem; therefore, the lack of receptors of glycoprotein Ib is probably only important in the context of multiple haemostatic abnormalities occurring in relation to extracorporeal surgery.

Anticoagulant action — the contact system

The activated clotting time is prolonged in the presence of aprotinin due to the inhibition of factor XIIa, XIa and, to a minor extent, factor Xa. The anticoagulant action is weak, but it is additional to the heparin-antithrombin III complex mechanism of inhibition. Remember that surgery is a balance between bleeding and clotting. If you abolish clotting completely, the patient is going to bleed profusely, so you do not want to use excess anticoagulant; if you add aprotinin you have to reduce the heparin dosage. Heparin dosage in the presence of aprotinin should be reduced to keep the activated clotting time at about 400 s; if you drop below this you can get fibrin formation in the extracorporeal circulation. Do not worry about levels of FDP dimer or thrombin-antithrombin complexes. They are interesting for haemostatic experts to think about, but not terribly important in the context of the surgeon. They are not a guide to telling us if we have got the right dose of aprotinin.

The kallikrein-complement system needs further attention as aprotinin is a powerful kallikrein inhibitor. The complement system activates the leucocyte, although I am not sure, haemostatically, that this is very important, because the leukocyte acts rather slowly, mediating the delayed inflammatory response. Is the leukocyte really capable of causing a major haemostatic defect in the 1 h on bypass or 1 h afterwards? There are also peptides produced by monocytes such as tumour necrosis factor. These can, in the laboratory, suppress fibrinolysis. What the relevance of this is in the body, I do not know.

Platelet defect

Concerning the platelet defect there is variable thrombocytopenia. Technological advances in oxygenators mean that this is not really a problem unless you are carrying out a prolonged operation. Not only do you have to worry about the number of platelets, but also the health of the platelets as well. We have been presented with much information about the fragmentation of the platelets. These are mostly seen in artificial extracorporeal circulations, and how much damage platelet membranes and fragments cause to the microcirculation is not certain. We need more good electromicrophotographs of the filters in humans to find out how many platelet fragments are being formed. The ristocetin defect which identifies the von Willebrand binding site on glycoprotein Ib is, apparently, the major platelet defect. The question is, what really causes this? Is it neutrophil elastase, or is it plasmin in the circulation? I am not convinced that we have now identified the enzyme that cleaves the glycoprotein Ib, and possibly other unidentified receptors on the platelets. The platelets appear to be relatively healthy in responding to ADP aggregation, but certainly, the platelet-membrane defect is important. Glycoproteins IIb/IIIa are probably not degraded. We have discussed extracorporeal bypass surgery, but I would like to see some equally good data done on major surgery without a bypass. That might tell us how much of the platelet deterioration is due to the bypass and how much is due to the operation process itself. 'What happens to glycoprotein Ib in non-bypass surgery?' Let us have some more information on this and get a comparison. Although you cannot use high-dose prostacyclin, because you get vasodilatation, perhaps a small amount of prostacyclin in conjunction with heparin would be useful in that you preserve platelet function as the platelets go through the oxygenator. Thus, the haemostatic problem may be due largely to the effect on platelets although, clearly, the inhibition of fibrinolysis could be synergistic. The anticoagulant action of aprotinin is helpful in that it prevents fibrin formation in the oxygenator and the artificial bypass, but, of course, if you use too much anticoagulant you have excessive bleeding because thrombin is not formed during the operation. The kallikrein complement situation needs further evaluation. Whether this reflects something that is truly happening in the circulation I am not sure.

It has been suggested that the best antithrombic and haemostatic regime is a combination of heparin, aprotinin and aspirin. This seems to preserve platelet function; if one of these is left out, the platelets might be degraded. Before advocating this, I would first like to see good clinical evidence showing that aspirin during surgery prevents re-occlusion at a later date. I am not convinced about this; I think this is going to need a well controlled clinical trial. Aspirin, if started post-operatively, is beneficial in that there is a 15—20% reduction in occlusion within 6 months after coronary artery bypass. If you give it during the operation you may get an even bigger reduction, but also, the danger of intra-operative haemorrhage increases.

Other factors affecting haemostasis after extracorporeal circulation

a) Membrane oxygenators which produce bubbles predispose to a haemostatic defect and it appears that the gentler the oxygenator the less haemostatic disturbance. b) Controlled suction appears to be better than uncontrolled suction and I would like to see some repetition of the very interesting work from Groningen. Let us have some more controlled clinical trials, as one clinical trial is never totally conclusive. c) The effect of hypothermia, I do not think we have sufficient information about hypothermia. Blood is cooled through these heat exchangers at temperatures down to 25—28 °C, and perhaps this cooling is an important aspect which we have not looked at sufficiently. Let us have more tests of coagulation and haemostasis at different temperatures. d) Finally, we get to the question I am still asking myself — how much post-operative haemorrhage is due to the extracorporeal circulation and how many of these haemostatic problems are due to long operations in ill people. After a major abdominal operation a patient will receive 10—12 pints of blood ; therefore is it really the extracorporeal circulation that mainly determines post-operative bleeding, or is it just the length and extent of the operation?

Future considerations

I have mentioned the various mechanisms that are important: the contact system, kallikrein formation, factor XI and XII activation, as well as the anticoagulant and antiplasmin effect of aprotinin. So, what dose of aprotinin do we use? The Scottish surgeons used a lower dose of aprotinin than most other groups but it did not seem to be sufficent to prevent post-operative blood loss. But I do think we need to have more dose-ranging studies at a clinical level. Do you need a plasma kallikrein inhibitory dose or not? I think we will only get the answers when we carry out different dose-ranging trials and see what the blood loss is. Therefore, when you consider doing some more studies on aprotinin to prevent surgical blood loss, you need a preliminary list of questions. Typical example questions would be as follows. What is of significance in the bypass? Clearly the longer the bypass surgical time, the more haemostatic defects you get. What is the role of the oxygenator type? (Membrane oxygenators are better than bubble oxygenators.) What is the role of cooling? The plasma expanders, such as Haemaccel and Hespan, have an inhibitory action on haemostasis in themselves, and may cause a friable fibrin structure. And finally, there is the question of the individual surgeon; clearly the haemostatic mechanism is not going to succeed if there is a large vessel bleeding in the thorax.

Author's address:
Prof. Dr. med. C. Prentice
Leeds General Infirmary
Great George Street
Leeds 691 3EX
Great Britain

56

II. Epidemiology — The Size of the Clinical Problem

Homologous Blood Use in Cardiac Surgery

M. A. Fox

The Regional Adult Cardiothoracic Unit Broadgreen Hospital, Liverpool,
England

Introduction

Fifteen years ago patients undergoing open heart surgery typically received 8 units
of homologous blood during their hospital stay [4]. Since that time there has been
a general decrease in blood consumption: however, there is little information regarding overall blood transfusion requirements from differing cardiac surgical units.

Review of Blood Usage

It is generally accepted that transfusion of homologous blood is undesirable. Therefore, centres that transfuse large quantities of blood tend not to publicise the fact.
Information regarding overall consumption of homologous blood must be sought
from independent survey or gleaned from whatever is published. Typically, papers
describing blood consumption are also concerned with blood conservation and
might be expected to represent those centres with the lowest blood consumption.
Extrapolation of this data to other centres should be done with considerable caution
to avoid underestimating the homologous blood consumption for the whole cardiac
surgical community.

U.S. Blood Usage

Cosgrove [1] has demonstrated it is possible to perform elective coronary artery
bypass surgery using the minimum of homologous blood (0.3 units per patient). In
his control group Love [3], describing autologous blood donation, revealed an homologous blood consumption of 2 units per patient, in patients presenting for a
variety of elective open heart surgical procedures. More recently, Giordano [2] reported a blood consumption of 8 units of homologous blood for an unselected group
of patients presenting for cardiac surgery, a total he was able to reduce to 3.69 units
per patient by intensive cell-saving techniques.

U.K. Blood Usage

Prompted by the lack of information concerning homologous blood consumption
in the United Kingdom, Russell [5] surveyed blood consumption and blood conservation techniques in the cardiac surgical centres in Britain, confining enquiries
to adult patients. From Fig. 1 it can be seen that the average homologous blood
consumption was 5.07 units per patient, but with four centres regularly transfusing
7 units. This sort of data is still rather crude, and takes no account of individual

surgical practice. Fig. 2 shows the homologous blood consumption of all patients undergoing open heart surgery, under the care of four surgeons from a single centre. Even within a single centre, with the same facilities, there is a two-fold difference in transfusion requirements between patient groups.

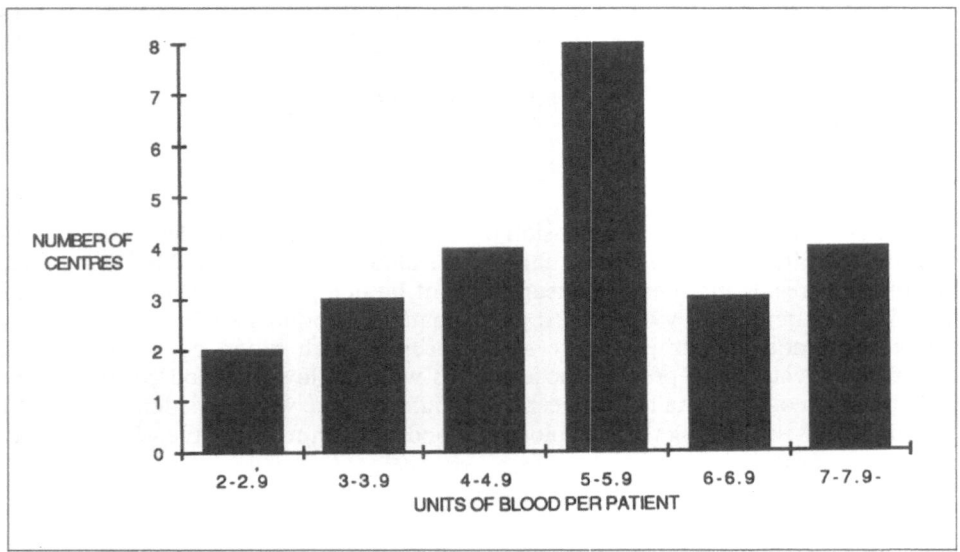

Fig. 1. Homologous blood usage in the United Kingdom.

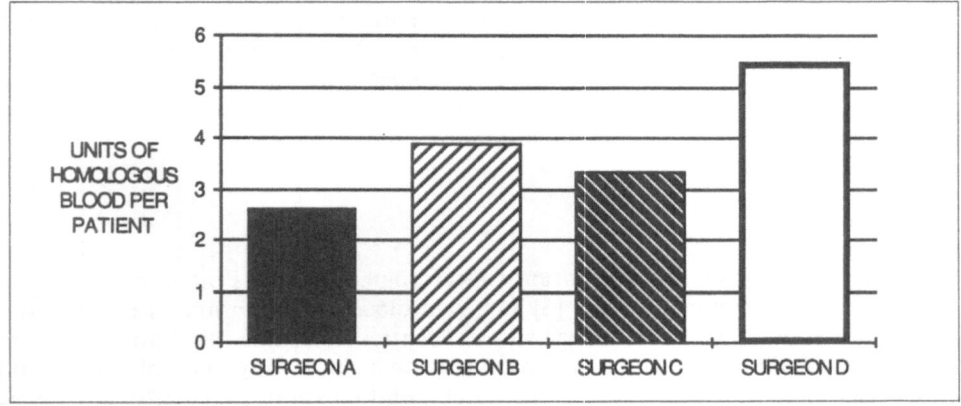

Fig. 2. Homologous blood usage by surgeon.

60

What dictates homologous blood consumption?

Why should there be an over 20-fold difference in the blood consumption between patients in the Cleveland Clinic [1] and four centres in Britain? An explanation of this difference may be found by considering the elementary and self-evident relationship of three factors concerned in the transfusion requirements for any surgical procedure. These are:
1.) The initial red cell mass;
2.) perioperative blood loss;
3.) ideal red cell mass.

Initial red cell mass

The initial red cell mass is the patients' haematocrit related to their body mass, prior to surgery. Clearly, a large patient with a high haematocrit can withstand a greater blood loss than a smaller patient with either a comparable or lower haematocrit. By rigorously controlling all other factors, Cosgrove [1] found indicators of initial red cell mass to be primary determinants of transfusion in patients undergoing coronary artery surgery.

Perioperative blood loss

This is the total amount of blood lost by the patient, during both the perioperative and postoperative phases of treatment.

"Ideal" red cell mass

This unsatisfactory term describes the haematocrit (related to the body mass) that a clinician designates as being acceptable for his patients in the postoperative phase of treatment.

These three terms are linked in the following way to determine transfusion requirements:
Initial red cell mass — Perioperative blood loss = Postoperative red cell mass
Postoperative red cell mass + X units of Blood = "Ideal" red cell mass

Blood-conserving techniques are typically concentrated in the perioperative period. From the above analysis of the determinants of transfusion requirements it can be seen that the initial red cell mass and the minimum acceptable haematocrit are also of considerable significance. Perhaps more attention should be paid to maximising the initial red cell mass by appropriate use of haematinics or autologous predonation of blood, and accepting the lowest patient haematocrit associated with an uncomplicated recovery.

Undoubtedly, implementing these two aspects of blood conservation will result in a reduction of homologous blood consumption at a fraction of the cost of some of the mechanical methods of blood salvage.

The work of a few centres demonstrate that, for the majority of patients, cardiac surgery without exposure to homologous blood or blood products is possible. It is for the rest of us to try and emulate these centres.

References

1. Cosgrove DM, Loop FD, Lytle BW, Gill CC, Golding LR, Taylor PC, Forsythe SB (1985) Determinants of blood utilization during myocardial revascularization. Ann Thoracic Surg 40: 380—384
2. Giordano GF, Rivers SL, Chung GKT, Mammana RB, Marco JD, Raczkowski AR, Sabbagh A, Sanderson RG, Strug BS (1988) Autologous platelet-rich plasma in cardiac surgery: Effect on Intraoperative and Postoperative Transfusion Requirements. Ann Thoracic Surg 46: 416—419
3. Love TR, Hendren WG, O'Keefe DD, Daggett WM (1987) Transfusion of predonated blood in elective cardiac surgery. Ann Thoracic Surg 43: 508—512
4. Roche JK, Stengle JM (1973) Open-heart surgery and the demand for blood. JAMA 225: 1516—1522
5. Russell GN, Peterson S, Harper SJ, Fox MA (1988) Homologous blood use and conservation techniques for cardiac surgery in the United Kingdom. Br Med J 297: 1390—1391

Author's adress:
Dr. M.A. Fox, Consultant Anaesthetist,
R.A.C.T.U.,
Broadgreen Hospital,
Thomas Drive ,
Liverpool L14 3LB,
England

Blood Use in Cardiac Surgery — A Transfusionist's Viewpoint

R. Eckstein

Funktionsbereich Transfusionsmedizin, Universitätsklinikum Rudolf Virchow, Standort Charlottenburg, Freie Universität Berlin, FRG

Introduction

Since the introduction of cardiopulmonary bypass and open-heart surgery into routine clinical use in the 1950s, dramatic changes have evolved in transfusion therapy of patients undergoing heart surgery. Early workers considered it beneficial that these patients receive fresh whole blood. It was, therefore, not unusual to collect blood on the morning of surgery from donors already precrossmatched with the patient. The standard practice was to collect the blood into heparin as the anticoagulant, markedly reducing its shelf-life if it was not used during the cardiac surgery. Furthermore, the blood bank was expected to crossmatch each of the units of blood with all other units, as well as with the recipient, for interdonor compatibility. It was not unusual to collect more than 10 units of blood routinely for each case. The strain of resources and the expense were inordinate.

Fresh whole blood

The reason for the requirement of "fresh whole blood" has been the belief that blood less than 24-h old has hemostatic properties superior to those of combinations of appropriate components. Therefore, similar strategies are occasionally advocated as desperation measures in cases of uncontrolled bleeding, whether surgical in nature or not. Although personal anecdotes about the greater hemostatic effectiveness of "fresh" whole blood are common, no controlled study has ever proven this contention and, in at least one study, outcomes were worse in patients receiving "fresh" blood than those receiving blood that was 3 to 4 days old [2, 6, 7].

It does not seem prudent, therefore, to expend resources to provide a modality of no proven merit, expecially as many of these practices became recognized as ineffective or superfluous with changes in cardiopulmonary bypass apparatuses, pump primes, intracardiac blood salvage, cardioplegic solutions, and improvements in postoperative care.

Packed red cells

Although certain transfusion problems seem unique to the heart surgery patient, their management increasingly conforms in general to the same principles that govern the diagnosis and treatment of other bleeding patients today. The conservative use of blood, with less concern about the level of hematocrit in hemodynamically stable open-heart surgical patients, and the use of erythrocytes alone instead of whole blood units accompanied with careful volume replacement by crystalloid or colloid solutions or fresh frozen plasma, is a reasonable and safe program to follow.

As the functional quality of red blood cells refers to their ability to bind and release oxygen in the most efficient manner, due to the intraerythrocytic concentration of 2,3-diphosphoglycerate, the application of blood units of no more than a few days of age with high levels of that factor should be preferred [10, 12].

Autologous blood

Even the best allogeneic transfusion programs are problematic with regard to the highest risk of homologous blood use— the transmission of infectious diseases. The array of possible transmissible microorganisms is at least the same for patients undergoing cardiac surgery as for any other category of patient. Of the commonly used transfusion modalities, all but albumin are capable of transmitting blood-borne infectious diseases harbored by the blood donor [3, 4].

The best homologous transfusion practice is to completely avoid homologous transfusion; autologous programs should be preferred whenever possible.

Autologous blood represents the safest source for transfusion and it eliminates disadvantages of homologous blood such as the transmission of infectious diseases, the risk of alloimmunization to red blood cells, platelets, and leukocyte antigens, and the risk of hemolytic, febrile, allergic, and graft vs host reaction. Furthermore, it can provide a source of blood for persons who have rare blood types or antibodies that make it difficult to find compatible blood (Table 1).

Autologous blood donation

Autologous transfusion can occur intraoperatively, prior to surgery associated with artificial hemodilution, and as part of intraoperative blood salvage done by clinical physicians, or preoperatively, best done by blood bank physicians in anticipation of elective surgery. All patients who must undergo elective cardiac surgical procedures for which blood replacement is anticipated should be considered candidates for predeposit blood donation.

Participants should be familiar with all aspects of a predeposit autologous donation program and must understand that involvement in such a program does not guarantee transfusion with only their own blood. Some reasons are listed in Table

Table 1. Autologous transfusion eliminates.

1) Transmission of infectious diseases
2) Alloimmunization
3) Hemolytic transfusion reactions
4) Febrile transfusion reactions
5) Allergic transfusion reactions
6) Graft vs host reaction (GvHD)

2. More blood may be required than was previously collected, as a result of unexpected blood loss or inability to collect the desired number of units. Some reasons why this goal may be unobtainable are, for example, insufficient time intervals available for collections, inadequate number of units ordered, limitation of storage interval and or surgical cancellation or postponement . Not all patients will be acceptable candidates for predeposit autologous donation because of concurrent medical problems and/or insufficient erythropoietic response. But when patients are suitable donors every effort should be made to have them provide for their total red blood cell needs.

Coronary artery disease is normally no contraindication for autologous blood predonation. Donors with abnormal pulse and blood pressure are not automatically excluded and must be evaluated individually. There are no weight requirements. There is no age limit for autologous donation, unlike volunteer blood donation, and children below the traditional minimum age of 17 years should be considered eligible. Studies have confirmed the safety of this practice in children as young as 8 years old [9]. But also donors over 66 years of age can be accepted, in most cases, at the discretion of the blood bank physican in accordance with their biological age [8].

The hemoglobin level should be not less than 11.0g/dl prior to donation, which corresponds with a hematocrit of 34 %. First-time autologous donors whose hemoglobin and hematocrit levels are below the normal range must be evaluated by the blood bank physician to determine if the degree of anemia has been observed before and is consistent with the requested reason for autologous donation. If not, the patient should be appropriately evaluated immediately.

Intravenous application of recombinant human erythropoietin — 600 units per kilogram of body weight twice a week during the donation period — increases the ability of patients about to undergo elective surgery to donate autologous blood. No adverse effects are attributed to the erythropoietin and, especially, patients with smaller blood volumes, e.g., women and children, and those who are anemic will most benefit from the ability of erythropoietin to enhance red cell production [5].

As the donation of every blood unit is accompanied by an iron loss of 250 mg, patients requiring multiple autologous units of blood should be placed on oral iron replacement therapy with iron sulfates or gluconates.

According to these multiple clinical implications (Table 3) predeposit autologous donations should best be made at hospital associated blood banks, but should also be possible in regional blood centers, depending on the convenience for the patient.

Table 2. Reasons for homologous blood use during autologous programs.

1) Unexpected blood losses
2) Insufficient number of previously collected units
3) Insufficient time intervals for collection
4) Inadequate number of units ordered
5) Limitation of storage interval
6) Surgical cancellation or postponement
7) Concurrent medical problems
8) Insufficient erythropoietic response

In any case, it is still desirable to collect as much blood as possible, as each auto-logous unit means potentially one less allogeneic unit.

Collection and storage of autologous blood

The number of predeposited units available for surgery is closely related to the maximum allowable storage time which is defined by the requirement for 70 % recovery at 24 h, i.e., at least 70 % of the transfused cells remain in the recipients circulation 24 h after transfusion. Transfused red blood cells that circulate after 24 h will have a normal survival curve in the recipient [11].

Blood collected in today's standard anticoagulant preservative CPDA-1 may be stored up to 35 days. Additive solution systems, approved only for red cell storage, permit a 49-day storage period that enables the preparation of at least 5 to 7 units.

Conventional Storage: Autologous blood units are usually stored as packed cells in the liquid state at 4 °C. For the preparation of those units it is desirable to use blood-collection units with integrally attached transfer containers. Cells and plasma should be separated by centrifugation some time up to the date of expiration of the whole blood. After the plasma and the buffy coat have been harvested in different transfer containers, red blood cells must be refrigerated at 4 °C. Buffy-coat free conservation improves their storage conditions; the buffy coat is discarded.

Optimally the plasma should be rapidly frozen in a methanol bath at − 50 °C and stored at − 30 °C or colder. Stored at or below these temperatures fresh frozen plasma has high Factor-VIII concentrations and the quality of the original unit of blood for a period of 12 months (Table 4). This kind of conservation enables auto-logous transfusion with optimal blood products, e.g., in orthopedic and plastic surgery for the vast majority of patients and should be a reasonable program to follow in cardiac surgery, as well.

Table 3. Clinical implications in autologous blood predonation programs in cardiac surgery.

1) Coronary artery disease
2) Abnormal pulse
3) Abnormal blood pressure
4) Body weight
5) Age
6) Hematocrit
7) Erythropoietin and iron application

Table 4. Storage conditions of autologous blood.

1) Conventional Storage
   Packed red cells (4° C; liquid state)
   Fresh frozen plasma (−30° C or below)

2) Cryopreservation
   Low-glycerol units (−150° C; liquid nitrogen)
   High-glycerol units (−80° C)

66

Cryopreservation: If more prolonged storage or more units are needed, they can be frozen when initially collected, either according to the low - or to the high - glycerol techniques which permit a storage under liquid nitrogen or at − 80 °C (Table 4). The procedure is time-consuming, expensive, and with respect to thawing and deglycerolization, is not without problems as regards the quality of erythrocytes, especially as wash protocols with hypertonic solutions are required. Moreover, deglycerolized red blood cells can be stored for only 24 h at 4 °C. Because deglycerolizing requires entering the container, it is considered an "open" system and bacterial contamination is possible [1, 12].

Therefore, the preparation of frozen units should be restricted to special indications as a sufficient source of blood for persons who have rare blood types or antibodies that make it difficult to find compatible homologous donors if unexpected blood losses occur.

Conclusions

Underutilization of predeposited autologous blood for transfusion is undoubtedly widespread, not only in cardiac surgery. This is so despite support for these programs throughout the scientific literature and intensive public awareness about transfusion-transmitted diseases, which results in pressure to avoid homologous blood transfusion. This problem should gradually be corrected.

However, any transfusion, whether autologous or allogeneic, has a risk of complications. Because of this small, but definite risk, patients should only receive transfusions, even with autologous blood, when absolutely indicated.

References

1. Bakker JC, Krijnen HW (1988) Kryokonservierung von Blutzellen. In: Mueller-Eckhardt C(Hrsg.) Transfusionsmedizin. Springer Verlag, Berlin, pp 194—202
2. Brismer B, Gullbring B, Olsson P (1978) Effects of stored fresh blood transfusion on postoperative function. Eur Surg Res 10: pp 153—164
3. Eckstein R (1988) Bluttransfusion und Infektionskrankheiten. Biotest, Dreieich
4. Eckstein R (1989) Immunhämatologie und Transfusionsmedizin. Gustav Fischer Verlag, Stuttgart, New York
5. Goodnough LT, Rudnick S, Price TH, Ballas SK, Collins ML, Crowley JP, Kosmin M, Kruskall MS, Lenes BA, Menitove JE, Silberstein LE, Smith KJ, Wallas CH, Abels R, von Tress M (1989) Increased preoperative collection of autologous blood with recombinant human erythropoietin therapy. New Engl. J. Med. 321: pp 1163—1168
6. Huestis DW (1974) Fresh blood; fact and fancy. In: Seminar on Current Topics. Am Assoc Blood Banks, Washington DC, p 117
7. International Forum (1976) Fresh blood - a myth or a real need? Vox Sang. 31: pp 368—379
8. Kurtz SR (1988) Blood donation. In: Churchill WH, Kurtz SR, (eds.) Transfusion Medicine. Blackwell Scientific Publications, Boston, pp 15—32
9. Silvergleid AJ (1987) Safety and effectiveness of predeposit autologous transfusions in preteen and adolescent children. JAMA 257: pp 3403—3404
10. Umlas J (1988) Transfusion therapy of patients undergoing cardiopulmonary bypass. In: Churchill WH, Kurtz SR (eds) Transfusion Medicine. Blackwell Scientific Publications, Boston pp 249—264

11. Valeri CR (1971) Viability and function of preserved red cells. New Engl J Med 284: pp 81—88
12. Valeri CR (1976) Blood banking and the use of frozen blood products. CRC Press, Cleveland p 46 and pp 109—118

Author's address:
Prof. Dr. Reinhold Eckstein
Abteilung Innere Medizin und Poliklinik
Universitätsklinikum Rudolf Virchow
Standort Charlottenburg
Spandauer Damm 130
1000 Berlin 19

Current Risks of Blood Transfusion

H. G. Klein

Department of Tranfusion Medicine, Warren Grant Magnuson Clinical Center, National Institutes of Health, Bethesda, Maryland USA

Introduction

Blood transfusion services play a critical role in modern cardiac surgery. Although current surgical techniques, careful attention to blood loss, and intraoperative blood salvage decrease the need for transfusion, few patients and fewer surgeons would consent to an operation if sufficient, safe blood components were not readily available. "Safe", however, is a relative term. Just a few years ago, the general public, and many experienced physicians, believed somewhat naively that compatible blood transfusions were entirely safe and certainly far less risky than almost any surgical procedure. The AIDS epidemic dispelled this illusion. Ironically, homologous blood transfusion is safer than ever before, and transfusion-associated AIDS is far from its most significant risk. A sober assessment of the risks of transfusion should help develop improved strategies for managing surgical patients.

Major risks of transfusion

The major risks of blood transfusion are listed in order of importance in Table 1. Transfusion-transmitted infectious diseases clearly overshadow all other complications of transfusion. North American and European physicians tend to concentrate on the risks of hepatitis viruses and retroviruses, but in many parts of the world other infectious agents are a far greater concern. Malarial parasites remain the major risk of red cell transfusions in most tropical Third-World countries; more than 15 % of the donor pool is infected in some endemic areas of Africa [2]. Chagas disease, caused by the blood-transmitted parasite T. cruzi, results in substantial morbidity and mortality in South and Central America and has been recently recognized as a growing problem in the United States [7]. No practical techniques have been found for screening prospective donors, and patients infected with these parasites are becoming increasingly difficult to treat.

Table 1. Major risks of blood transfusion.

Transmission of infectious agents
Hemolytic reactions
Alloimmunization
Immune suppression
Febrile reactions
Other allergic reactions
Graft-vs-host disease

Approximate risks of transfusion per unit transfused in the USA are listed in Table 2. While minor allergic reactions are common, they are seldom more than an inconvenience for patient and physician. Once recognized, simple fever and chill reactions can usually be well managed by removing contaminating leukocytes from the transfusion component, and urticarial reactions can be prevented by pretreating susceptible patients with antihistamines. Most hemolytic reactions result from clerical errors, giving the wrong blood to the wrong patient, rather than from technical errors. A variety of "failsafe" systems are commercially available, but none has yet proved effective in eliminating this risk. Fortunately, fatalities related to hemolytic transfusion reactions are rare.

Posttransfusion hepatitis

There have been no recent prospective studies of posttransfusion hepatitis (PTH) in the United States, however best estimates place the risk at about 5 % per patient transfused [5]. More than 90 % of these hepatitis cases are thought to be caused by so-called non-A, non-B (NANB) hepatitis viruses, about 2 % by hepatitis B virus (HBV), and the remainder by a variety of agents including cytomegalovirus (CMV), Epstein-Barr virus, and extremely rarely by hepatitis A virus. The risk of PTH will likely be further reduced by the introduction of a new laboratory screening test for hepatitis C virus (HCV), an agent that appears to account for 80 % or more of NANB hepatitis [8]. Since this assay detects an antibody, anti-HCV, there will still be a "window" period during which a blood donor may be infectious, yet anti-HCV negative. Preliminary studies suggest that the window period may be a year or longer for some donors. Nevertheless, widespread use of this screening test may eliminate as much as 50 % of PTH.

In the past, physicians have questioned the importance of PTH as a health hazard. In fact, most acute PTH infections are either clinically mild or inapparent. However, as many as one-third of such cases progress to chronic liver disease, and a significant number of these patients, perhaps as many as 20 %, eventually develop cirrhosis. Furthermore, both HBV and HCV have strong associations with hepatocellular carcinoma, thus adding cancer to the list of complications of blood transfusion [6].

Retroviruses

Retroviruses remain the most feared transfusion-transmitted infectious agents. HIV-1 probably accounts for about one infection per 150,000 units transfused in

Table 2. Relative risks of transfusion per unit in the United States (1989).

Minor allergic reactions	1:100
Viral Hepatitis	1:200
Hemolytic transfusion reaction	1:6000
Fatal Hemolytic Reaction	1:100,000
HIV infection (ultimately AIDS)	1:150,000

the USA [4]. More than 90 % of infected blood components infect the recipient and it appears that virtually all of these patients will eventually develop AIDS. HIV-2, a related agent as yet rare in the United States, can also cause AIDS, and other similar agents will undoubtedly be identified, making the task of laboratory screening increasingly difficult. Another retrovirus, HTLV-1, endemic in southwest Japan and in the Caribbean basin, has been transmitted by transfusion of cellular blood components. This virus is associated with T-cell leukemia; the incubation time appears to be measured in years. No cases of leukemia related to transfusion have been reported yet. A myelopathy known as tropical spastic paraparesis can also follow HTLV-1 infection and a small number of these cases has been traced to infected transfusions [3]. Currently all cellular blood components in the USA are tested for the presence of antibody to HTLV-1 and positive units are discarded.

Donor screening and laboratory testing have been effective methods of lowering the risk of blood transfusion, but neither technique will eliminate the risk. Major infectious agents still elude the most senstitive assays, while less common infections such as parvoviruses, spirochetes, babesial parasites, bacteria, and possibly slow viruses cannot conceivably be eliminated by practical screening methods. Until methods of inactivating infectious agents in blood components become available, transfusion-transmissible infection will continue to be a major hazard and the emergence of new agents a potential threat to public health [11].

Other complications

For the sake of completeness, three other complications of blood transfusion are worth mentioning: alloimmunization, immunosuppression, and graft-vs-host disease. Alloimmunization after transfusion occurs often, but is usually clinically inconsequential. Red cell antibodies occur at a frequency of about 1 % per unit transfused, but many of these antibodies are not clinically significant [10]. Very rarely do transfusion services fail to locate compatible red cells because a patient has multiple alloantibodies. In contrast, as many as 30 % of patients who receive chronic platelet transfusions become refractory to further platelet transfusion because of alloimmunization ot platelet-related antigens. This complication is potentially lethal for thrombocytopenic patients, although the actual number of such patients that die from hemorrhage in the USA each year appears to be small. Prevention of platelet alloimmunization is an area of intense, but as yet unsuccessful, research [1]. Finally, alloimmunization from plasma proteins occurs, but, with the exception of the rare appearance of anti-IgA, these alloantibodies do not appear to account for singnificant clinical problems.

Transfusion-associated immunosuppression

There is currently great debate in the transfusion community about the existence or importance of transfusion-associated immunosuppression. Reports of more frequent postoperative infections and increased cancer recurrence in heavily transfused patients have stimulated a great deal of interest, especially in light of the apparent immunosuppressive effect that transfusion confers on renal transplant recipients

[2]. The importance of transfusion-related immunosuppression remains to be determined.

Finally, the immunosuppressed patient is at a small but finite risk of developing graft-vs-host disease from foreign lymphocytes contained in the transfused component. While rare, this complication is invariably fatal, and the frequency appears to be increasing as more tissue-compatible family members direct their blood donations to first-degree relatives. Low dose gamma irradiation of blood components is an effective, though often logistically difficult, preventive measure for susceptible patients [9].

Substantial progress has been made in decreasing the infectious complications of blood. Disposable equipment, improved screening and testing, and increasingly prudent use of red cells have all contributed to this goal. Too often, however, the surgeon seems to forget that components other than red cells and whole blood can transmit infectious disease. Although a few infectious agents such as CMV and HTLV-1 seem to be confined to cellular components (including platelets), HIV-1 and the hepatitis viruses are as readily transmitted by plasma and cryoprecipitate. The success achieved in pasteurizing albumin and fractionated clotting-factor concentrates has not been matched by efforts to inactivate viruses in cellular blood components.

Improving transfusion safety

The best way to improve transfusion safety is to avoid exposure to blood or at least to homologous blood components. Programs for preoperative autologous red cell, plasma, and even platelet donations have grown dramatically during the last decade. Operations that are likely to require large volumes of blood now frequently take advantage of intraoperative salvage and hemodilution techniques. Unfortunately, practical substitutes for red cells are still years away and there is little immediate promise for platelet or leukocyte substitutes. Too often, however, physicians overlook existing alternatives that decrease the need for blood. Bloodless volume expanders, such as hydroxyethyl starch and crystalloid solutions, and adjuncts to hemostasis, such as epsilon aminocaproic acid and desmopressin acetate, are available in the pharmacy and are safe and effective in many clinical situations where blood is presently transfused. Recombinant growth factors such as erythropoietin have already decreased transfusion requirements for patients with chronic renal failure and may soon be available to the cardiac surgeon. Aprotinin, whatever its mode of action, may further obviate the need for transfusion in cardiac surgery patients. While completely safe blood transfusion may not be achievable in this century, judicious use of transfusion, autologous blood, and adjunctive agents can certainly decrease the current level of risk.

References

1. Aster RH (1988) New approaches to an old problem refractoriness to platelet transfusions. Transfusion 28: 95—96
2. Blumberg N, Heal JM (1989) Transfusion and host defenses against cancer and infection. Transfusion 29: 236—246
3. Bove JR (1988) HTLV-1 and blood transfusion. Transfusion 28: 93—94

4. Cumming PD, Wallace EL, Schorr JB, Dodd RY (1989) Expcsure of transfused patients to human immunodeficiency virus through the transfusion of blood components that test antibody-negative. N Engl J Med 321: 941—946

5. Dienstag J, Alter HJ (1986) Non-A, Non-B hepatitis: Evolving epidemiologic and clinical perspective. Seminars in Liver Disease 6: 67—81

6. Gillian JH, Geisinger KR, Richter JE (1984) Primary hepatocellular carcinoma after chronic non-A, non-B posttransfusion hepatitis. Ann Int Med 101: 794—795

7. Kirchhoff LV (1989) Is Trypanosoma cruzi a new threat to our blood supply? Ann Int Med 111: 773—775

8. Kuo G, Choo Q-L, Alter HJ, et al. (1989) An assay for circulation antibodies to a major etiologic virus of non-A, non-B hepatitis. Science 244: 362—464

9. Leitman SF, Holland PV (1985) Irradiation of blood products: Indications and guidelines. Transfusion 25: 293—300

10. Lostumbo MM, Holland PV, Schmidt PJ (1966) Isoimmunizatiɔn after multiple transfusions. N Engl J Med 275: 141—144

11. Produz KN, Fratantoni JC (1988) Inactivation of virus in blood products. Transfusion 28: 2—3

12. Wells L, Ala FA (1985) Malaria and blood transfusion. Lancet 1 1317—1319

Author's address:
Harvey G. Klein, M.D.
Chief, Department of Transfusion Medicine,
Warren Grant Magnuson Clinical Center,
National Institutes of Health,
Bethesda, Maryland 20892
USA

Blood Use in Adult Cardiac Surgery — Extrapolations from the Carola data base

R. C. G. Gallandat Huet, A. F. de Geus[1], H. E. Mungroop, N. G. Borgstein, T. Keane, J. T. M. Pierce, G. F. Karliczek[2], A. Eijgelaar[3]

Department of Anesthesiology, Section of Thoracic Anesthesia, State University Hospital Groningen, The Netherlands
[1] Department of Medical Information Science, State University Groningen, The Netherlands
[2] Kerkhoff Klinik, Department of Cardioanesthesia, Bad Nauheim, FRG
[3] Thoraxcentre Department of Thoracic Surgery, State University Hospital Groningen, The Netherlands

Introduction

The current climate has given new impetus to minimize blood usage during cardiac operations. In the literature, however, data about blood loss and blood use for valve replacements or combined procedures is sparse, usually only elective coronary revascularization procedures are studied. To facilitate debate as to which patient group would probably benefit most from blood-loss reducing strategies in cardiac surgery, we investigated retrospectively blood loss and blood usage in several patient groups collected in our database from 1985 onwards.

Material and methods

We examined 1886 operations for coronary revascularization and valve replacement (76% of database population). Rethoracotomies within 24 h and emergency valve replacements were excluded. The remaining 1755 operations were distributed as follows: 701 elective CABG patients, only vein grafts (514 males and 187 females); 386 combined IMA and CABG operations, 177 emergency CABG operations (including 24 failed PTCA procedures), 171 internal mammary artery grafts (IMA), 152 aortic valve operations, 63 combined CABG/valve operations, 47 CABG re-operations operations, 45 mitral valve replacements, and 13 combined valve (AVR/MVR) operations. The failed PTCA procedures (dissections) were considered separately.

Database entries for blood loss in the operating room (OR) and intensive care (ICU), and the use of donor blood products in the OR, the ICU, and on the ward were analyzed. Blood absorbed into the drapes and swabs was not documented.

Every operation was performed with a membrane oxygenator primed with 2 l of colloid; 1—2 l of crystalloid cardioplegia were infused initially. Lactated Ringers fluid, used for heart-surface cooling, was drained to the heart-lung machine; the total machine prime was eventually reinfused. Heparin regimen consisted of initial 3 mg/kg^{-1}, followed by hourly top-ups if necessary. Protamine 3 mg/kg^{-1} was given to reverse heparin effects.

A cell-saver was not used, but in indicated cases a hemofilter was used to restore Hb level at the end of bypass. Diuresis was increased, if necessary with frusemide. Preoperative autologous blood harvesting was not performed.

Indications for donor blood were a hemoglobin of 65 g.l^{-1} at the end of bypass or a persistent Hb of 85 g.l^{-1} after 6 h on the ICU in spite of adequate diuresis. The influence of preoperative Hb level on blood donor requirement was checked.

Possible contributary factors for increased blood loss were evaluated in the coronary revascularization group. The influence of age, sex, operation time, and duration of cardiopulmonary bypass on blood loss was assessed. Increase in blood loss as a result of diabetic vasculopathy (insulin treated patients) or vasodilator therapy (nitroglycerin treated patients) was also estimated.

The data was analyzed with χ-square test, by multiple regression, by Kruskal Wallis one-way analysis, and the Mann-Whitney pairs test.

Results

Average blood loss in the OR and ICU ranged between 0.4 l to 1.5 l in all groups, with some differences ($p < 0.005$; Table 1). Total blood loss in elective and emergency CABG operations was equal (not shown), but increased in other groups ($p < 0.001$). Failed PTCA patients tended to bleed more, all received heparin, aspirin, and 25% received streptokinase. Preoperative blood loss was recorded in 50% (CABG) to 85% (combined valve procedures) of the cases. In the ICU, chest-drain blood loss was retrieved in 99% of the cases. There was no influence of age, sex, operation time, and duration of bypass on blood loss. Blood loss was not influenced by vasodilator therapy or diabetic vasculopathy (22 patients).

Table 1. Blood loss.

Groups	OR. average (SEM) ml.	OR. range	ICU. average (SEM) ml.	ICU. range	Total average (SEM) ml.	Total range
CABG	423 (29.7)	100—8405	429 (12.5)	75—6110	864 (36.9)	290—10101
re CABG	599 (101.0)	100— 2900	565 (49.5)	109—1650	1171 (118.4)	385— 3780
CABG/IMA	402 (30.0)	100— 4300	676 (24.6)*	130—6354	1085 (47.6)	345— 7254
Failed PTCA	1143 (781.2)	150—10500	495 (92.7)	156—1340	2061 (1109.0)	450—10840
IMA	420 (32.4)	100— 1500	624 (28.1)*	100—1900	1002 (54.7)	275— 3330
CABG/VALVE	873 (160.8)	159— 4150	544 (67.0)	150—3350	1420 (190.2)	390— 4850
AVR	722 (99.2)	100— 7250	418 (30.3)*	80—3440	1163 (124.3)	315— 9595
MVR	544 (104.5)	120— 2000	398 (54.7)	50—1630	1048 (140.4)	150— 2730
AVR/MVR	1721 (565.1)	400— 5780	527 (148.2)	150—1890	2320 (694.0)	680— 7670

Abbreviations: RBC/VB = packed cells or full blood; FFP = fresh frozen plasma; IMA = internal mammary artery; AVR = aortic valve replacement; MVR = mitral valve replacement. Tables 1 and 2 both data of 701 CABG operations, 47 reoperations, 386 combined IMA/CABG operations, 24 failed PT CA operations, 171 IMA grafts, 63 CABG/valve operations, 152 aorta valve operations, 45 mitral valve replacements, 13 double valve operations.
* $P < 0.005$, signifies differences between OR and ICU blood loss.

75

In 43% of CABG patients no blood cells were given. In all other patient groups this percentage was less. The blood requirement for CABG procedurs and valve operations was similar, and increased for combined procedures. Although platelet function is seriously affected during bypass, only 2% of the elective CABG patients required platelet infusion. Patients with reoperations, failed PTCA procedures, combined CABG/valve procedures, and double-valve procedures needed more (Table 2).

Hemoglobin level was comparable in all groups before and after operation, after the ICU period, and on the ward. Preoperative hemoglobin level was not related to blood use. Hemoglobin level at the end of the operation ranged from 80.6 to 86.7 g.l^{-1}, and prior to discharge from ICU, from 108.7 to 114.0 g.l^{-1}.

Discussion

The percentage of patients who received no blood products is comparable with percentages given in other studies, ranging between 18% and 46% [1, 3]. The amount of donor blood used is rather low by comparison with that reported in recent literature [2, 4—6]. Blood-use reducing strategies such as the use of a cell-saver [4], reinfusion of shed mediastinal blood (our policy), infusion of fresh blood [7], or the use of predonated blood, will influence these figures. But valid comparisons between workers is difficult to make as they seldom state what type of oxygenator was used [2, 5—7], and it is well known that platelet function is better preserved with the use of membrane oxygenators. We believe that the type of oxygenator should be mentioned as a factor for determining blood loss, and blood use. As far as platelet use is concerned our study supports strategies to preserve platelet function during bypass in reoperations (CABG), for failed PTCA procedures, for double valves and combined CABG/valve operations.

Table 2. Blood use.

	OR.	ICU.	Total		% of Patients		
	average (SEM) units	average (SEM) units	average (SEM) units	range	RBC/VB	FFP percentage	Platelets
CABG	0.5 (0.03)	0.8 (0.03)	1.58 (0.08)	0—28	56.8	2.1	1.4
re CABG	0.95 (0.11)	1.42 (0.15)	2.76 (0.35)	0—9	78.7	12.8	6.4
CABG/IMA	0.57 (0.06)	1.32 (0.08)	2.0 (0.13)	0—21	67.9	1.3	1.0
Failed PTCA	2.10 (0.66)	2.81 (0.75)	4.2 (1.5)	0—36	94.4	16.7	4.2
IMA	0.38 (0.03)	1.1 (0.07)	1.5 (0.13)	0—10	62.4	—	0.58
CABG/VALVE	1.30 (0.13)	1.45 (0.15)	3.01 (0.36)	0—13	76.2	14.3	6.4
AVR	0.84 (0.07)	0.99 (0.08)	1.99 (0.19)	0—18	67.8	5.2	1.9
MVR	0.61 (0.11)	0.92 (0.11)	1.17 (0.25)	0—6	66.7	4.4	—
AVR/MVR	2.75 (1.3)	2.85 (0.83)	5.5 (1.7)	0—20	76.9	23.1	30.7

Abbreviations same as in Table 1.

In studies of blood-use reducing strategies, patients are sometimes selected by excluding IMA procedures, long bypass times, or females [2]. In our study, blood loss and blood use was not influenced by emergencies, bypass times, age, gender, and the prevalence of IMA grafting. This is controversial because Ferraris and Gildengorin found gender to be an important discriminator between high and low users, whilst Davies et al. found that IMA procedures increased blood loss. Perhaps surprisingly, Hackmann et al., were unable to demonstrate an association between surgical skills and blood loss. Bleeding time, another reported factor for discriminating excessive blood loss was not assessed in our study.

Conclusion

In routine coronary bypass and valve replacement procedures an average of 2 units of donor blood were used per patient during hospitalization. This is a low figure but comparison with the literature is difficult due to differences in techniques. No donor blood was used in 43% of the routine coronary bypass procedures and in, respectively, 25% and 33% of the aorta valve and mitral valve replacement procedures. Blood use doubled in combined procedures. Patients with a double-valve replacement received an average of 5—6 units of donor blood cells. Blood loss was not related to cardiopulmonary bypass duration, operation time, and sex in 1482 coronary patients.

References

1. Davies MJ, Picken J, Buxton BF, Fuller JA (1988) Blood-conservation techniques for coronary-artery bypass surgery at a private hospital. Med J Aust 149: 517—19
2. Dietrich W, Barankay A, Dilthey G, Mitto H, Richter JA (1989) Reduction of blood utilization during myocardial revascularization. J Thorac Cardiovasc Surg 97: 213—9
3. Diedrich W, Barankay A, Dilthey G, Henze R, Niekau E, Sebening F, Richter JA (1989) Reduction of homologous blood requirement in cardiac surgery by intraoperative aprotinin application. J Thorac Cardiovasc Surg 4; 37 (2): p 92—8
4. Ferraris VA, Gildengorin V (1989) Predictors of excessive blood use after coronary artery bypass grafting. J Thorac Cardiovasc Surg 98: 492—7
5. Hackmann T, Gascoyne RD, Naiman SC, Growe GH, Burchill L, et al. (1989) A trial of Desmopressin to reduce blood loss in uncomplicated cardiac surgery. NEJM 321: 1437—43
6. Lee KF, Mandell J, Rankin JS, Muhlbaier LH, Wechsler AS (1988) Immediate versus delayed coronary grafting after streptokinase treatment. J Thorac Cardiovasc Surg 95: 216—22
7. Mohr R, Martinowitz U, Lavee J, Amroch D, Ramot B, Goor DA (1988) The hemostatic effect of transfusing fresh whole blood versus platelet concentrates after cardiac operations. J Thorac Cardiovasc Surg 96: 530—4

Author's address:
R. C. G. Gallandat Huet
Department of Anesthesiology,
Section for Thoracic Anesthesia
State University Hospital Groningen
Oostersingel 59
7913 EZ Groningen
The Netherlands

Evolution of Requirements to Replace Blood and Plasma in Cardiac Surgery

G. Marggraf, M. Schax, H. Trübenbach, M. Brand, K. R. Flechsenhar,
N. Doetsch

Department of Thoracic and Cardiovascular Surgery, University Medical School,
Essen, FRG (Dir.: Prof. Dr. J. Chr. Reidemeister)

Introduction

Increasing knowledge about immunological [6, 18], oncological [4, 5. 17], and infectious [2, 12, 19] risks when transfusing blood have altered attitudes and indications of blood-transfusions as well as the effort to reduce the loss of blood intraoperatively and postaperatively [1]. Recently, attention has been particularly focussed on the potential risk of HIV-infection. The high risk of hepatitis infection after transfusion is well-known; it amounts to 4 %, corresponding to 25. 000 infected patients in the Federal Republic of Germany annually [13, 15].

Materials and methods

General methods of blood saving

Autotransfusion: A sufficient number of autologous blood-units can be harvestet in a select group of patients over an extended period. Traditional storage with stabilizing agents, so far used on a routine-basis, is not feasible due to the long time-interval required for storage. Thus, in our department, between 1982 and 1984, we used the so-called low-glycerol-rapid-freezing technique in order to produce packs of red blood cells that were deep-frozen and available for an unlimited period of time [11, 14]. This method is time-consuming, cost-intensive, and requires numerous personnel, it was therefore confined for special indications, such as rare blood-types, irregular antibodies, etc. Another method that focuses on utilization of autologous blood, is the retransfusion of blood lost through mediastinal drains to filtrating systems. No anticoagulating agents have to be added to the defibrinated blood. Any negative effects on coagulation-specific physiological characteristics could be excluded according to our own investigations [10]. The risk of infection, potential transfusion of cellular split-products, free hemoglobin, and microscopic particles, and the diminished blood-loss in the first postoperative hours leading to an insufficient quantity for retransfusion, have all eliminated retransfusion in the clinical routine apart from a small number of cases.

Hemodilution: For a long time in cardiac surgery, the concentration of hemoglobin was maintained at a comparatively high level between 12 and 14 g/dl by utilization of 13.1 units of bank blood on the average (intra- and postperatively) because of the hypothesis that patients with particularly severe coronary artery disease may benefit from a high number of red blood cells in order to maximize myocardial oxygenation. Knowledge about satisfactory myocardial oxygenation above a concentration of 8 g/dl of hemoglobin, as well as the realization in vascular surgery about amelioration of perfusion and microcirculation by modification of flow-properties of blood have entirely changend our attitude about the perioperative level of hemoglobin [16]. The first conclusion that we drew from this fact in our own department was the use of a blood-free and protein-free prime-volume of the heart-lung-machine (HLM) in the adult patient [9]. Further hemodilution inevitably entails systemic uptake of the cardioplegic solution since we introduced cannulation with a single large cavoatrial (two-stage) venous catheter in left-heart surgery [3, 7, 8]. During the surgical procedure, hemoglobin-levels below 7 g/dl are tolerated under the conditions of extracorporeal circulation and cardiac arrest. Stimulating the diuresis, spontaneous hemoconcentration up to 8 g/dl at the end of extracorporeal circulation and further hemoconcentration up to 9 or 10 g/dl at the end of the surgical procedure is easily achieved without any replacement of bank blood in more than 50 % of patients.

Reduction of postoperative hemorrhage: The improvement of the HLM-equipment with exclusive use of membrane-oxygenators, the shortening of the total time of operation and, particularly, of the duration of extracorporeal circulation have considerably diminished the harmful effects of extensive perfusion-time on the coagulation-system. Additionally, by the routine-use of aprotinin in the dosage-schedule of 2 million units initially, 2 million units at the onset of extracorporeal circulation, 500.000 units/h as continuous infusion until the end of the operation, our own investigations showed lowering of the average hemorrhage through the mediastinal drains from 723 ml to 274 ml.

Retrospective analysis

Blood-saving methods were verified retrospectively from 1979 until 1988 by comparing representative patient-groups and correlating these with the methods, used (Fig. 1). Data are based on 6466 patients, who underwent cardiac surgery with cardiopulmonary bypass.

Results

Phase I: No blood-saving methods

The first period was designated as a comparative phase representing the philosophy of high hemoglobin demand. No pharmacological and technical methods were realized to save bank blood. Thus, that period can be characterized for its high requirement of bank blood and fresh frozen plasmas.

Phase II: Transfusion of autologous blood, priming-composition

In the period 1982—1984, in a select group of patients, we supported the autologous blood donation prior to elective cardiac surgery. Additionally, the cardiotomy

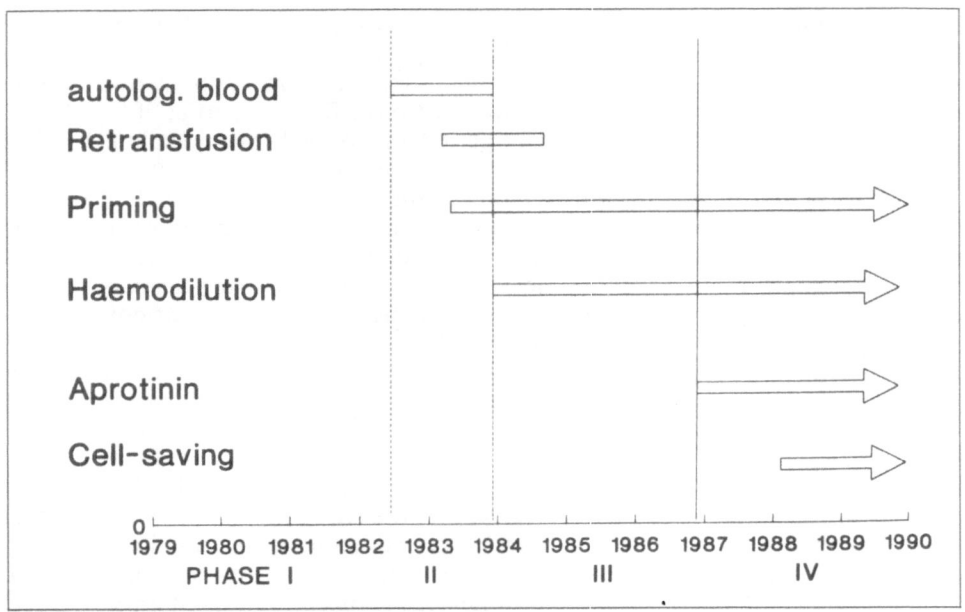

Fig. 1. Methods of blood saving.

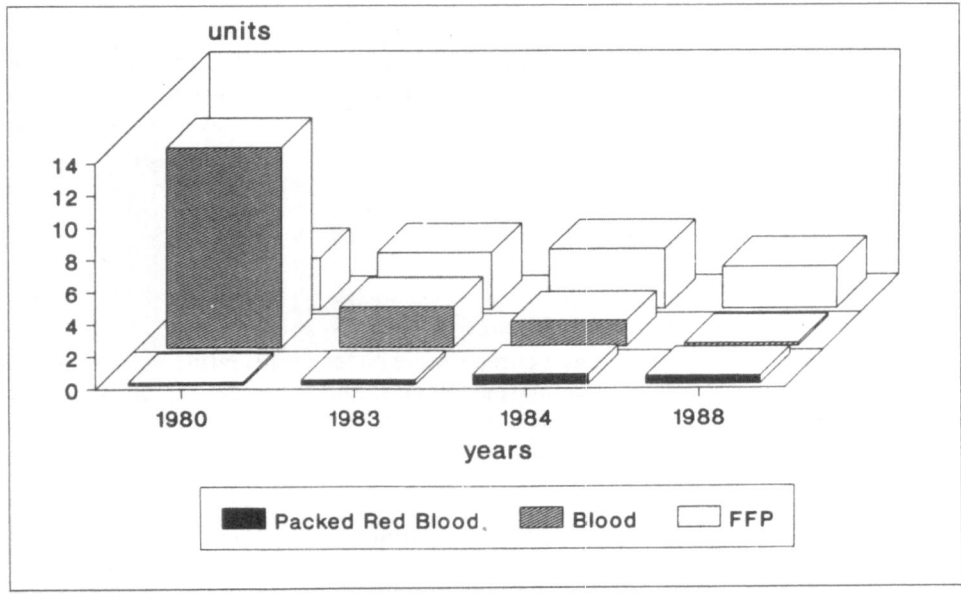

Fig. 2. Development of blood use in cardiac surgery.

reservoir was used as a drain collector and, whenever necessary, the filtered blood was retransfused. At the same time, our attitude about the intraoperative and post-operative hematocrit demand changed. Thus, we first excluded any bank blood, later any protein-containing solutions from priming-volume. This led to a considerable reduction in the demand of bank blood, amounting to 2.5 units of whole blood on the average with the requirement of packed red blood cells and fresh frozen plasma remaining nearly unchanged.

Phase III: Hemodilution

A further increase of hemodilution was achieved by systemic uptake of cardioplegic solution (HTK according to Bretschneider) avoiding suction of the right atrium during cardioplegic perfusion. Thus, we reduced intraoperative blood loss, resulting in a diminished demand of 2.2. units per patient. However, the demand for fresh frozen plasma remained equal.

Phase IV: Reduction of postoperative hemorrhage

The routine use of a aprotinin with ensuing lowering of postoperative hemorrhage has resulted in a further considerable reduction of use of bank blood, amounting to 0.17 packs of whole blood on the average. The prevailing philosophy of extensive hemodilution still forces us to substitute packed red blood cells as replacement of first choice in case of demand. For the first time, we noticed a decrease of the average-requirement of fresh frozen plasma. We consider this to be an effect of improved coagulability and reduced fibrinolysis depending on aprotinin.

Conclusion

Further reduction of bank-blood demand can be accomplished by retransfusion of the volume remaining in the oxygenator. Due to the shortened time of operation and extracorporeal circulation, stimulated diuresis is not sufficient to compensate for the entire extracorporeal volume-overload. The remaining volume undoubtedly may be retransfused directly, or later during intensive care. One of the main dis-advantages is a low hematocrit that does not provide the desired increase in the number of oxygen delivering particles. Furthermore, the high content of heparin of this blood leads again to an inhibiting effect upon coagulation. Since 1988, sepa-ration of red blood cells from the remaining volume utilizing a compact cell-saver system has been performed, in order to make high-quality concentrates of red blood cells available. Further reduction of plasma that bears an identical risk-reduction of infection can be expected by further improvements in reducing the damage of co-agulation components under the conditions of extracorporeal circulation. Innova-tions in HLM-techniques, further reduction of surgical extracorporeal ciruclation, as well as the decrease of endogenous hyperfibrinolysis depending on aprotinin may be contributing factors. New systems for a possible out-patient clinic-based harvest of autologous fresh plasma are already in clinical practice and may increase the use of autologous fresh plasma in the future. This may help to cover the requirement to improve coagulability or to increase oncotic pressure while avoiding homologous blood products.

References

1. vBormann B, Ratthey K (1988) Indikation zur Autotransfusion an einem Groß-Klinikum. Lab med 12: 414
2. vBormann B, Schleinzer W (1987) Die akute normovolämische Hämodilution als Fremdblutsparendes Verfahren. Wissenschaftliche Informationen Fresenius Stiftung 1: 186—204
3. Doetsch N, Zerkowski HR, Wolfhard U, Schmidt H, Sauerland N (1988) Monoatriale oder biatriale Kanülierung? Vorteile und Nachteile des HLM-Anschlusses mit venösem Zweistufenkatheter. Thorac cardiovasc Surgeon 36, Suppl I: 32
4. Hermanek Pjr, Guggenmoos-Holzmann I, Schricker KT, Resch T, Freuden K, Neidhardt P, Gall FP (1989) Der Einfluß der Transfusion von Blut und Haemoderivaten auf die Prognose des colorectalen Carcinoms Langenbecks Arch Chir 374: 118—124
5. Hodgson WJB, Lowenfels AB (1982) Blood transfusions and recurrence rates in colonic malignancy Lancet 2: 1047
6. Mueller-Eckert C (1980) Gefahren bei der Transfusionsmedizin Anästh Intensivther Notfallmed. 15: 179—188
7. Rohm N, Bayindir O, Doetsch N, Barbboutas M, Zerkowski HR (1985) Reduktion des Blutverbrauches bei Operationen am Herzen mit der Herz-Lungen-Maschine durch zusätzliche Hämodilution mit kardioplegischer Lösung nach Bretschneider. In: Dudziak R, Reuter HD, Kirchhoff PG, Schuman F (eds) Proteolysen und Proteinaseninhibition in der Herz- und Gefäßchirurgie Schattauer, Stuttgart—New York pp 303—307
8. Rohm N, Doetsch N, Zerkowski HR, Olivier L, Reidemeister JC (1986) Klinische Erfahrungen in der Herzchirurgie mit der intraoperativen Haemodilution. In: Heilmann L, Beez M (eds) Neuere klinische Aspekte zur Haemodilution Schattauer, Stuttgart—New York pp 237—241
9. Sauerland N, Doetsch N (1987) Einflüsse der Hydroxyaethylstärke im Prime-Volumen der Herz-Lungen-Maschine auf den Haemoglobingehalt und den kolloidosmotischen Druck. Kardiotechnik 10, 157—160
10. Sauerland N. Doetsch N, Zerkowski HR, Brand M (1988) Blutsparende Maßnahmen in der Herzchirurgie - Auswirkungen der Retransfusion des postoperativen Drainageblutes. Kardiotechnik 11, 112—117
11. Schax M, Rohm N, Hammad-Zulfoghari D, Luboldt W (1987) Autologes Transfusionsprogramm in der Herzchirurgie. In: Kretschmer V, Stangel W (eds) Transfusionsmedizin 1986 - Infektionen, Autotransfusion, Lymphokine. Beiträge zu "Infusionstherapie und klinische Ernährung", Bd. 18 Karger, Basel pp 72—75
12. Schleinzer W, Mehrkens HH, Weindler M, Wollinsky K, Pohland H (1987) Klinisches Konzept der autologen Transfusion: Hämodilution, maschinelle Autotransfusion, Plasmapherese, Eigenblutspende. Anästh Intensivmed 28: 235—241
13. Schricker KT, Ryba W (1970) Ikterische und anikterische Transfusionshepatitis. Fortschr Med 88: 1371
14. Schricker Kt, Schricker E (1984) Tiefkühlkonsevierung von autologen Erythrozyten und Frischplasma. In: Lawin P, Paravinici D (eds) Hämodilution und Autotransfusion in der perioperativen Phase. Schriftenreihe Intensivmedizin Notfallmedizin Anästhesiologie Bd. 49. Thieme, Stuttgart—New York pp 12
15. Sugg U (1987) Die Risiken der Transfusion von Blut und Blutderivaten. 17. Bayerische Anästhesistentag. 08.—09.05.1987, Nürnberg
16. Sunder-Plassmann L (1984) Pathophysiologische Grundlagen der akuten, isovolämischen Hämodilution. In: Lawin P, Paravinici D (eds) Hämodilution und Autotransfusion in der perioperativen Phase. Schriftenreihe Intensivmedizin Notfallmedizin Anästhesiologie, Bd. 49 Thieme, Stuttgart—New York pp 23
17. Tartter PL, Burrows L, Kirschner P (1984) Perioperative blood transfusion adversely affects prognosis after resection of stage I (subset NO) non-oat lung cancer. J Thorac Cardiovasc Surg 88: 659

18. Trobisch H (1988) Nebenwirkungen homologer Blutderivate. Optimierte Transfusionstherapie. Lab med 12: 426
19. Winter J, Preuße CJ, Schulte HD (1989) Spezielle Aspekte fremdblutsparender und blutstillender Maßnahmen in der Thorax- und Kardiovaskularchirurgie. Akt Chir 24: 181—184

Authors' address:
Dr. G. Marggraf
Dep. Thoracic Cardiovasc. Surg.
University Medical School
Hufelandstr. 55
D-4300 Essen 1
FRG

AIDS and Surgery: On the Need to Reduce the Risks of HIV Infection

Pitfalls and Perspectives of a Tardive Epidemic

M. G. Koch, Karlsborg, Sweden

The virus

We are confronted today with a new, serious disease of pandemic proportions, the first lentivirus infection that we know to have struck man. In the course of nearly 10 years' intensive research we have learnt enough about this pathogen to understand the resulting epidemic [27, 39, 40]. The time has come for a resumé of the first decade with AIDS.

The causative agent of AIDS, the Human Immunodeficiency Virus (25, 26), HIV (Fig. 1), invades specifically those cell types which are of crucial importance for the efficiency (macrophages) and coordination (T-helper cells) of our immune system. Moreover, the virus infects several other important cells (e.g., immature T-cells, hematopoetic cells, certain cells in the brain and other organs) and leads to functional impairment of B-cells, killer cells, and other important (trophic?) cells in various tissues.

The virus has many unusual porperties [27, 30, 31] among which the following are remarkable:
1. Rapid antigenic shift
2. Antigen shedding from mature virus particles
3. Molecular homologies between viral structural proteins and cellular antigens or receptors
4. A predominantly intracellular existence and the ability to pass from one cell to another through intercellular cytoplasmic bridges
5. The ability to cause syncytia formation leading to cell death
6. A sophisticated regulation of its own replication, including self-inhibition
7. The ability to survive in macrophages
8. The assistance (opsonisation) of antibody-complement complexes which mediate the invasion of certain cells (antibody-dependent virus enhancement, ADE).

The short-term consequences of these properties are:

(1) prevents a fully developed immunity by rapidly changing viral envelope characteristics,

(2) withdraws the virus from neutralizing antibodies and possibly directs such antibodies towards immunologically active host cells,

(3) enables the virus to bypass the common immunological alarms and gives rise to various auto-immune reactions; there may even, in time, by cumulative selection, occur an adaptation to the individual HLA-makeup and other host factors,

(4) allows the virus to spread without being vulnerable to circulating antibodies,

(5) leads to the destruction even of uninfected cells,

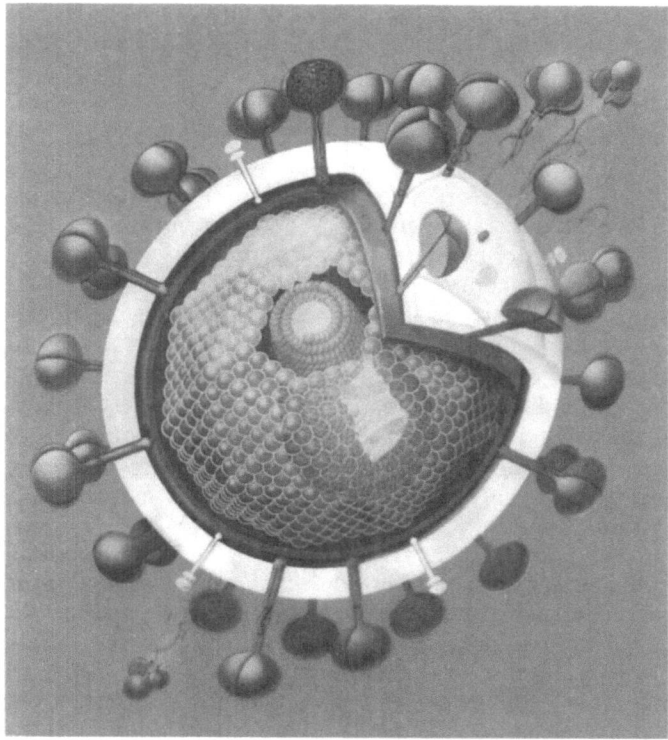

Fig. 1. Model of a mature HIV particle; M. G. Koch, VåC Karlsborg, on the basis of information, electron micrographs and computer graphic constructions by H. R. Gelderblom, M. Özel, G. Pauli, Robert-Koch-Institut, Berlin; P. A. Marx, R. J. Munn, K. I. Joy, University of California, Davis, USA; H. Frank, W. Schäfer, H. Schwarz, Max-Planck-Institut, Tübingen; J. C. Chermann, F. Barré-Sinoussi, C. Dauguet, P. Picouet, L. Montagnier, Institut Pasteur, Paris; A. Karpas, W. Gillson, Dept. of Haematology, University of Cambridge, UK; P.M. Feorino, E. Palmer, CDC, Atlanta; L. Nilsson, J. Lindberg, Karolinska Institut, Stockholm; H. Wolf, S. Modrow, Max-von-Pettenkofer-Institut, München; J. A. Levy, L. Oshiro, Cancer Research Center, Universitiy of California, San Francisco; A. M. P. Bouillant, S. A. W. Becker, Animal Disease Research Institut, Nepean, Canada, S. Höglund, B. Morein, B. Strandberg, L. Liljas, Biomed. Centrum, Uppsala, A. F. Bykovsky, Gamaleya-Institut, Moskow; (art work: GRAPHICO, Hamburg).

(6) provides for inactive proviruses a long period of latent ("dormant") intracellular existence, without evoking antibodies, and grants the host a long period of silent infection, thus prolonging the time for survival and virus spread within the host organism and among individuals by up to 20 years,

(7) turns the ability of the host to find and to incorporate pathogens into an advantage for HIV in reaching its target cells, and

(8) uses the normal immunological response for enhanced invasion of phagocytes, which harbour the virus for a long time and permanent spread it within the host.

These uncommon features lead to the following long-term outcome:

1. While other epidemics regularly recede, automatically limited by increasing immunity in the population, HIV spread will go on and AIDS will be with us for a very long time - if not forever.
2. Normal efforts of our immune system lead inevitably to its burn-out, thus causing disease.
3. Infection will usually occur unnoticed and at least some HIV proviruses will initially remain immunologically "invisible", but later lead to a confusing variety of symptoms.

4. Even if immunization should be possible some time in the future, there will be a certain fraction of virus particles that are not physically accessible to antibodies or a multitude of drugs.
5. Damage to the organism widely excceds the break-down of infected cells alone.
6. Delayed detection of infected persons makes epidemiological observations of necessity provisional, so that the outer limits of HIV spread, cannot be seen and public and political reactions will, therefore, even in the future, be guided by the number of AIDS cases rather than by the decisive underlying number of HIV infections. That "freezes" a delay in health policies of about 10 years and will considerably hamper our chances to contain HIV spread.

Just these features mirror the "lenti" principle, the crucial condition causing a "tardive" epidemic with all its natural pitfalls, biases, and misconceptions.

7. The virus can infect through healthy mucosal membranes, making HIV infection an effective sexually transmitted disease with some features of hepatitis B. Such diseases tend to maintain a certain level of prevalence within large populations.
8. Some very important efforts towards immunization are turned into a hazard, jeopardizing conventional clinical trials on human patients. Apes as subsitutes will become increasingly rare.

Thus the so-called "negative", "inhibitory", "suppressive", or "down"-regulation of the viral replication processes, be it of "weak" or "defective" virus strains, turns out as a very "positive" quality for virus spread and survival. That way lentiviruses do not immediately express viral antigens or replicate in all cells, thus partly avoiding the normal awareness, alarm, and response of our immune system [18, 19, 43]. This "lenti" strategy makes DNA probes the only adequate test to prove infection and seems to have opened a new niche for the virus to persist in large populations without risk of eradicating the host species.

HIV's lentivirus-specific affinity for, and resistance to, macrophages (cells that are designed to destroy pathogens by incorporation and lytic activity) has many severe consequences and may turn out to be the key problem of this type of infection. It also undermines the concept of a "minimal infectious dose" and may be lead to a total failure of vaccination efforts. Antibodies, by propagating virus recyling within the phagocytic system may partly be useless and even jeopardize an immunological silence which would extend the period of clinical latency and host survival.

The isolation of about, 8,000 strains of HIV, which all seem to differ from one another, up to 17 virus variants isolated from one single patient, and the tendency to develop both drug resistance and increasing virulence over the course of some years, give an idea of the variability of HIV. The significantly different type HIV-2 has more recently started to spread from West Africa and has by now reached at least Europe and the Americas. HIV's closest relative, SIV in monkeys, has after just one year in cell culture suddenly developed a new genetic variant with changed tropism, causing an intestinal disease fatal within some weeks. It is quite obvious that we are not dealing with a single virus. HIV behaves more like a moving target, a comet, the tail of which rapidly broadens, fan-like, into a multitude of genetically different variants.

By integrating into the chromosome of the infected cell, HIV can save a copy of its genetic information, which effectively "vanishes" in the host cell's genome (Fig. 2). There it cannot be selectively destroyed by conventional drugs. The virus is very difficult to recognize until viral antigens are produced. Infection is thus initially

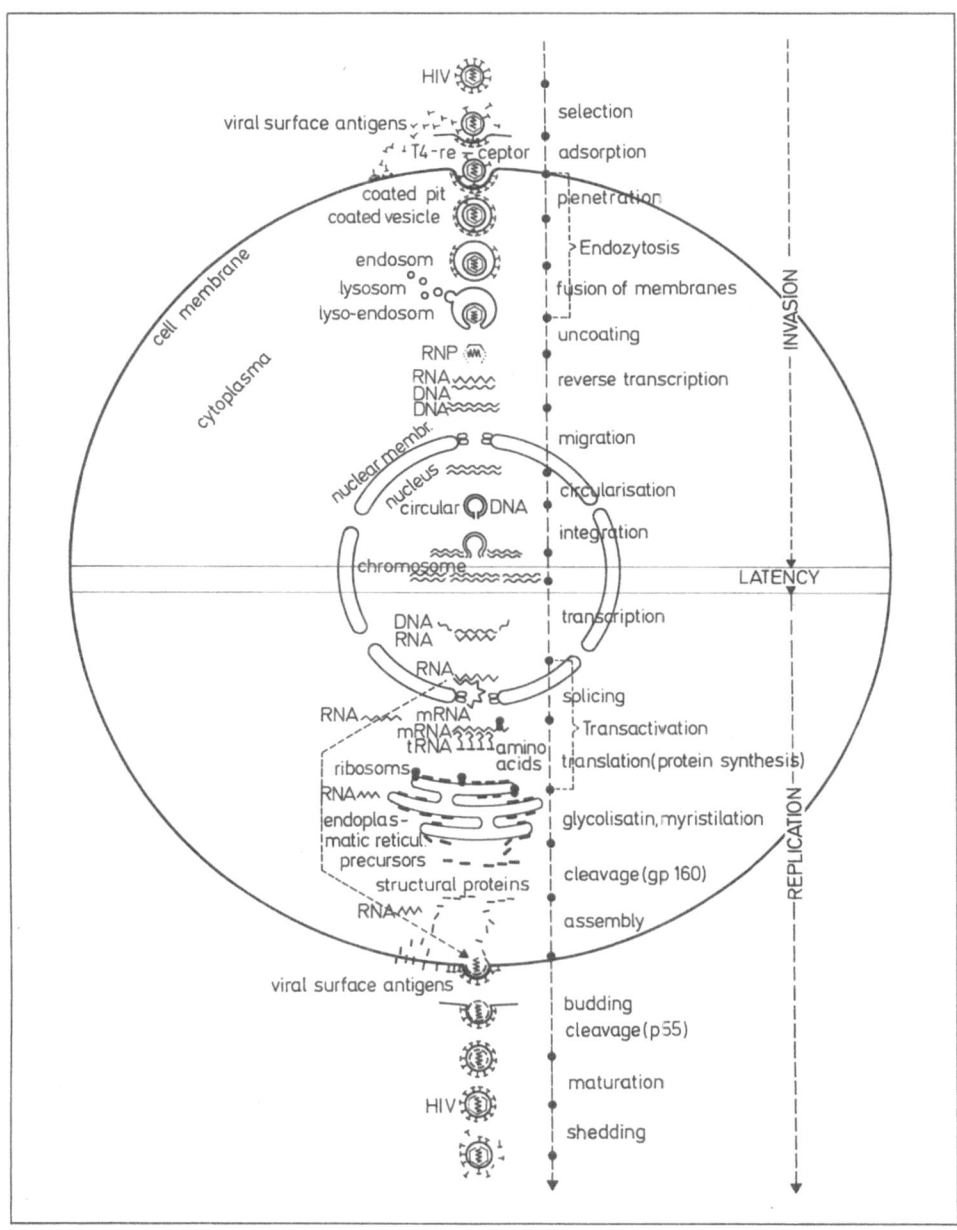

Fig. 2. Life cycle of HIV, showing the single steps of invasion and replication (From M. G. Koch: "AIDS — Vom Molekül zur Pandemie", Copyright: Spektrum der Wissenschaft, Heidelberg 1989).

"silent", but persistent, and the contagiousness lifelong, as is the necessity for any conventional therapy. Frequent "vertical infection" gives the virus direct access to the next generation, which then must be treated as well.

The combination of "lenti-features with other properties of retroviruses give HIV the qualities of a "smart", insidious, and well adapted intracellular parasite, which to combat requires more skills and intelligence than our immune system has developed over millions of years. The long incubation time, by optimizing its spread, compensates for the inevitably lethal outcome, which otherwise would be a handicap in the competitive straggle for virus survival. Therefore, this epidemic is not self-limiting by its high mortality, as is the case for many others (e.g. Marburg disease, Ebola fever) nor is it undergoing changes towards a more benign course.

On the contrary, intraindividually there is a tendency towards increasing virulence by means of cumulative selection of HIV variants with a higher replication rate and cytotoxicity. This may explain why there is no life-long symbiosis between HIV and its host organism. That tendency, however, is balanced interindividually by decreasing transmission rates during shorter survival.

Due to the circumstances described above, we will for a considerable time lack both effective therapy and a protective vaccine. We have to plan, not for years, but for decades. During this period, risk-reducing advice will be our main prophylaxis. In other words, we must vaccinate the susceptibles with information.

The disease

The acquired immunodeficiency syndrome, AIDS, is the irreversible final stage of a chronic progressive infection with HIV. The disease is characterized by cellular immune deficiency, life-threatening secondary infections by opportunistic pathogens, certain malignancies, various trophic and neurological disturbances, and auto-immune reactions.

The mortality of AIDS is about 80 % after two years, about 98 % after three years. The average survival time after diagnosis is about 400 days, much of which is spent in hospital. None of more than 170,000 patients in USA and Europe has ever recovered from AIDS, a circumstance that is, even by historical standards, exceptional.

Infected persons are persistent HIV carriers and seem to develop AIDS at an increasing rate over time. There are strong indications that most or all of them will progress to disease in the course of a long observation time, and several ongoing clinical follow-up studies show increasing evidence for such a serious final outcome.

AIDS is only a defined late stage of a *disease that has no proper name yet* (we use, in analogy to tuberculosis, salmonellosis, toxoplasmosis, cryptococcosis, cryptosporiodiosis, shigellosis, leishmaniosis, legionellosis, brucellosis, filariosis, babesiosis or rickettsiosis, the therm **"human lentivirosis"** [42]). It shows a tremendous variety of prodromal stages (LAS, ARC) and other clinical pictures (ITP, LIP, AIP, HIV enterocolitis, wasting), some of which, though lethal, do not always fulfill the CDC's AIDS case definition. In addition, HIV infection facilitates the development and aggravates the course of more common bacterial diseases such as tuberculosis, salmonellosis, skin infections, or septicemia of various origins. The basic immune deficiency seems to trigger an ever widening variety of infections, malignancies, auto-immune diseases and other unusual conditions, often in combination with each other.

The affinity of HIV for the brain [36] and other parts of the central nervous system (CNS), another typical feature of lentiviruses, becomes ever more obvious (AIDS dementia complex, ADC). HIV infection sometimes leads to brain disease and death before the immune system becomes markedly damaged.

Many complicated functions in the human organism are not really appreciated until their breakdown unveils their importance. The AIDS condition makes manifest and dangerous that abundance of microbial species, against which we incessantly have to fight for survival. The HIV-infected patient, whose immune system is continnous deteriorating, must do this under a gradually diminishing and finally vanishing protection.

The epidemic

The epidemic probably started in the 1950s in the region of Central Africa [23] and has spread at an alarming rate. Many million people in more than 100 countries on all continents had already been infected when the first AIDS cases were detected in 1981 — a magnificent start for a sexually transmitted disease. That means that the first decade with AIDS has been the third or fourth decade with HIV. Today this virus is found all over the world and more than 150 countries are reporting AIDS cases (see Table 1). Even Canadian Inuit Eskimos, Navajo indians, Australian aborigines and people from Greenland, the South American jungle, and remote Pacific islands are affected. In spite of repeated messages about the epidemic "levelling off" the situation is continuously worsening world-wide (Figs. 3 and 4). There is so far no proven way to contain the further spread of the virus.

The situation in some Central African countries and in certain parts of the Caribbean is fundamentally disastrous [4, 44, 45, 48]. There are urban populations among whom HIV prevalence is rising by 1—4 % annually. A similar development seems to take place outside Africa in certain urban regions with large slum areas (e.g., in Latin America). How to stop the spread of this virus in slum populations is hard to cuvisage. Man's mind may balk at the implications of this development and therefore hesitate to project the course of the epidemic in the future. Nature, however, does not, and next decade's epidemiological development in terms of AIDS cases is already determined.

The real number of infected persons is difficult to ascertain due to the presence of antibody negative virus carriers. Their existence confounds effective screening as it may take several years before specific anti-HIV antibodies can be detected in blood [22, 33, 35]. The necessary techniques to clear this "blind spot" (PCR and other tests for viral DNA) have not yet been sufficiently developed for general screening.

The obvious concentration of AIDS patients within certain risk groups does not imply definite restriction of its future spread. The term "risk group" may be useful for discussion and epidemiological surveillance, but should not induce unfounded complacency outside these groups: in reality, HIV crossed their boundaries many years ago. There are no really distinct risk groups, but there is risky behaviour that may cluster within certain sections of the population. The virus takes advantage of every chance it gets. Thus our message must be that everybody in the vicinity of

HIV ought to reduce these chances by all means and, in fact, independent of his sexual preference, life style, and religious or political convictions.

Most asymptomic virus carriers are today completely unaware of their condition. They contribute unwitlingly and incessantly to the further spread of HIV [34]. Due to the time lag between infection and disease, AIDS statistics are HIV archeology and definitely inappropriate for the surveillance of this epidemic and for the monitoring of our interventions' efficiency.

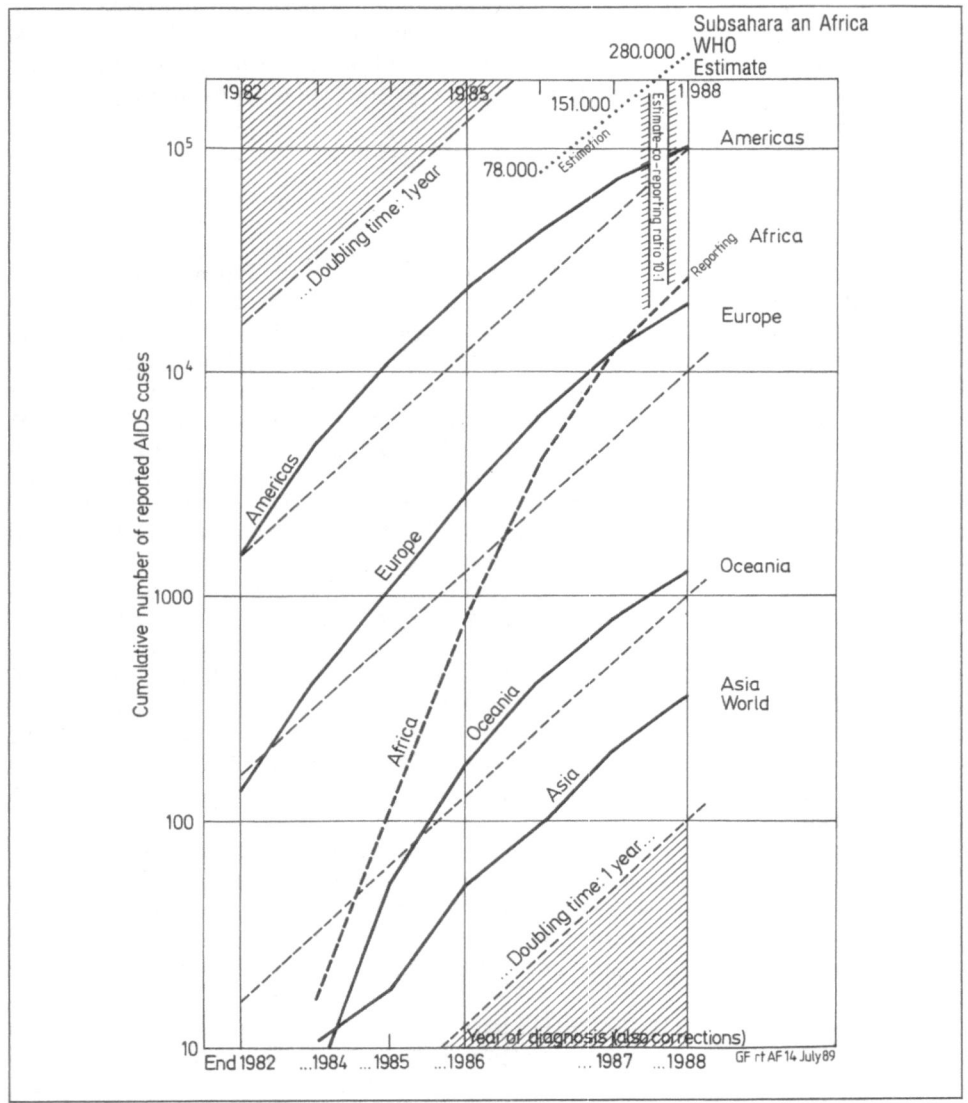

Fig. 3. AIDS cases in different regions of the world, semilogarithmical. Very similar epidemiological features are seen with marked differences in the time of onset and an obvious delay in reporting from Central Africa. The dotted curve above represents actual WHO estimates (R.P.Bernard, AIDS Feedback, AF 0689, Genf 1989).

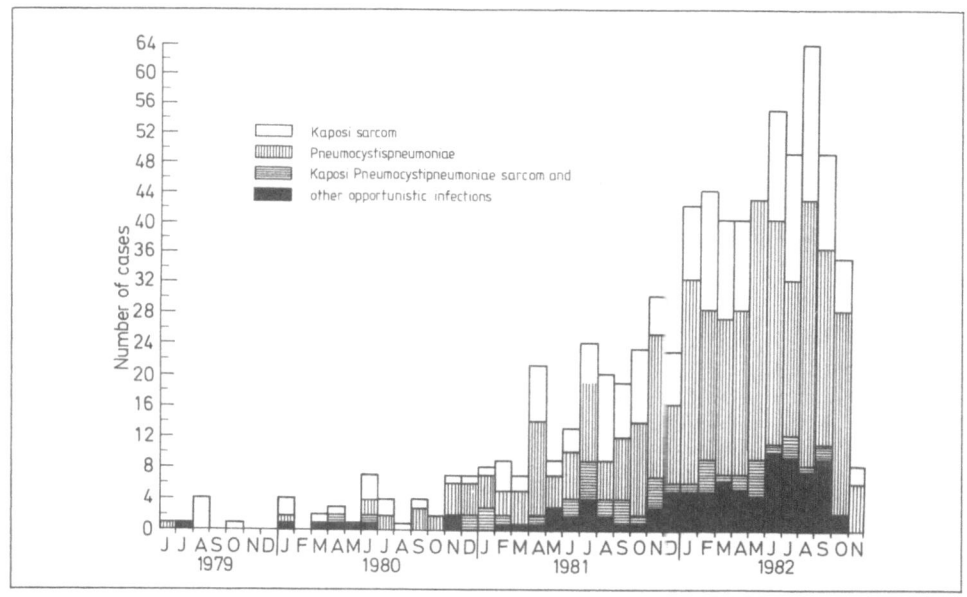

Fig. 4. Monthly AIDS cases in the USA until 1982, not cumulative, mainly diagnosed retrospectively, D. N. Lawrence, CDC, 1983. From M. G. Koch: AIDS - vom Molekül zur Pandemie, Spektrum der Wissenschaft, Heidelberg 1987, 1989).

Political considerations often create smoke screens around the true epidemiological situation. We know quite a lot about AIDS cases. We have some knowledge about the symptomatic HIV carriers and much less about the asymptomatic ones. However, we have no real insight into the actual dynamics of HIV spread, partly due to the lack of decisive will to gain this knowledge. Therefore the mutual accusations of over- or under-reaction will continue.

The epidemic has, after a gentle beginning, become rampant. Starting with unalarming case rates in the early 1980's, the yearly loss of life in America will soon exceed that during the whole Vietnam war (55,000). Even the losses of World War I could once be surpassed. The crucial point one has to bear in mind is that these figures are not markedly influenced by the number of currently acquired infections [38, 39]. The projection above would come true, even if, tonight, 1 million drug addicts suddenly became concerned about their health, if several million prostitutes started retraining for new careers, if many millions of their customers preferred to stay at home, and if millions of journeys from and to the USA were cancelled. The patients of tomorrow are the HIV carriers of yesterday. Most of them just do not know that they have been on their way towards disease for several years.

It might help us to imagine this epidemic correctly if we take a good look at Fig. 4, which shows the AIDS cases in the USA (partly retrospectively) noted until 1982. How would this diagram look today in its updated from? Instead of 60 cases a month, now 600—800 cases are diagnosed weekly. The column for early 1990 would, instead of 12 cm, be about 5 m high. The curve, after all, developed as might have been assumed.

Astonished? There is worse to come, illustrating the need of avoiding surprises. The magnitude of the actual epidemiological problem, of course, is not constituted by the AIDS patients known today, but by the (mainly still invisible) "reserve" of HIV carriers. Their current number, referring to the cautious estimate of the CDC, 1—1½ million, would then correspond to a height of 2—3 km. This "wall" of future patients, some of whom tumble down every month according to the CDC AIDS case definition, has to be thought of as standing behind the cases of disease manifest today. It is this high "wall" that respresents the real size of the HIV problem, the potential of further virus spread. The epidemic, surely, is not over. At least 90—95 % of the problem is still to come; in Latin America and Africa a great deal more.

The transmission

Virus spread is linked to the two fluids that sustain life: blood and semen, and to behaviour that is difficult to change: transmission occurs through sexual contact, by contaminated paraphernalia for drug abuse or paramedical activities, through blood and blood products, and by transplanted organs, tissues, or donated semen. Donor screening is crucial.

Macrophages in general (e.g., Langerhans cells in the skin and macrophages in the lung, the brain, and other tissues) seem to provide a widespread vector (passing even the blood-testis and blood-brain barrier: "trojan horse theory") as well as a reservoir for virus persistence. Their frequent infection indicates an unexpectedly high virus load in the HIV carrier. This feature, too, is known for other lentiviruses.

Recent studies have shown the existence of T4-positive, locally adapted macrophages (the infection of which may also occur by other "gates" than the T4 receptor) in healthy mucosa of the oral, vaginal, cervical and rectal regions; these cells are found to be susceptible to HIV and are infected early. Thus the assumption that open wounds must be present for virus transmission is no longer valid. This is confirmed by experiments with simian lentivirus (SIV) [32]. Infection through normal mucosa (e.g., sexual contacts) may occur frequently, superficial macrophages being the primary target cells.

The latter mode of infection could give rise to long seroconversion latency and incubation periods, accompanied by a consequential delay in infectivity and in the development of measurable amounts of HIV-specific antibodies (seroconversion). The frequent detection of long-term seronegative virus carriers, particularily among heterosexual partners, represents an additional, yet "invisible", part of the epidemic, the consequences of which (i.e., the manifestation of the accumulated potential of infectiousness) would be considerably delayed. The contagiousness of recently infected virus carriers seems not to be fully developed until many years later.

AIDS is spread as a sexually transmitted disease, with some of the same properties as hepatitis B. In the initial phase of every epidemic, however, we only see the main routes of transmission. Small alternative pathways of contagion will either be insignificant or become relevant only when the epidemic spread has reached a certain magnitude. The very high frequncy of sexual contacts might obscure for a long time uncommon modes of transmission.

It is not yet possible to specifiy finally the infectiousness of HIV. Transmission to health-care and laboratory workers, though infrequent, has occured in about 100 reported cases, even by blood splashes without injuries [13, 20]. Due to the possibility of longer seroconversion latency in cases with a low initial infection dose, our actual knowledge is incomplete and our conclusions are, of necessity, preliminary.

The detection of HIV in cockroaches, mosquitoes, tsetse flies, ticks, and other insects from two central African high-risk areas, the proven survival of the virus in the common bedbug, as well as the documented spread of the equine lentivirus EIAV between horses by biting stable flies, raises questions about the possibility of virus spread by biting insects (not just mosquitoes) as mechanical vectors, which by now are difficult to answer. There is, however, no indication at all that any insect would act as a biological vector for lentiviruses.

In general, we have to consider that the route and the initial dose of infection may be crucial for the duration of both the seroconversion latency and the incubation period. Initially, we see mainly fast-developing cases, so we are prone to a recurrent underestimation of its true length. Those patients who are repeatedly and massively infected could today (misleadingly) predominate among the actually manifest AIDS cases.

Within less than 10 years, AIDS has, in the statistics on notifiable infectious diseases in the USA [6, 8, 9, 10, 12], already surpassed 28 of 30 diseases, which have had opportunities to spread for centuries. In the USSR one infected man returning form Africa has given rise to at least 69 secondary cases (61 children and 8 mothers [3]), in India among 129 blood donors 97 (75 %!) were found infected (supposedly by contaminated equipment of the blood centre [2]). Romania has thousands of children infected on similar routes. Therefore it seems unwise to talk about a "very low infectiousness". The actual, rather short, observation time of about 9 years (to be compared to the natural history of this infection of up to 20 or more years) should make us cautious [47]. By unwillingness to think, or wishful thinking, our lack of detailed knowledge and other uncertainties are often converted into unwarranted optimism leading to premature and tendentious statements.

Posttransfusion infections and nosocomial risks

It has been known since 1982 that recipients of blood products are at risk for HIV infection. There are more pathogens than HIV that can be transferred by blood products, e.g., HTLV-1, -2, delta-HBV, NANBH (HCV), and several unconventional ("slow") viruses. Even mandatory screening of blood donors, as repeatedly reported, cannot completely avoid HIV infections due to the existence of seronegative virus carriers. The seroconversion latency period seems, in at least some cases, to last up to several (4 or more) years, and the prevalence of this condition is not yet finally known. Unlike antibody tests, antigen tests, virus culture, and even electron microscopy, hybridisation tests of the PCR type are the only appropriate means of finding early HIV infection, when provirus copies integrated in host chromosomes remain predominantly inactive (dormant). Not before such gene probes are reliable and widely used in the future we will be able to answer some essential questions.

Therefore, preventing posttransfusion infections by blood saving strategies and autologous blood transfusion has become crucial. There are several effective and proven strategies for blood saving under surgery which today should be used as far as possible. There will, however, always remain a certain requirement for fresh blood and erythrocyte transfusion.

Legislation makes it mandatory for the physician to chose the treatment which includes the lowest possible risks for his patient. West German courts have decided that the physician thus must inform his patients clearly and thoroughly about the

Table. 1. Reported AIDS cases, based on national reporting systems, on the WHO's Weekly Epid. Record, and on the CDC's MMWR, for most of the developed countries until March/April 1990, for some developing contries with one or more years' delay.

Country	inhabitants (mill.)	AIDS cases	Country	inhabitants (mill.)	AIDS cases
Austria	7.6	415	Angola	9.0	104
Belgium	9.9	563	Benin	4.6	36
Denmark	5.1	470	Burkina Faso	8.3	555
Finland	5.0	49	Burundi	5.2	3100
France	56.0	8025	Central African Rep.	3.0	662
FRG	61.6	4749	Congo	2.0	1250
Greece	10.1	249	Egypt	55.0	8
Iceland	0.25	13	Ethiopia	48.0	193
Ireland	3.7	108	Gambia	0.8	62
Italy	57.5	6100	Ghana	14.8	921
Luxembourg	0.38	20	Ivory Coast	11.8	250
Malta	0.36	14	Kenya	23.7	6004
Monaco	0.03	6	Malawi	8.1	2586
Netherlands	14.7	983	Mozambique	15.3	48
Norway	4.2	139	Niger	7.5	56
Portugal	10.3	306	Nigeria	115	35
San Marino	0.03	1	Rwanda	7.3	1302
Spain	39.8	5020	Senegal	7.7	207
Sweden	8.4	406	South Afrika	25.7	310
Switzerland	6.6	1255	Sudan	25.0	113
U.K.	56.9	3157	Tanzania	24.8	4158
			Uganda	16.8	7375
Bulgaria	9.0	6	Zaire	34.0	11732
Czechoslovakia	15.7	18	Zambia	7.8	1892
GDR	16.4	17	Zimbabwe	10.0	1148
Hungary	10.6	33			
Poland	38.4	22	Argentina	33.0	377
Rumania	23.2	74	Bahamas	0.25	350
USSR	28.7	26	Barbados	0.26	93
Yugoslavia	24.0	111	Bermuda	0.06	122
			Bolivia	6.9	16
Australia	16.2	1760	Brazil	154	10200
Canada	26.3	3557	Chile	13.0	149
Cyprus	0.7	14	Colombia	31.8	471
Israel	4.5	110	Costa Rica	2.9	113
New Zealand	3.4	156	Cuba	10.6	61
USA	251	128319	Dominican. Republ.	7.3	1028
			Haiti	6.2	2215
China	1070	3	Honduras	5.1	344
Hong Kong	5.7	22	Jamaica	2.4	121
India	835	32	Mexico	88.1	3100
Japan	123	108	Panama	2.4	84
Philippines	62.0	26	Paraguay	4.5	12
Thailand	55.0	25	Peru	21.8	210
Turkey	55.4	28	Puerto Rico	3.7	3400
			Trinidad and Tobago	1.3	456
			Uruguay	3.0	66
			Venezuela	19.3	419

Total of AIDS cases as of 31. March 1990 reported to the WHO:	252 000
WHO's estimate of the real case load, world-wide:	650 000

residual risks posed by a blood transfusion (in spite of donor testing) and the currently available means to avoid them. Autologous blood transfusion is today the safest way of meeting these demands, and nearly all planned surgery (i.e., 55—80 % of all surgery) can be supplied by autologous blood. There are, in Europe at least, some well qualified and experienced blood banks for storage and distribution of autologous blood (e.g., in Düsseldorf and Munich, FRG), and to avoid legal troubles in the future the physician must be able to prove that he has undertaken maximum efforts to provide that safe procedure to his patients. Otherwise the patient should sign a paper freeing his physician from responsibility for future harm due to conventional blood transfusion.

The risks for nosocomial infections also require a re-evaluation of routines in surgery and patient care. Precautions as recommended by the CDC [5, 7], the San Francisco General Hospital Operating Room Committee [46], and the revised guidelines for CPR recently issued by the Emergency Cardiac Care Committee of the American Heart Association [1] should, indeed, be followed carefully.

Problems of time lag

The incubation period is unusually long and not yet finally known. This gives rise to a surprising and treacherous gap between what is visible and the underlying reality, leading to a lack of alertness and motivation in public health policies. In fact, much published excitement has turned out to be no more than the storm before the lull.

The incubation period is also extremely variable, which results in uncommon "smearing effects" and a biasing acceleration in the number of AIDS cases appearing initially, called "transients" (recently analyzed by González et al. [16, 17, 37] are insidious in that their passing mimics a slow-down of the epidemic and thus may give rise to unfounded optimism. Positive transients fade away after 5—10 years and are followed by "negative transients" due to a diminishing number of susceptible, but not yet infected, persons within certain groups at risk. This saturation effect continues to distort the curve of the epidemic and to prolong the strong (but spurious) impression of a reduction in its spread. Such changes are generally perceived, but hardly understood by the public.

The slow rise in infectiousness of HIV carriers leads tu unusual retarding effects in the sexual virus spread, known as "tardants" or "amplified delay" [15]. They, too, characterize the nature of a "tardive" epidemic and tend to obscure the accumulating potential of future HIV spread in the heterosexual population.

Retrospective studies have unearthed sporadic AIDS cases dating back to the 1960s [21] the earliest proven cases from Norway in 1966 [14], the earliest positive serum confirmed by Western Blot from Kinshasa in 1959. These findings have evoked the question, "Why didn't the epidemic start then, rather than as late as 1981?". The answer, of course, is that it **did** start then. To understand a lentivirus infection is to realize that the long, unnoticed slope of a slow exponential spread necessarily extends back into the past for several decades. Any other finding would be a miracle. The state of disease spread today, therefore, merely reflects the infection spread some 10 years ago. By the same token, the situation of infection spread today will not become visible until 2000 or later. This means that, at any given moment, we are always at a later stage than is apparent.

Lentivirus infection thus gives rise to lenti-observation, lenti-comprehension, and lenti-reaction, and, consequently, to a 10-year "incubation period" also for our errors in AIDS policies. Certain mistakes are very likely to be made and common erroors to remain unrecognized for a whole decade, until their consequences become difficult to ignore. We do not perceive continuously growing changes unless their speed exceeds certain thresholds. The lenti-principle in terms of micromolecular events and genomic regulation is mirrored on the macro-scale of the epidemiological outcome: just as HIV slips in under the threshold of our immune response by its lenti-properties, this tardive epidemic does not evoke adequate reactions in health policies until late in its course.

Problems of intervention

Intimate contacts have always proved to be refractory to legislation and to elude any form of control. Drug abuse, too, does not seem to be particularly susceptible to advice or legal surveillance. Moreover, especially in certain risk groups such as intravenous drug addicts and prostitutes, not every virus carrier shares a sense of — usually unquestioned — loyalty towards the community at large. Some irresponsible persons will deliberately carry on spreading the virus and thus aggravate the problems we have to face. Other risk groups such as homosexuals and highly promiscuous people often fight quixotically, and, in fact, sametimes successfully, many reasonable approaches to contain HIV spread or even to uncover the facts [35]. Thus, in a longer perspective, they strongly counteract their own true interests.

The public has forgotten what an epidemic means and how it is fought. Old lessons must be relearned (although they can be found recorded in the annals of medicine, plagues, laws, and history - books that reflect mankind's experience) and will subsequently lead us back to well known principles: **find the sources, understand the ways of spread - and interfere with both as fast as possible** [28, 29].

There is a wealth of experience in other countries, from which we may derive great benefit. This chance, however, is often blocked by "opportunistic inertia", territorial imperatives, internecine squabbles, and a widespread reluctance to overcome prejudices and to reconsider premature convictions. Bavaria, for example, is today rather notorious, isolated, and criticized for its health politics. Is that a good criterion of truth? More and more countries begin to arrive at similar conclusions. Bavarian health politics (e.g., certain vaccinations, X-ray screening, teaching venereology) in the good tradition of Max von Pettenkofer and other renowned scientists, have in the course of history often initially been criticized by most other countries. Seven to 20 years later the world has, as a rule, followed Bavaria's example finally sharing the underlying considerations. Will this happen again in the time of AIDS? Today, Japan, Iceland, Finland, India, GDR and many other countries apply similar strategies; several US states are beginning to do the same - and many more countries will follow within the next decade [29].

The scope of the problem

Our society has repeatedly shown its lack of ability to deal with — even major — hidden and "creeping" disasters [24, 37]. The complex and dynamic structure of this problem has all the properties, which, throughout the history of mankind, have regularly led to a persistent deficiency of intentional awareness and a consequential delay in action. It is just the sort of problem we are prone to muddle with rather than to master.

The prospects for therapy are hardly more promising. We have not succeeded in fighting cancer, virus infection, chromosomal damage, auto-immune disease, immune deficiency, infections of the CNS, and brain atrophy. AIDS is a combination of these seven unsolved problems; thus, of course, any real solution is far away.

HIV infection is extending throughout the world, invisibly and ineluctably, a silent explosion in slow motion. Like a delayed rumble from a distance, AIDS cases appear around us, lit from long-smouldering HIV infections. It is crucial to understand AIDS as merely the final flash-into-fire of a virus that arrived 10 years before. As yet, we have no real idea how long this fire will be nourished.

Omitted actions sometimes give rise to a catastrophic lack of consequences
(S. Lec).

Summary

Molecular biology has revealed specific lentivirus features of the HIV genome implying self-regulation by inhibitory shackles, i.e., suppressing ("down-regulating") production of viral antigens and even virus replication for long periods. This so-called "negative" regulatory control seems, however, to constitute a considerable advantage in the niche of intracellular persistence, for it avoids arousing the immune system's awareness, alarm, and response. This grants the host organism a long time span of survival and provides the virus with an equally long period of silent spread within and between individuals. This process seems to be mirrored on the macro-scale of epidemiology.

The unusually long incubation period of up to 19 years or more (with an average of about 10 years) gives rise to unusual phenomena such as "transients", "tardants", cumulative selection of more malignant virus variants, and a general delay of various dynamic effects. Even the visible outcome of saturation kinetics and the fully developed potential of infectivity, supposedly increasing under several years of infection, is considerably postponed.

Due to the resulting treacherous gap between what is visible and what is hidden in the course of HIV spread, society reacts to the epidemiological situation only in proportion to the actual number of AIDS cases, that it, constantly with a 10-year delay. The real state of HIV spread, however, should be measured by the number and regional distribution of virus carriers, mainly inaccessible to immediate surveillance. Lentivirus infection gives rise to lenti-observation, lenti-comprehension, and lenti-reaction, and, thus, to a 10-year "incubation period", even for erroneous judgements in AIDS policies. Common errors and mistakes are likely to occur and to remain unrecognized for a whole decade, until their consequences become difficult to ignore. We do not perceive continuous changes unless their speed exceeds certain levels. Just as HIV slips in under the threshold of our immune response by its "lenti"-properties, this lenti-epidemic does not prompt adequate reactions in health policies until late in its course.

It has been known since 1982 that recipients of blood products are at risk for HIV infection. Even mandatory screening of blood donors, as repeatedly reported, cannot completely avoid HIV infections due to the existence of seronegative virus carriers. The seroconversion latency period seems, in at least some cases, to last up to several (4 or more) years, and the prevalence of this condition is not yet finally known. Hybridisation tests of the PCR type are the only appropriate means of finding early HIV infection, when provirus copies integrated in host chromosomes remain predominantly inactive (dormant). Not before such gene probes are reliable and widely used in the future we will be able to answer some very crucial questions.

There are several effective and proven strategies for blood saving under surgery which today should be used as far as possible. There will, however, remain a certain requirement for fresh blood and erythrocyte transfusion, where autologous blood transfusuion is the safest way to avoid infections of all kinds. Nearly all planned surgery (i.e., 55—80 % of all surgery) can be supplied by autologous blood.

The risks for nosocomial infections also require a re-evaluation of routines in surgery and patient care. Precautions as recommended by the CDC, the San Francisco General Hospital Operating Room Committee, and the revised guidelines for CPR recently issued by the Emergency Cardiac Care Committee of the American Heart Association should, indeed, be followed carefully.

Literature

1. American Heart Association (1989) Revised guidelines for cardiopulmonary resuscitation JAMA, Nov 17
2. Banerjee K, Rodrigues J, Israel Z, Kulkarni S, Thakar M (1989) Outbreak of HIV seropositivity among commercial plasma donors in Pune, India. Lancet, July 15: 166
3. Belitsky V (1989) Children infect mothers in AIDS outbreak at a Soviet hospital. Nature 337: 493
4. Bernard R P (1989) End April 1989 Global Status of Reported AIDS Cases and 1987 WHO/GPA Estimates for Subsaharan Africa (Calculations, Rankings, Documented Illustrations). Pre-World Health Assembly Meeting of the HGO-PHC Group, Geneva 1989, May 8, AF 0489: 1—10
5. CDC (1987) Recommendations for prevention of HIV transmission in health-care settings. MMWR 36 (Suppl 2S, Aug 21)
6. CDC (1988) Update AIDS och HIV infection among health-care workers. MMWR 37: 229—34, 239
7. CDC (1988) Update: Universal precautions for prevention of transmission of HIV, hepatitis B virus, and other bloodborne pathogens in health-care settings. MMWR 37/24: 377—88
8. CDC (1988) Trends in HIV infection among civilian applicants for military service. US, Oct 1985 — Mar 1988. MMWR 37: 677—9
9. CDC (1988) Distribution of AIDS cases, by racial/ethnic group and exposure category, US, Jun 1, 1981 — Jul 4 1988. MMWR 37, S. 3: 1—10
10. CDC (1989) Update: AIDS - US, 1981—1988. MMWR 38(14): 239—236
11. CDC (1989) Guidelines for prevention of transmission of HIV and HBV to health-care and publicsafety workers. MMWR 38, S-6: 1—37
12. CDC (1989) AIDS cases reported through Sept. 1989. HIV/AIDS Surveillance 1989, Oct: 15 pp
13. Cronstedt J (1988) Wie minimal ist das Risiko der HIV-Übertragung im Kontakt mit Patienten? Verdauungskrankh 6(4):153—7
14. Fröland SS, Jenum P, Lindboe CF, Wefring KW, Linnestadt PJ, Böhmer T (1988) HIV-1 infection in Norwegian family before 1970. Lancet June 11: 1344—5
15. González JJ, Davidsen P, Moe CE, Koch MG (1988) The initial non-infectious period and the seroconversion latency period are critical parameters for HIV spread. EC Workshop on Quantitative Analyses of AIDS, Bilthoven 1988, July 6—8, Abstracts
16. González JJ, Koch MG (1986) On the role of transients for the prognostic analysis of AIDS and the anciennity distribution of AIDS patients. AIFO 1(9): 621—30

17. González JJ, Koch MG (1987) On the role of transients (biasing transitional effects) for the prognostic analysis of the AIDS epidemic. Am J Epidemiol 126 (6): 985—1005
18. Haase AT (1986) The pathogenesis of slow virus infections: molecular analyses. J Infect Dis 153: 441—7
19. Haase AT (1986) Pathogenesis of lentivirus infections. Nature 322: 130—6
20. Hickl EJ, Koch MG (198) Die Entwicklung der AIDS-Epidemie und ihre Bedeutung für Geburtshilfe und Gynäkologie. Geburtsheilk 49: 313—27
21. Huminer D, Rosenfeld JB, Pitlik SD (1987) AIDS in the pre-AIDS era. Rev Inf Dis 9: 1102—8
22. Imagawa DT, Lee MH, Wolinsky SM, Sano K, Morales F, Kwok S, Sninsky JJ, Nishanian PG, Giorgi J, Fahey JL, Dudley J, Visscher BR, Detels R (1989) HIV-1 infection in homosexual men who remain seronegative for prolonged periods. N Engl J Med 320: 1458—62
23. Karpas A (1987) Origin of the AIDS virus explained? New Scientist Jul 16: 67
24. Koch MG (1987) AIDS - die verdrängte Lentivirus-Pandemie. Spektrum d Wiss 10: 12—14
25. Koch MG (1987) The anatomy of the virus. New Scientist Mar 26: 46—51
26. Koch MG (1987) HIV - die unvollendete Geschichte einer Virusentdeckung. Spektrum d Wiss 7: 14—5
27. Koch MG (1987) AIDS - vom Molekül zur Pandemie. Spektrum der Wissenschaft, Heidelberg; reprint 1989, 306 pp
28. Koch MG (1988) Erst in zweiter Linie ein psychosoziales Problem. Ärztl Praxis 40: 1598—1600
29. Koch MG (1988) AIDS - die lautlose Explosion. Nomos, Baden-Baden
30. Koch MG (1988) Prinzipien der antiviralen Therapie - In: L'age-Stehr J, Helm EB, Koch MG (eds) AIDS und die Vorstadien, Sekt IV, Kap 1. Springer, Berlin, Heidelberg, New York, Tokyo
31. Koch MG (1988) Impfstoffentwicklung. In: L'age-Stehr J, Helm EB, Koch MG (eds): AIDS und die Vorstadien, Sekt IV, Kap 1. Springer, Berlin, Heidelberg, New York, Tokyo
32. Koch MG (1988) AIDS-Converence Stockholm: Critical appraisal and reports onn the most important news. AIFO 3: 579—84
33. Koch MG (1989) Congress Reports: 2 Deutscher AIDS-Kongreß in Berlin, 23—24. Jan. 1989, Bericht 2. AIFO 4: 206—8
34. Koch MG (1989) An ivisible underground network. AIDS Insurance Reports 7(13): 97—104
35. Koch MG (1989) Congress Reports: V. Internationale AIDS-Konferenz in Montreal, June 4—9 1989. AIFO 4 (8 and in prep., engl.: in prep)
36. Koch MG (1988) Vom Lentivirus zum Slow Toxin - an der Schwelle neuer Erkenntnisse im Bereich der Neuropathologie. 61 Jahrestagung der Deutschen Gesellschaft für Neurologie, Frankfurt 22—24 Sept. 1988. Verhandlungsband Nr. 5, in press
37. Koch MG, González JJ (1987) Transiente Phänomene - ein Exkurs über Aufmerksamkeitsfallen. AIFO 2: 553—8
38. Koch MG, L'age-Stehr J(1987) Möglichkeiten der Prognose im Rahmen der AIDS-Epidemiologie. AIFO 2(2):94—9
39. Koch MG, L'age-Stehr J, González JJ, Dörner D (1988) Epidemiologie von AIDS. Spektrum d Wiss 1987 (Aug): 38—51; reprint April 1988
40. Koch MG, L'age-Stehr J, González JJ, Dörner D (1988) The Epidemiology of AIDS. AIDS Insurance Reports 7(9): 65—72
41. Koch MG, L'age-Stehr J, González JJ, Dörner D (1988) Modeling the AIDS epidemic. AIDS Insurance Reports 7(10):73—80
42. L'age-Stehr J, Helm EB, Koch MG (eds) (1988) AIDS und die Vorstadien. Springer Berlin, Heidelberg New York, Tokyo
43. Levy JA (1988) Mysteries of HIV: challenges for therapy and prevention. Nature 333: 519—22
44. Piot P, Plummer FA, Rey MA et al (1987) Retrospective seroepidemiology of AIDS virus infection in Nairobi populations. J Infect Dis 155,6: 1108—12
45. Reeve PA, (1989) HIV infection in patients admitted to a general hospital in Malawi. BMJ 1989, 298 1567—8
46. Schecter WP, Chambers HR, Crombleholme W, Dailey P, Hadley K, Lusby G, McAnish JW, Sooy D, Tarkington A, Williams J (1988) Surgical care in the era cf AIDS infection. Report from the San Francisco General Hospital Operating Room Committee 1988, Mai 10

47. Tessmann I (1989) Limited significance of null results. Lancet 1989, Oct 21: 982
48. WHO (1989) AIDS - Situation 30. Sept. 1989. Weekly Epidemiol Rec, Genf 64, No 40

Authors' address:
Michael G. Koch, M.D.
VåC, S-54600 Karlsberg, Sweden
P.L. 9471

Epidemiology — Screening for Infectious Diseases Transmitted Through Blood and Blood Products

S. Seidl[1], and P. Kühnl[2]

[1] Dept. of Immunohematology, University of Frankfurt, Red Cross Donor Service, Hessen, FRG
[2] Dept. of Transfusionmedicine, University of Hamburg, FRG

Introduction

A major risk of blood transfusion is transmission of infectious diseases. The pattern of these diseases varies in different parts of the world, but hepatitis, AIDS, and CMV-infection are considered to be the most important ones. In recent years blood banks have introduced several screening tests to detect these diseases. Apart from these procedures, the most effective "screening method" is adequate selection of donors, ensuring that they are in good health and that their history does not indicate risk of transmitting a disease.

Table 1 shows remarkable differences among these three diseases: The prevalence of infectious agents is extremely low in HIV infection, whereas approximately 50% of the donor population is CMV-antibody positive. Hepatitis B antigen (HBsAg) has been observed in approximately 0.5% of blood donors in central Europe. Results recently obtained with a new screening test for hepatitis C (hepatitis nonA,nonB) show positivity rates between 0.5 and 1.0%. The clinical significance of these infections is different: HIV-infection will cause (after a period of several years) AIDS, and thus, the death of the recipient. Hepatitis infection may cause post-transfusion hepatitis (PTH) and may also lead to chronic hepatitis or liver cirrhosis. CMV infection, however, is of particular importance in immunocompromised patients, i.e., patients undergoing bone marrow transplantation or leukemia patients receiving chemotherapy.

Post-transfusion hepatitis

The disease was originally described as "serum hepatitis" but was later modified to post-transfusion hepatitis (PTH). There are at least two hepatitis viruses known to be transmitted through blood and blood products: Hepatitis B virus (HBV) and the infectious agent of hepatitis nonA,nonB (HNANB), hepatitis C virus (HCV). Hepatitis A Virus is seldom transmitted, because viremia is extremely rare. In recent years the results of several prospective studies performed in open-heart surgery patients have been published. Table 2 summarizes the data. These studies include a total of 2207 patients receiving on average 8.6 units of blood per patient. PTH was observed in 166 patients (7.5%) with a wide (geographical) range: 2.1% to 20%. Only a few PTH-cases were caused by CMV (3.6%) or HBV (9.6%); the majority of all cases (86.7%) were due to infection by the HNANB-agent. Similar results have also been observed in the TTV (transfusion transmitted virus) Study [1]. Among the four participating centers (New York, St. Louis, Houston, and Los Angeles) the highest incidence of PTH was observed in Houston (18%), whereas in St. Louis only 4% contracted PTH, thus also underlining geographical differences. Since most of these studies were performed in the years between 1981 and 1983, i.e., before several measures were introduced to prevent blood donation from individuals being at high risk, the overall percentages of PTH might be much lower today.

In several studies a correlation has been observed between increased ALT (SGPT)-levels and/or presence of anti-HBc in the donor and the incidence of PTH in recipients. The results of two ALT-studies from the United States clearly indicate that transfusion of donor blood with elevated ALT-levels resulted in a higher percentage of PTH than donor blood with normal or slightly increased ALT-concentrations. The anti-HBc status of the donor blood and the incidence of PTH in the recipient are shown in Table 3. After transfusion of anti-HBV-negative blood PTH in recipients occurred in 9.4%, but increased to 20.4% after transfusion of anti-HBc positive blood [9]. ALT (SGPT) screening is performed in West-Germany and in other European countries (Italy, Switzerland, Austria, and France).

Table 1. Screening for infectious Diseases.

HBV	HBsAg	0.5%	Chron. Hepatitis
HCV (HNANB)	HCV-Ab.	0.5—1.0%	Cirrhosis
CMV	CMV-Ab.	50%	Immunsuppr. Pat.
HIV	HIV-Ab.	$\leq 0.001\%$	AIDS

Table 2. Incidence of post-transfusion hepatitis. Eight prospective studies in patients undergoing open-heart surgery.

Patients	Transfused. units/Pat.	Post-transfusion Hepatitis total	caused by	
2.207	8.6 (4—12)	166 7.5% (2.1—20.0%)	6 CMV 16 Hep. B 144 Hep. NANB	3,6% 9.6% 86.7%

Table 3. HBV Antibodies in blood donors and PTH NANB in recipients (9).

Donor HBV- Antibodies	Donors n	Donors assoc. with PTH NANB in Recipients	P value
negative	3974	373 (9.4%)	—
Anti-HBs	109	12 (11.0%)	—
Anti-HBs+ Anti-HBc	171	31 (18.1%)	< 0.001
Anti-HBc	49	10 (20.4%)	< 0.01

102

In the United States, both tests (ALT and anti-HBc) have been recently recommended by the AABB (American Association of Blood Banks) for use as as "surrogate tests". It might well be that this screening will continue after the introduction of hepatitis C screening, because of the long "window period" and the strong correlation observed between surrogate markers and anti-HCV positivity [2].

The recent development of a specific test to detect HNANB is a breakthrough in HNANB-research. Utilizing recombinant technology an antigen has been produced that detects antibodies in HNANB patients. The infectious agent, though not yet known, is termed hepatitis C virus (HCV) and is probably a member of the Flavivirus family. HCV can be separated from another HNANB-virus that has caused several hepatitis epidemics in Southeast Asia, and elsewhere (Table 4); it is provisionally termed hepatitis E virus (HEV), since the suffix D is already been used to designate Hepatitis D Virus (Delta agent). HCV is parenterally transmitted through blood or blood products (transfusion associated PTH), but also through other routes (sporadic infection), whereas HEV is enterically transmitted. This virus most probably belongs to the Calicivirus group.

The prevalence of anti-HCV among the German blood donor population has been studied in a multicenter trial: 3123 blood donors were tested by ELISA, 18 initially reacted positive (0.58 %), 13 remained HCV-antibody positive after repeat testing (0.42%). This percentage fits well with the average percentage (0.51%) observed in more than 50 000 European blood donors (published at the First Hepatitis-C congress in Rome, in 1989). The anti-HCV prevalence varies in various parts of the world; also a North-South tendency has been observed, similar to the HBsAg prevalence. Anti-HCV prevalence ranges from 0.2 to 0.3% in Scandinavia, whereas in South Europe more than 1% of the donor population is anti-HCV positive (Barcelona 1.13%). A correlation has been observed between "surrogate markers" and anti-HCV positivity in patients suffering from transfusion-associated HNANB [2]. In this study, 88 % of the blood donors involved in PTH were anti-HCV positive, 33% of them also had increased ALT-level, whereas anti-HBc could be demonstrated in more than 50% of these HCV-antibody-positive donors. In several European studies a weak correlation in donor blood was observed between anti-HCV positivity and elevated ALT-levels and/or anti-HBc positivity. In West Germany, anti-HCV was found in 2.2% of sera with an increased ALT-level, and in 1.7% of sera that were

Table 4. Hepatitis non-A, non-B (4).

Hepatitis C Virus (HCV)	Hepatitis E Virus (HEV)
Parenterally transmitt.	Enterically transmitt. (Burma, Mexico, Russia, etc.)
< 80 nm ≥ 10 000 nucleotides single-strand RNA	27—38 nm single-strand RNA
Flavivirus	Calicivirus-like
HCV-Ab assay (ELISA)	HEV-Ag assay (IF)

also positive for anti-HBc. In other European countries these percentages varied between 4% and 9% (for ALT) and 2%—9% (for anti-HBc), but the number of investigated sera is still rather small.

In an American study [2] anti-HCV has been found in almost all cases of transfusion-associated chronic PTH, but only in 60% of acute PTH. In a study from West Germany, patients with acute or chronic hepatitis (post-transfusion or sporadic) were screened for anti-HCV. Forty-five % of acute hepatitis patients and 74% of patients suffering from chronic hepatitis were found to be anti-HCV positive. A high anti-HCV prevalence has also been observed in hemophiliacs, ranging from 30% to 90%, and a wide range of anti-HCV positivity among dialysis patients (4—60%). Anti-HCV is detectable 15 to 20 weeks after transfusion of anti-HCV-positive donor blood, i.e., a long "window period" exists, but by continuing "surrogate testing" a certain number of anti-HCV-positive donors will be detected earlier and thus, withdrawn from the donor pool. It is still not yet clear whether all anti-HCV-positive donors are infectious or not. In a study from the USA, 88% of anti-HCV-positive chronic hepatitis patients had been transfused with anti-HCV-positive blood [2]. This percentage is not confirmed by a Dutch study in which only one-third of anti-HCV-positive donors caused hepatitis [11]. Although several questions remain, there is no doubt that routine donor screening for anti-HCV will prevent a certain number of PTH.

Transfusion-associated AIDS (TAA)

Acquired immunodeficiency syndrome (AIDS) is the most severe manifestation of an infection with the retroviruses HIV 1 or HIV 2. Since the publication of the first AIDS-cases in the USA, many thousands of AIDS cases have been reported, observed mainly in homosexual (or bisexual) men or in i.v. drug users. Also, a small proportion of transfusion recipients or hemophiliacs have been infected by HIV-contaminated blood or blood products, i.e., coagulation factor concentrates. In most countries routine screening for HIV-antibodies was introduced in 1985, and donor blood that is anti-HIV positive is discarded. Despite HIV-screening, TAA cases have slightly increased in recent years (Table 5), reaching similar percentages in the United States and in West Germany. This increase is explained by the long incubation period of the disease. It has been shown [8] that in recent years TAA cases were diagnosed with a rather short incubation period in contrast to TAA cases that had been transfused between 1978 and 1983. HIV infection is followed by a several months incubation period (demonstrating HIV antigen) before antibodies are detectable. Therefore, an individual might be infectious before HIV antibodies appear. A commercially available HIV-antigen test has been evaluated in Europe and in USA. Approximately 500 000 blood donors were investigated by blood centers in Austria and Bavaria, and no serum could be detected that was HIV-antibody *neg-*

Table 5. TAA (transfusion-associated AIDS).

	1984	1985	1986	1987	1988
West Germany	—	0.5%	1.9%	2.4%	2.6%
USA	1.1%	1.9%	1.8%	2.1%	2.7%

104

Table 6. Red cross donor service, Hessen, FRG, HIV-positive blood donors (1985–1988) n = 37.

	1985	1986	1987	1988	Total	%
1. Homosexual (or bisexual)	11	7	1	1	20	54
2. i.v. Drug users	1	2	–	–	3	8.1
3. Transf. AIDS	1	–	–	–	1	2.7
4. Heterosexual	1	–	1	–	2	5.4
5. unknown	6	3	1	1	11	29.7
	20	12	3	2	37	99.9

ative, but reacted positive in the HIV antigen test [3]. The data from the USA confirm these results, thus indicating that HIV-antigen screening provides no additional benefit, at least at this time.

Besides HIV-antibody screening other measures have also been introduced. Since 1983, persons belonging to so-called "high-risk groups" are not accepted as donors. They are informed by a leaflet before donating blood. An additional "confidential donor self-exclusion" procedure has been introduced by which the donor is confidentially asked whether his/her blood should be used for transfusion or only for laboratory use. A few cases of HIV infection after transfusion with HIV-screened blood have been reported [12]. Nevertheless, there is general agreement that the blood supply is extremely safe today! The risk of transmitting HIV infection through screened blood is 1 : 1 million or less. Each year a few blood donors are identified who are HIV-positive. Table 6 shows the analysis of these HIV-positive donors and clearly indicates that donors still come to the donor session although they belong to "high-risk" groups.

As in other countries also in W-Germany the prevalence of HIV-positive blood donors has decreased remarkably. The percentage of HIV-positive donors was high in 1985 (55/100 000), i.e., in the beginning of HIV-screening; thereafter it decreased to 6/100 000 in 1987, and in 1988, only one HIV-positive donor among 100 000 screened was observed. Also, attempts have been made to calculate the number of HIV-positives among the general population. After introducing the laboratory reporting system (Labor-Berichtspflicht), in W-Germany all HIV-positive (WB-pos.) individuals are reported anonymously to the Reference laboratory in Berlin. The first analysis revealed 32 779 HIV-positive individuals. When compared with the total population of 61 million the percentage is 0.05%. The true figure might be either greater (because not all HIV-positive individuals have been tested so far) or smaller (because of double-reporting).

The prevalence of HIV-positivity in patients suffering from severe hemophilia ranges from 70% to 90%. It has been demonstrated that HIV infection in hemophiliacs started as early as 1980 in W-Germany (Munich), and then gradually increased to 50% in 1985. However, there are still three European countries (Norway, Belgium, and Finland) with a very low incidence of HIV-infectivity among their hemophiliacs (4–8%). This is explained by the fact that in these countries coagulation factors are prepared predominantly from domestic sources. In a survey of the Council of Europe (conducted in 1986/87) a correlation between HIV-antibody prevalence and the percentage of imported F VIII has been demonstrated. Countries with a high percentage of imported F VIII (mainly from the USA) have a high incidence of seropositivity among their hemophilia patients.

Recently, a new retrovirus, HIV 2 has been described, which also causes AIDS. Although the prevalence of HIV-2 infected people is extremely low (and all HIV-2-positives can so far be traced back to West Africa) blood banks in West-Germany have decided to screen for both viruses, utilizing a combi-test (HIV 1/HIV 2).

Another retrovirus, *human T-lymphotropic virus type I* (HTLV I) represents the first human retrovirus closely linked to a particular form of T-cell malignancy, the adult T-cell leukemia (ATL); HTLV I antibodies were detected in almost all ATL cases in the United States and in Japan. Important modes of transmission are by sexual intercourse, perinatally from mother to child, and by blood transfusion. After transfusion of HTLV-I-positive blood (whole blood, packed red cells) seroconversion was observed in more than 60% of recipients [7], but HTLV-I transmission did not occur after transfusion of HTLV-I-positive fresh frozen plasma. However, no case of ATL due to HTLV-I infection aquired by blood transfusion has been reported to date, possibly due to the very long latent period ($> 10-20$ years). In some endemic areas in Japan, a HTLV I-seroprevalence of $1-2\%$ has been found and routine blood-donor screening is performed. HTLV-I screening has also been introduced in the USA because HTLV-I infections have been reported. The positivity rates are markedly influenced by social class. In West Germany, the present epidemiological situation does not require HTLV-I screening of blood donors.

Cytomegalovirus infection

Human cytomegalovirus (CMV) is a member of the herpes virus group, it is transmitted vertically and horizontally by sexual contact, blood transfusion, organ transplants, or from mother to child, and it can persist life-long as a latent, sometimes reactivated infection. CMV disease can occur as a primary infection, which can be symptomatic in seronegative recipients of latently or actively infected donor blood or as reactivated infectious, largely asymptomatic in seropositive recipients of a seropositive or seronegative blood unit; in reinfection with a CMV strain different from the one originally infecting the recipient (Table 7) CMV-antibody-prevalence studies in the adult population have shown that approximately 50% of the donor population is infected (Table 8). Most blood transfusion services screen part of their blood supply in order to provide CMV-negative blood for neonates or immunocompromised patients.

Table 7. Three forms of post-transfusion CMV infections (immunocompetent recipients).

1. Primary infection	May be symptomatic in seronegative recipients of a CMV-infected blood	IgM, IgG response
2. Secondary infections		
reactivation	Largely asymptomatic in seropositive recipients of seropositive **or** neg. blood (donor WBC trigger-allograft reaction, reactivating latent, endogenous CMV of the recipient)	IgG ↑ 4× no IgM
re-infection	CMV strain different from the one originally infecting the recipient (restriction endonuclease analysis of CMV-DNA for strain discrimination)	IgM response possible

Significant morbity and mortality were noted in studies, particularly among infants weighing 1500 g or less, when CMV-positive blood was given; the extremely low risk of CMV-negative blood has also been confirmed. Immunocompromised transplant patients may be easily infected from a transplanted organ. The donor kidney has been identified as the major vehicle for CMV transmission to CMV-seronegative recipients. Also in other immunocompromised patients (patients undergoing bone marrow transplantation, patients with malignancies, AIDS, etc.) a higher risk of CMV infection after blood transfusion has been observed.

Laboratory diagnosis of CMV infection can be established by several methods; blood-donor screening for CMV antibodies is commonly used by blood transfusion services. The effectiveness of donor screening has been established in several studies, summarized in Table 9. After transfusion with CMV-negative blood only 1/289 neonates was infected, whereas CMV-positive blood resulted in 8.8% CMV infection (26/294), of which 17 were symptomatic; in nine cases death of the neonate was the final outcome. CMV infection can also be prevented by transfusion of filtered blood because leucocytes harbor CMV. Data of a recent study [5] have shown that no CMV infection occurred in 42 neonates transfused with filtered (CMV-positive and CMV-negative) blood, but nine CMV infections were observed in 59 neonates transfused with unfiltered (CMV-positive and CMV-negative) blood. Another way of preventing CMV-transmission is the use of frozen, deglycerolized, washed red cells. The efficacy of prophylactic anti-CMV immunoglobulin administration was evaluated in kidney transplants. Passive immunization completely prevented CMV related death, although it did not reduce the incidence of CMV isolation, viremia, or disease.

Table 8. Prevalence of CMV-antibodies (blood donors).

Country		CMV-seropositive			
	n	n	%	m. %	f. %
West Germany	450	253	56	56	56
Switzerland	100	44	44	46	42
Belgium	31	11	35	23	36
USA (New York)	944	636	64	64	64

Table 9. Effectiveness of CMV-donor screening. Comparison of several trials in CMV-seronegative neonates

Transfusion with CMV *negative* blood

n	infected
289	1 (0.3%)

Transfusion with CMV *positive* blood

n	infected
294	26 (8.8%) 17 (65%) Symptomatic 9 (35%) Deaths

References

1. Aach RD, Szmuness W, Mosley JW, Hollinger FB, Kahn RA, Stevens CE, Edwards VM, Werch J (1981) Serum alanine aminotransferase of donors in relation to the risk of nonA,nonB hepatitis in recipients. The transfusion-transmitted viruses study. N Engl J Med 304: 989—992
2. Alter HJ, Runge RH, Shich JW, Melpolder JC, Houghton M, Qui-Lim C, Kuo G (1989) Detection of antibody to hepatitis-C-virus in prospectively followed transfusion recipients with acute and chronic nonA,nonB hepatitis. N Engl J Med 321: 1494—1498
3. Bäcker U, Weinauer F, Gathof AG, Gossrau E, Eberle J, Deinhardt F. HIV Antigen Screening in Blood Donors. Abstr., AIDS-Congress Stockholm, June 12—16, 1988
4. Bradley DW. The Viruses of nonA,nonB Hepatitis, Enterically and Parenterally Transmitted. EASL, 24th Meeting, Munich, August 30—September 2, 1989
5. Gilbert GL, Hayes K, Hudson IL, James I (1989) Prevention of Transfusion-Acquired Cytomegalovirus Infection in Infants by Blood Filtration to Remove Leucocytes. Lancet, I: 1228—1231
6. Kühnl P, Sibrowski W, Böhm BO, Seidl S (1989) HIV-Epidemiologie im Hinblick auf Bluttransfusionen. Hefte zur Unfallheilkunde, Heft 207: 347—366
7. Okochi K and Sato H. Blood transfusion related transmission of HTLV-1 (ATLV). Abstract, XIX Congr. Int Soc Blood Transfusion, Sydney, May 11—16, 1986
8. Peterman TA (1987) Transfusion-Associated Acquired Immunodeficiency Syndrome. World J. Surg. 11: 36—40
9. Stevens CE, Aach RD, Hollinger FB, Mosley JW, Szmuness W, Kahn R, Werch J, Edwards V (1984) Relation to HBV antibody status of blood donors to the occurrence of nonA,nonB hepatitits in their recipients. Ann Intern Med 101: 733—741
10. Tegtmeier G, 1987 Blood Transfusion and the Transmission of Cytomegalovirus (1987) In: Moore SB (ed) Transfusion-Transmitted Viral Diseases. Amer Ass Blood Banks, Arlington VA pp 87—108
11. Van der Poel CL and Reesink HW: Infectivity of Anti-HCV Positive Blood. Poster 1st Hepatitis-C Meeting, Rome, September 11—16, 1989
12. Ward JW, Homberg SD, Allen JR, Cohn DL, Critchley SE, Kleinmann SH, Lenes BA, Ravenholt O, Davis JR, Quinn MG, Jaffe HW (1988) Transmission of human immunodeficiency virus (HIV) by blood transfusions screened as negative for HIV antibody. New Engl J Med 318: 473—479

Authors' addresses:
Prof. Dr. S. Seidl,
Dept of Immunhematology University Frankfurt,
Red Cross Donor Service Hessen,
Sandhofstr. 1
6000 Frankfurt/M.

Prof. Dr. P. Kühnl
Dept. of Transfusionmedicine,
University Hamburg
Martinistr. 52
2000 Hamburg 20

III: Non-Pharmacological Methods for the Reduction of Blood Use in Cardiac Surgery

Autologous Blood Predonation

H. Kuppe[1], Th. Breitfeld[2] and P. Schmucker[1]

[1] Institute of Anaesthesiology, German Heart Institute, Berlin
[2] Seroplas Company, Berlin

In cardiac surgery, ten and more years ago, it was current practice to use homologous blood as a routine priming component of the extracorporeal system. In addition, after weaning from extracorporeal circulation, hemoglobin values were transfused in patients up to values between 10—12 g Hb/100 ml, since the oxygen transport capacity reaches its maximum at approx. 12 g/100 ml. There is, however, no reason why a Hb-value of 10 or even less should not be accepted, at least in patients following uneventful operations.

Table 1 shows the Hb-values and the transfused units of red cells and fresh frozen plasma in the first 20 patients undergoing orthotopic heart transplantation in Berlin in early 1986, as compared to 20 patients transplanted in late 1988. Obviously, the total amount of transfused blood components has been considerably reduced by the mere acceptance of a lower Hb-value.

The mean transfused units are shown in Table 1. In fact, only seven out of 20 patients in the 1988 group received homologous blood transfusions. Our current practice is to take into consideration the transfusion of homologous blood with a Hb-value of 7 and less. As can be expected, this procedure is not completely without problems.

Figure 1 shows the total peripheral resistance during aortocoronary bypass-operation in 12 patients with good left ventricular function and in 12 patients with impaired left ventricular function. T1—T5 are the values prior to extracorporeal circulation, T6 and T7 show the values immediately after extracorporeal circulation, and before the end of the operation, respectively. The total peripheral resistance in these patients is obviously reduced after weaning from extracorporeal circulation. A number of our patients actually require vasoconstrictive treatment after weaning from extracorporeal circulation. This reduction in peripheral vascular resistance is

Table 1. Transfusion of units of homologous packed red cells and of homologous fresh frozen plasma in 20 patients undergoing orthotopic heart transplantation at the German Heart Institute, Berlin, in early 1986, as compared to 20 patients in late 1988. The first column shows the mean hemoglobin value subsequent to surgery; the second column, the amount of packed red cells; the third column shows the amount of units of fresh frozen plasma.

	Hb (g/100 ml) at the end of operation	Red cells transfused (units)	Fresh frozen plasma transfused (units)
1986 (n = 20)	10.4	3.35	3.6
1988 (n = 20)	8.3	1.14	0.95

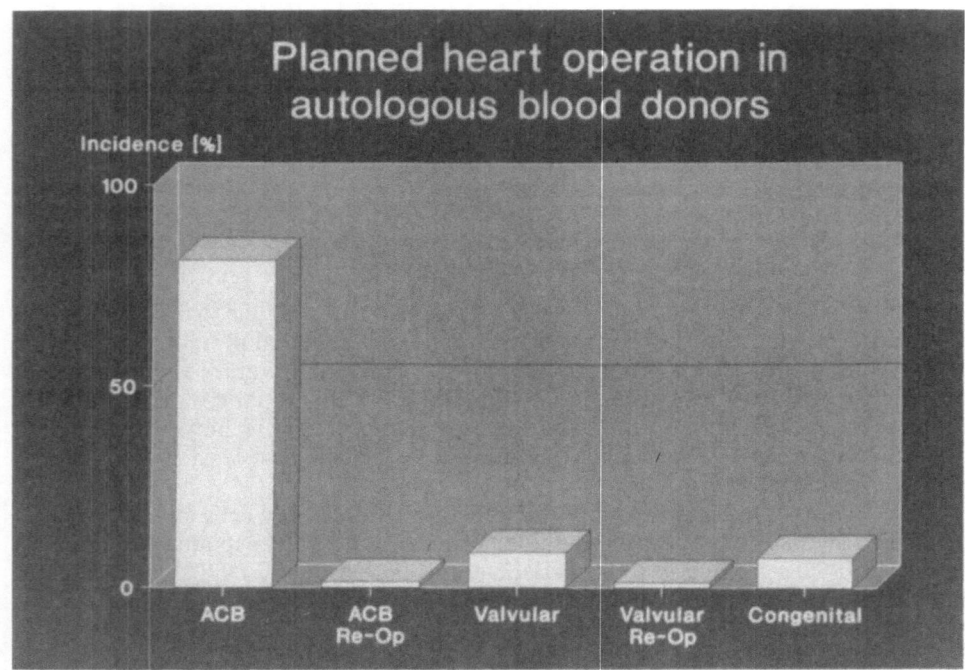

Fig. 1. Planned heart operations in 230 patients taking part in the autologous blood predonation program at the German Heart Institute, Berlin.

at least partially due to a reduced blood viscosity, as a consequence of a relatively low Hb-value. One could define this phenomenon by stating that we are, in fact, replacing red cells with noradrenaline. So far no infections havebeen transferred by noradrenaline infusion, in contrast to blood transfusions. The tolerance of a relatively low Hb-value is, of course, limited by a hemoglobin value of 7 in the majority of patients.

Therefore, in 1987 an outpatient autologous blood predonation program was initiated at the German Heart Institute Berlin, in order to reduce the utilization of homologous blood even more. From January 1988 through August 1989, 379 outpatients scheduled for cardiac surgery were included in this program, resulting in a total of 843 autologous blood donations.

The data of 230 unselected patients, giving a total of 549 donations, have been studied; 188 (n = 81.7%) were male and 42 (n = 18.3%) female. The patients were aged 54.0 ± 10.5 years (18—77). The fact that the majority of patients are male is explained by the prevalence of coronary artery disease leading to surgical intervention, as shown in Fig. 2.

Together with information regarding the planned operation date, all patients also received information regarding the possibility of autologous blood donation; they were also informed about the risks and possible problems. Patients who were willing to take part in the program were asked to contact the Seroplas-Company and arrange a date for the first donation, which was set approximately 4 weeks prior to the planned operation date.

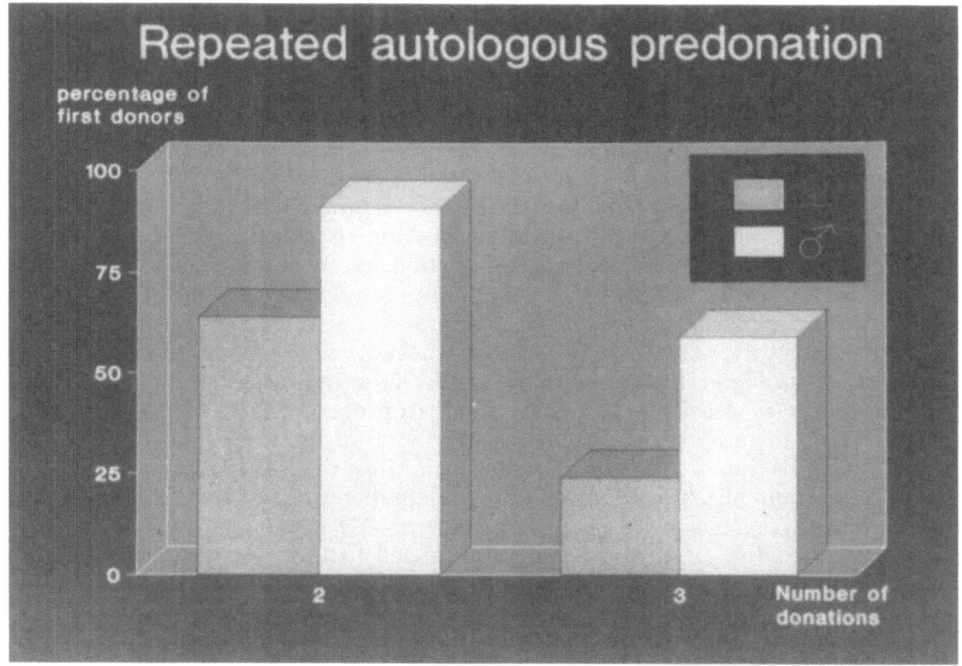

Fig. 2. Percentage of 230 patients included in the autologous blood predonation program (n = 100%) who were able to give a second and third autologous blood predonation, respectively.

Following evaluation of case history and physical examination, patients gave written informed consent and were included in the program unless one of the exclusion criteria listed in Table 2 was applicable. Some of these criteria seem rather arbitrary.

In particular, patients with a left-ventricular ejection fraction of less than 45% and a proximal stenosis of the left coronary artery of more than 40%, and patients with a maximum exercise tolerance of less than 50 W were excluded from the predonation program.

Table 2. Exclusion criteria for the preoperative autologous blood donation program used by the German Heart Institute, Berlin, and the Seroplas Company, Berlin, 1988—1989.

— body weight < 50 kg
— poor general health
— infectious disease
— history of epilepsy
— anemia (Hb < 12.5 g/100 ml prior to scheduled donation)
— unstable angina pectoris
— aortic stenosis
— LVEF < 45%
— maximum exercise tolerance < 50 W
— 100 mm Hg < SAP < 180 mm Hg
— 50/min < HR < 100/min
— severe arrhythmia
— AVC-conduction-disorder

Since patients suffering from cardiac disease are inclined to be more subject to undesirable side-effects following blood predonation, the normal procedure was modified. The actual hemoglobin value was determined after the opening of a peripheral venous way, if there was more than 12.5 g/100/ml, the venous way was connected to an infusion system.

At the next stage, a second venous way was opened for collection of the blood donation. In order to maintain approximate isovolemic conditions during the collection (which took approx. 15 min) 500 ml Ringer's solution was infused. If a decrease in blood pressure occurred, hydroxyethyl starch was administered. Before, during, and 30 min subsequent to blood donation, heart rate and ST-segment were controlled by a continuous ECG. Blood pressure was also repeatedly controlled.

Figure 3 shows the percentage of patients who were able to donate a second and third unit of autologous blood, respectively. Out of a total of 230 patients included in the study (defined as 100%), 198 were able to proceed to the second stage, and 121 were able to make a third donation. The reason for the exclusion from the second and third donations, respectively, was in most cases a Hb-value below 12.5 g/100/ml. As could be expected, more women than men were excluded from a repeat donation for this reason.

Table 3 shows the number of patients admitted to the first, second, and third donations, respectively, together with the mean hemoglobin-values. Please note that patients with a hemoglobin lower than 12.5 g/% had already been excluded from the donation, which indicates that, in all patients, hemoglobin decreased more rapidly than shown in Table 3.

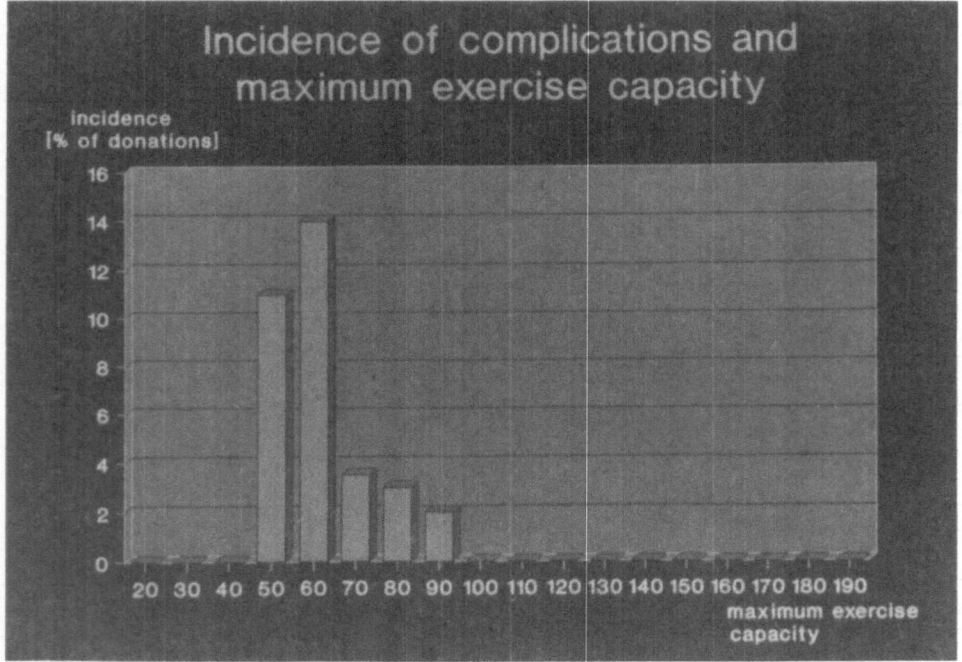

Fig. 3. Incidence of complication during 549 autologous blood predonations in 230 patients scheduled for cardiac surgery on the ordinate against maximum exercise tolerance on the abscissa.

114

Table 3. Number of repeat autologous blood predonations in 230 patients scheduled for cardiac surgery and hemoglobin value prior to the first, second, and third donations, respectively.

1st donation	n = 230	Hb = 14.8 ± 2.1 (12.5 − 18.7)
2nd donation	b = 198	Hb = 14.4 ± 0.9 (12.5 − 16.5)
3rd donation	n = 121	Hb = 13.2 ± 0.9 (12.5 − 18.2)
Total donations	n = 549	

Immediately following the donation the whole blood was centrifuged and fractionated into packed red cells and fresh frozen plasma. The blood components were stored as usual until the operation.

In order to evaluate the ratio of risks and benefits of the procedure more thoroughly, particular attention was paid to complications during and after blood donation.

Complications observed during and after autologous blood donation can be divided into the categories as shown in Table 4. Table 5 shows the hemodynamic complications during and immediately after blood donation. It is clear that the incidences of bradycardia and hypertension are relatively low. Therapeutic interventions were necessary only in 15 cases, when hemodynamic complications were associated with nausea or with precordial pain. The most serious complication was one case of epileptic seizure in a patient with a history of epilepsy, about which we had not been informed. There was no case of preoperative death.

Patients with complications leading to therapeutic intervention, during or immediately after blood donation, were excluded from the program and not admitted to the second and third donations, respectively. Twelve patients were excluded from the program due to an increase in precordial pain during the interval between the donations.

Table 4. Definition of complications observed during and immediately after 549 autologous blood predonations in 230 patients scheduled for cardiac surgery.

Bradycardia	(< 45/min)
Hypotension	(SAP < 100 mmHg)
Precordial pain	
Nausea	
Epileptic seizure	

Table 5. Incidence of bradycardia and hypotension, as well as the incidence of therapeutic intervention during autologous blood predonation.

Bradycardia	1.1%		0.5%
Hypotension	4.5%		4.3%
Therapeutic intervention		2.37%	
n = 549	during		after

So far, the complication rate of 2.4% donations requiring therapeutic interventions is relatively high, as compared to normal homologous blood donors, in whom the complication rate is considered to be lower than 1%. Exclusion criteria had been defined at the commencement of the program. On account of the relatively low incidence of complications, we attempted to perform variance analysis as far as possible, in order to evaluate the factors influencing the incidence of complications more thoroughly.

Table 6. Correlation between the incidence of complications during 549 autologous blood predonations in 230 patients scheduled for cardiac surgery, together with preoperative data evaluated by means of variance analysis.

LV ejection fraction	n.s.
Cardiac index	n.s.
Exercise performance < 75 W	$p < 0.05$
2 and more drugs	$p < 0.05$

Table 6 shows some presumed risk factors with regard to their influence on the incidence of complications. Complications could only be observed in patients scheduled for coronary bypass-operation. Since this is the case in the majority of patients, the aforementioned fact probably does not have any significance. The cardiac index and a left ventricular ejection fraction in a range of 45% and more, did not in any way influence the incidence of complications in patients included in the program. However, since patients with a left ventricular ejection fraction of less than 45% had been excluded from the program, there could well be a correlation between ejection fraction and complication incidence in an unselected total of patients, including patients with severely impaired left ventricular function and a left ventricular ejection fraction of less than 45%.

In contrast, there is a significant correlation between maximum exercise tolerance and complication incidence, and between the amount of drugs taken by the patients and the complication incidence. This means that patients taking two or three different drugs as therapy for cardiac disease are much more likely to be subject to complications during autologous blood donation than patients taking only one drug.

Figure 4 shows the incidence of complications, plotted against the maximal exercise tolerance. It is clear that complications during autologous blood donation requiring therapy are much more likely to occur in patients with a maximal exercise tolerance of less than 75 W, than in patients with a higher exercise tolerance.

From this point of view, the exclusion from the autologous predonation program of patients who had an exercise tolerance of less than 50 W appears to be justified. However the possibility of including patients with an ejection fraction of lower than 45% should be taken into consideration, since the ejection fraction seems to have no influence on the complication rate in our patients, which probably means that the borderline value was not reached at 45%.

After having defined the risk of blood predonation, what are the benefits?

Table 7 shows the amount of homologous packed red cells transfused in the unselected total of our patients in 1988, as compared to the 230 patients who predonated autologous blood. Approximately 46% of the unselected total of our patients

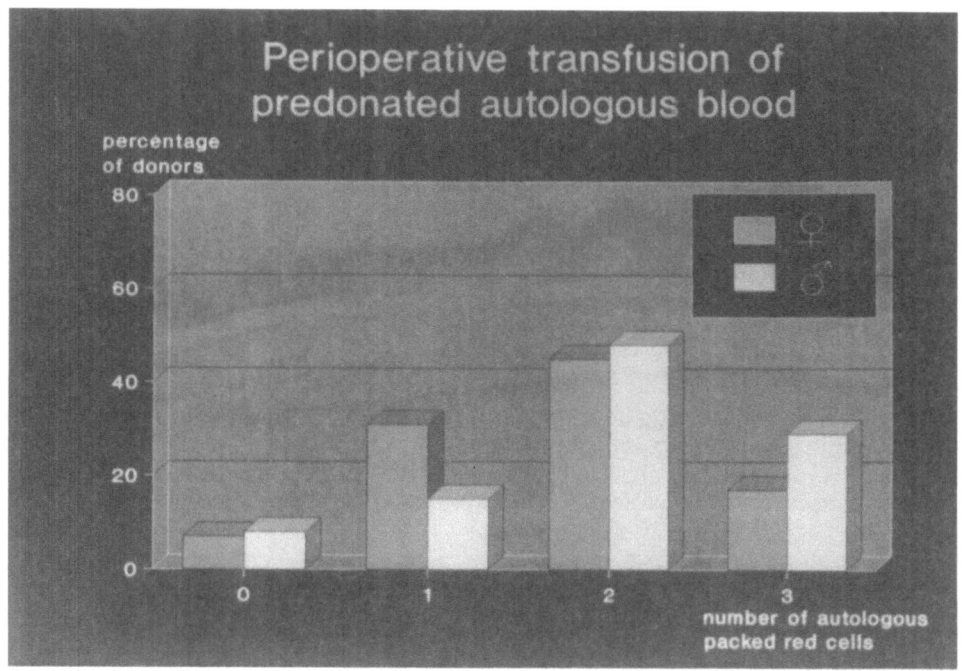

Fig. 4. Percentage of the number of autologous predonated blood units transfused perioperatively in the 230 patients included in the autologous predonation programme.

Table 7. Percentage of heart operations without transfusion of homologous blood, and average amount of units of transfused homologous packed red cells in the unselected total of patients who underwent surgery at the German Heart Institute, Berlin, in 1988 and in 230 patients included in the autologous blood predonation program.

Patients without transfused homologous red cells	69 %	45.6%
Units of transfused homologous red cells	1.05	3.6
	Pat. with autologous predonation	Total unselected Patients

and 69% of patients in our predonation program received no homologous blood. This difference does not seem to be very striking. The point is, however, that the total of unselected patients required transfusion of a mean of 3.6 units packed red cells, whereas the mean unit of packed red cells in patients taking part in the program was only approx. 1.0 units.

Figure 5 shows the amount of autologous blood units transfused perioperatively in patients included in the program. It is clear that less than 10% of patients do not require transfusion of either autologous or of homologous blood. This is probably due to the fact that autologous donors have a reduced red cell volume and a lower hemoglobin value at the beginning of the operation, as compared to the unselected total of patients scheduled for surgery. There could even be the effect four autologous transfusions being considered to be of less risk than homologous transfusions; the majority of patients are administered 2 units of autologous blood.

Conclusions

Firstly, it is clear that the incidence of homologous blood transfusion and the amount of homologous blood transfused in patients undergoing cardiac surgery is considerably reduced by outpatient autologous blood predonation.

Secondly, with the administration of intravenous fluids during the predonation of blood, complications during and immediately after autologous blood predonation requiring therapy were seen in only 2.4% of the donations. The control of ECG and blood-pressure monitoring during the donation is emphasized. In the event of complications, emergency equipment should be present, as well as skilled personnel.

Thirdly, patients with aortic stenosis and patients with a left ventricular ejection fraction of lower than 45% have been excluded from the program; it is not clear whether the exclusion of such patients is justified or not. An ejection fraction in the range of 45% and more does not appear to influence the complication rate. In contrast, complications during and immediately after autologous blood predonation seem to be more likely in patients regularly taking more than two cardiac drugs, and, particularly, in patients with a maximum exercise tolerance of less than 75 W.

References

1. Council on Scientific Affairs (1986) Autologous blood transfusions. JAMA 256: 2378—80
2. Perioperative red blood cell transfusion (1988) JAMA 260: 2700—3
3. Mempel, W. (1988) Autologe Transfusion. Anästh Intensivmed 29: 65—67
4. Riemer, J Höhne M (1988) Eigenblutspende, perioperative Hämodilution und intraoperative Autotransfusion aus der Sicht eines kleineren Krankenhauses. Anästh Intensivmed 29: 72—77
5. Goodnough LT, Rudnick S, Price TH et al. (1989) Increased preoperative Collection of Autologous Blood With Recombinant Human Erythropoietin Therapy. N Engl J Med 321: 1163—8

Author's address:
Prof. Dr. P. Schmucker
Institute of Anaesthesthesiology
Deutsches Herzzentrum Berlin
Augustenburger Platz 1
D-1000 Berlin 65, FRG

Resuscitation Fluids for the Treatment of Hemorrhagic Shock in Dogs: The Effects on Myocardial Blood Flow

A. R. Tait and L. O. Larson

Department of Anesthesiology, University of Michigan Medical Center, Ann Arbor, Michigan, USA

Introduction

The importance of plasma substitutes as an alternative or adjunct to blood has been well recognized for many years. Today, this importance is re-emphasized because of the AIDS epidemic and the increasing number of surgical procedures requiring large replacement volumes of blood.

The efficacy of the plasma substitutes in restoring blood volume following trauma or acute blood loss has been well documented [1—3], however, the hemodilution caused by administration of these fluids results in a decrease in oxygen content and, thus, a potential for reduced oxygen transport [4] particularly to the myocardium. Race et al [5] and Rosburg and Wulf [6] demonstrated a compensatory increase in myocardial pefusion following dextran-induced normovclemic hemodilution. Furthermore, Rosburg and Wulf showed that hypovolemia following hemodilution results in myocardial ischemia in dogs. No studies, however, demonstrating the effect of hemodilution on myocardial blood flow following a period of acute hemorrhage are available. The purpose of this preliminary study, therefore, was to investigate the effects of different plasma subsitites on myocardial blood flow (as measured by the radiolabeled microsphere technique) following hemorrhage in the dog.

Methods

This study was approved by our Institutional Review Board. Forty-one dogs of either sex and weighing between 20—25 kg were anesthetized with pentobarbital (30 mg/kg) and paralyzed with pancuronium (0.1 mg/kg). Following tracheal intubation the lungs were ventilated on oxygen to maintain the $PaCO_2$ between 35—40 mmHg. Arterial pH was adjusted to normal values (7.35—7.40) using 4.2 % sodium bicarbonate. The left femoral vein was cannulated for the administration of intravenous fluids as was the left femoral artery for the direct measurement of arterial pressure and arterial blood sampling. The right femoral artery was cannulated for withdrawal of reference arterial samples during the injection of radioactive microspheres. A pulmonary artery thermodilution catheter was inserted via the right external jugular vein for the measurement of pulmonary artery pressure (PAP), central venous pressure (CVP), capillary wedge pressure (CWP), and cardiac output (CO). Cardiac output was measured in triplicate by the thermodilution technique. Left ventricular pressure was measured using a Millar high fidelity micromanometer which was inserted into the left ventricle via the left carotid artery. Left ventricular pressure was differentiated to continuously measure dP/dt. The right carotid artery was also cannulated with a large-bore polyethylene catheter that was connected to a heparinized

Wigger's reservoir for collection of shed blood. A left-sided thoracotomy was performed and a left atrial catheter was placed for injection of radioactive microspheres. The lungs were re-expanded before closing the chest.

All animals were bled into the heparinized Wigger's reservoir and the height of the reservoir was adjusted to maintain mean arterial pressure (AP) at 35 mmHg for a period of 90 min. Following this period of hemorrhage the animals were reinfused with one of five fluid types, i.e., 1) Gelofusine (modified fluid gelatin); 2) Haemaccel — 35 (modified fluid gelatin); 3) Hespan (Hetastarch), 4) Lactated Ringers solution (LRS); and 5) reinfusion of shed blood. Assignment of animals to a fluid group was by random selection.

Hemodynamic, blood gas/electrolyte, and blood flow measurements were made at the following times: 1) initially, following a 30 min stabilization period (control); 2) following 90 min of controlled hemorrhage (shock, 90 min); 3) resuscitation of the animal to control capillary wedge pressures, and to control respiratory and metabolic parameters (0 min resuscitation); and 4) 90 min following initial resuscitation (90 min resuscitation).

Blood flow measurements

Regional myocardial blood flow was measured by the radiolabeled microsphere technique. Four measurements were taken per animal using one of six available isotopes for each flow determination. Microspheres were 15 μ in diameter and were isotopes for each flow determination. Microspheres were 15 μ in diameter and were 46_{Sc}. The order in which the individual isotopes were used was by random selection for each animal.

Prior to injection the microspheres were sonicated for 30 min and vortexed for 5 min to ensure adequate dispersal. Approximately 1—2 million microspheres were injected into the left atrium per measurement. Reference arterial blood was withdrawn from the femoral artery at a constant rate (7.0 ml/min). Withdrawals were initiated before injection and for a period of 2 min thereafter. At the end of the experiment each dogs was euthanized and the heart removed and placed in formaldehyde prior to sectioning. Radioactivity in the sectioned tissues and reference blood was measured in a gamma counter. Calculation of blood flows were made using a computer formula based on standard equations and correcting for background and overlapping counts. Blood flow was calculated from the equation:

$$Qm = \frac{(Cm \times Qr)}{Cr} \tag{1}$$

where Qm = myocardial blood flow (ml/min), Cm = counts/min in the tissue sample, Qr = withdrawal rate of the reference blood (ml/min), and Cr = counts/min in the reference blood. Intra-group comparisons were made using Paired t test with Bonferroni correction for multiple comparisons. A p-value of < 0.05 was considered significant.

120

Results

Heart rate was unchanged following hemorrhage and subsequent resuscitation in all groups. Capillary wedge pressure and pH dropped significantly following hemorrhage, but were subsequently returned to control values on resuscitation as per the protocol. Mean arterial blood pressure was reduced to 35 mmHg following hemorrhage in all groups. Subsequent resuscitation, however, showed that the mean blood pressures of animals resuscitated with either Gelofusine, Haemaccel or LRS were significantly lower than their corresponding control values, whereas animals treated with Hespan or reinfused blood had their mean pressures returned to near control values. Cardiac output data is shown in Table 1. The use of either Gelofusine, Haemaccel or Hespan following hemorrhage restored the cardiac output to control levels, whereas there was a significant reduction in cardiac output in animals treated with LRS or reinfused blood compared with control values.

Myocardial blood flow in the posterior papillary muscle and the anterior wall of the myocardium are presented in Tables 2 and 3. There was a significant drop in myocardial blood flow following hemorrhage in all groups, however, dogs resusci-

Table 1. Cardiac output (L/min).

	Gelofusine	Haemaccel	Hespan	LRS	Blood
Control	5.22±1.2	5.75±1.0	4.1±0.8	6.28±2.9	4.43±1.3
90-min Shock	1.02±0.3*	1.25±0.3*	0.99±0.3*	1.43±0.6*	0.72±0.2*
0-min Resus.	4.42±1.7	5.87±2.1	4.92±1.6	3.53±1.8*	3.74±1.6*
90-min Resus.	3.91±1.8	5.70±1.6	4.25±1.7	2.53±1.1	1.99±1.1**

Values mean ± S.D.; * $p < 0.05$ vs control; ** $p < 0.05$ vs 0 min resuscitation

Table 2. Posterior papillary muscle blood flow (ml/g/min).

	Gelofusine	Haemaccel	Hespan	LRS	Blood
Control	2.63±1.50	2.11±1.10	2.37±1.2	2.57±1.36	2.44±0.91
90-min Shock	0.59±0.25*	0.72±0.25*	0.78±0.27*	1.18±0.18*	0.85±0.49*
0-min Resus.	3.85±1.82	4.77±3.1	4.31±2.65	2.75±1.95	1.94±0.72
90-min Resus.	3.24±1.96	3.37±1.12	4.0±2.41	1.94±1.08	1.24±0.61

Values mean ± S.D.; * $p < 0.05$ vs control

Table 3. Anterior wall myocardial blood flow (ml/g/min).

	Gelofusine	Haemaccel	Hespan	LRS	Blood
Control	2.01±1.18	1.67±0.65	1.99±0.98	2.21±1.03	2.11±0.36
90-min Shock	0.63±0.24*	0.58±0.16*	0.67±0.22*	1.0 ±0.64*	0.73±0.49*
0-min Resus.	3.35±1.99*	4.02±2.34	3.91±2.48	2.05±1.39	1.51±0.42
90-min Resus.	3.24±1.99	2.46±0.32	3.90±2.68	1.55±0.94	1.48±0.69

Values mean ± S.D.; * $p < 0.05$ vs control

Table 4. Hematocrit (%).

	Gelofusine	Haemaccel	Hespan	LRS	Blood
Control	36.9	31.8	34.6	32.9	32.3
90-min Shock	40.3	36.5	37.3	35.6	34.3
0-min Resus.	21.2	18.2	17.5	22.5	34.1
90-min Resus.	15.0	13.3	13.4	18.0	32.4

Table 5. Myocardial oxygen Transport (ml/min/g).

	Gelofusine	Haemaccel	Hespan	LRS	Blood
Control	0.48	0.34	0.37	0.40	0.37
90-min Shock	0.11*	0.12*	0.13*	0.19*	0.13*
0-min Resus.	0.36	0.37	0.35	0.25*	0.31
90-min Resus.	0.24	0.23	0.26	0.19	0.19

* $p < 0.05$ vs control

tated with Gelofusine, Haemaccel or Hespan demonstrated an increased flow above that of their respective control values. On the other hand, dogs resuscitated with LRS or blood demonstrated flows that returned to levels at or slightly below control. At 90 min following resuscitation the flow in the colloid groups had decreased slightly, however, they were still maintained at above control levels. Interestingly enough, a similar blood flow pattern was observed in the kidneys.

The effect of hemodilution by the different fluid groups is shown by the hematocrit values in Table 4. All groups showed a significant degree of hemodilution except for the bloot group. Since there was a significant degree of hemodilution and alteration in the flow following resuscitation with the various fluid groups it was deemed important to determine the degree of oxygen delivery to the myocardium for each of the treatment groups. Myocardial oxygen transport values are described in Table 5.

It can be seen that myocardial oxygen delivery following resuscitation with Gelofusine, Haemaccel or Hespan was returned to control values and that the apparent hyperemia seen in these groups following resuscitation appears to have been in response to the decreased oxygen carrying capacity brought on by the marked hemodilution. Dogs treated with reinfused shed blood showed adequate oxygen transport to the myocardium. Since there was little diminution of oxygen-carrying capacity in this group there was no necessity for compensatory hyperemia.

Animals treated with LRS, however showed no hyperemia in response to the hemodilution and, consequently, myocardial oxygen transport was significantly decreased from control values upon resuscitation with this fluid.

Discussion and conclusion

This data suggests that the artificial colloids Gelofusine, Haemaccel, and Hespan compensate for the reduced oxygen-carrying capacity that their hemodilution causes by increasing perfusion to the myocardium and thus maintaining adequate oxygen delivery to the heart. This compares favorably with the oxygen delivery of reinfused blood. Lactated Ringers solution, however, did not increase perfusion in response to hemodilution, resulting in a decrease in oxygen supply to the myocardium. Although we did not measure oxygen uptake in these experiments (but will in future studies), these results, although preliminary, suggest an interesting difference between colloids and crystalloids with respect to the restoration of myocardial blood flow following hemorrhage.

References

1. Moss GS, Lowe RJ, Jilek J and Levine HD (1981) Colloid or crystalloid in the resuscitation of hemorrhagic shock, a controlled clinical trial. Surgery 89: 434
2. Poole GV, Meredith JW, Pennell T, and Mills SA (1982) Comparison of colloids and crystalloids in resuscitation from hemorrhagic shock. Surg Gynecol and Obstet 154: 577—586
3. Mishler JM (1984) Synthetic plasma volume expanders — Their pharmacology, safety and clinical efficacy. Clin in Haematol 13: 75—92
4. Gisselsson L, Rosberg B and Ericsson M (1982) Myocardial blood flow, oxygen uptake and carbon dioxide release of the human heart during hemodilution. Acta Anaesth Scand 26: 589—591
5. Race D, Dedichsen H and Schenk W (1967) Regional blood flow during dextran-induced normovolemic hemodilution in the dog. J Thorac Cardiovasc Surg 53: 578
6. Rosburg B and Wulff K (1979) Regional blood flow in normovolemic and hypovolemic hemodilution. Brit J Anaesth 51: 423

Authors' address:
Alan R. Tait, Ph. D.
Department of Anesthesiology
University of Michigan Medical Center
1500 E. Medical Center Drive
Ann Arbor, Michigan 48109 USA

Reduction of Blood Use in Cardiac Surgery by Topical Hemostasis Using Fibrin Sealant

A. Haverich

Hannover Medical School, Division of Thoracic and Cardiovascular Surgery, Hannover, FRG

Introduction

Fibrin sealant has been used in cardiovascular surgery in Europe for more than 10 years [1—5]. By mimicking the natural pathway of fibrin production, it allows for topical bleeding control [6—8] and for presealing of vascular prostheses [9—18]. When needed under extracorporeal circulation, the method has been found to be especially helpful in redo-operations and emergency resternotomies, as illustrated by a recent multicenter trial in the United States [20].

Material and methods

Fibrin adhesive consists of commercially available concentrated frozen cryoprecipitated or lyophilized fibrinogen of human origin that is prepared for use by either warming or dilution, respectively. The material is activated by thrombin (500 NIH units/ml), calcium chloride (40 mmol/l), and the antifibrinolytic agent aprotinin (3000 KIU/ml) [19]. The mode of action, transferring the fibrinogen into insoluable fibrin plus inhibiting fibrinolysis by aprotinin is depicted in Fig. 1. Using the fibrin adhesive as a hemostatic agent, only a small amount of fibrinogen is applied to a piece of collagen fleece or sponge; the thrombin solution is dripped onto the material, which is pressed onto the bleeding site for approximately 1 min. Alternatively, components can be sprayed onto oozing surfaces for control of bleeding. For sealing vascular prostheses, the fibrinogen is smeared onto the surface of the stretched fabric and, subsequently, the thrombin solution is massaged into the graft.

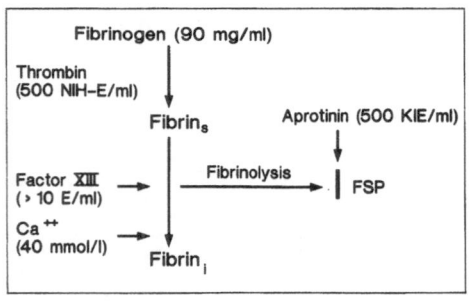

Fig. 1. Mode of action when using fibrin sealant for bleeding control (see text for further explanation).

Results

In our patient group we used presealed woven grafts, double Velour knitted grafts, and plain knitted grafts. The average amount of fibrinogen used for bleeding control was 0.8 ml (range 0.5—4 ml). Presealing prosthetic fabric required a mean of 1.3 ml (range 0.5 ml—6 ml) of adhesive.

Fibrin glue has been used in a total of 380 bleedings in the high-pressure system. There were only 13 failures (3.4%). The adhesive was used for arterial bleedings from aortic canulation sides, aortotomies, and coronary bypass anastomoses (Table 1).

In the low-pressure system, the adhesive was used in 376 cases and failed in only 1.9% of the applications (Table 2). Fibrin gluing appeared especially helpful in pediatric cardiac surgery for sealing suture lines in the atria, the caval veins, the right ventricle and pulmonary artery, including puncture hole bleeding from PTFE patches. In addition, the adhesive was effective in every case of diffuse epimyocardial bleeding resulting from separation of pericardial adhesions and in venous hemorrhages occurring at the sites of exposure of the coronary arteries.

Low-porosity, woven Dacron-grafts were presealed with fibrin glue and implanted in 99 patients under full heparinization and extracorporeal circulation. There was no incidence of early or late bleeding from the prosthetic fabric (Table 3). High-porosity knitted prostheses were used in 39 patients (Table 4) undergoing extracorporeal circulation. Except for two cases the sealing was successful. One of the failures was caused by delayed leakage occurring in the only non-Velour graft implanted.

Table 1. Bleeding control in the high-pressure system.

	Number of patients	Number of failures
Aorta	211	10
CAB proximal	65	2
CAB	93	1
IV	11	—
Total	380	13 (3.4%)

Table 2. Bleeding control in the low-pressure system.

	Number of patients	Number of failures
IVC, SVC, atrium	105	1
Coronary veins	39	—
RA, PA	27	3
RV patch (PTFE)	22	3
Epi-/myocardial	90	—
Fixation of CABG	93	—
Total	376	7 (1.9%)

Knitted prostheses (204) were implanted for descending aortic replacement, thoracoabdominal or infrarenal aortic replacement. Partial intravenous heparinization was used in all cases. Out of these, six grafts, which were primarily sealed with fibrin glue, showed transprosthetic blood loss (Table 5). In all these cases, severe hypovolemic shock symptoms due to ruptured aneurysms had preceded graft implantation.

Table 3. Results of fibrin presealing of woven grafts during ECC.

	Number of patients	Number of failures
Aortic arch	11	—
Ascending aorta	63	—
RV-PA conduit	11	—
RV patch	14	—
Total	99	—

Table 4. Results of fibrin presealing of knitted grafts during ECC.

	Number of patients	Number of failures
Ascending aorta	14	1*
RV-PA conduit	6	1
RV patch	14	—
LV patch	5	1
Total	39	2 (5.1%)

* delayed leackage occurred in the only non-velour graft

Table 5. Results of fibrin presealing of knitted grafts (with heparin).

	Number of patients	Number of failures
Descending aorta	42	1
Thoracoabdominal aorta	20	—
Ruptured	5	2
Infrarenal aorta	105	1
Ruptured	32	2
Total	204	6 (2.9%)

126

Discussion

Hemostatic gluing has been an interesting alternative to suturing ever since the introduction of synthetic tissue glues. Although most bleeding complications in cardiovascular operations can be controlled by conventional methods, such trials often result in continuing hemorrhage and circulatory depression. However, adhesives have been of little value in cardiovascular operations until now, because of their dependence on absolutely dry surfaces. In contrast to synthetic adhesives, fibrin glue, using a biological system, represents a reliable alternative for solving these problems. Optimal concentrations of the components of the glue have been studied in detail, as has the addition of substance to inhibit fibrinolytic activity [19]. Fibrin gluing is now employed routinely whenever suturing is impossible, difficult or dangerous. However, it may also be used to save waiting time for spontaneous hemostasis [3, 6].

The method is most effective for control of oozing, but it should also not be overextended in situations where brisk arterial bleeding sites are reserved for surgical closure. Fibrin glue has been applied in prophylactic sealing of suture lines and of puncture holes in PTFE patches. In addition, aortocoronary bypass grafts may be fixed on the cardiac surfaces to prevent any kinking of the graft (Table 2) [16]. The use of fibrin adhesive and presealing vascular prosthetic fabric appeared logical in view of the fact that even tightly woven material remained mandatory in the presence of full heparinization and extracorporeal circulation [17, 18]. Fibrin presealing, therefore, is now the preferred method for sealing woven prostheses and has also reduced the blood loss in complex cardiovascular proceduring involving insertion of prosthetic material. Fibrin sealing of knitted grafts has resulted in superior healing characteristics of the prostheses. This has been proven histologically in animal studies in which woven and knitted tubes have been inserted [9, 11].

Recently, a very important study on the efficacy of fibrin sealant for bleeding control in open-heart surgery has been published [20]. In a multicenter study involving eight US-centers enrolled for FDA approval of this agent in the USA, a randomized investigation comparing fibrin sealant with conventional agents for topical hemostasis (oxy cellulose, gelatine, and topical application of thrombin alone) was performed. This study was limited to reoperative cardiac surgery and emergency resternotomy. Under the adverse conditions in this patient population, significantly higher success rates were obtained with respect to bleeding control when using fibrin adhesive (92.6%) compared to conventional therapy (12.4%; $p < 0.005$). Moreover, application of fibrin glue following failure of conventional methods of topical hemostasis resulted in a cross-over success rate of 82% following subsequent use of fibrin sealant. Interestingly, significant improvement of postoperative blood loss and resternotomy rates were reported for the first time in a study designed in a randomized fashion ($p < 0.05$). These data [20] confirm earlier results from European studies that proved fibrin sealant to be effective with respect to reduction of perioperative blood loss in cardiac procedures irrespective of other blood-saving methods used in open-heart surgery.

In conclusion, 10 years after its introduction, fibrin sealant remains a useful tool of topical bleeding control under adverse conditions of extracorporeal circulation and full heparinization. Its use reduces postoperative blood loss and the rate of resternotomies. In conjuction with autotransfusion and antifibrinolytic treatment, use of donor blood in cardiac surgery can be restricted to a very limited number of patients.

References

1. Spängler HP, Holle H, Braun F (1973) Gewebeklebung mit Fibrin. Wr Klin Wschr 85: 827—829
2. Haverich A, Maatz W, Walterbusch G (1982) Evaluation of fibrin seal in animal experiments. Thorac Cardiovasc Surg 30: 215
3. Borst HG, Haverich A, Walterbusch G, Maatz W (1982) Fibrin adhesive: an important hemostatic adjunct in cardiovascular operations. J Thorac Cardiovasc Surg 84: 548
4. Wahlers Th, Haverich A, Borst HG (1986) Die Fibrinklebung und der Fibrinantibiotikumverbund in der Herz- und Gefäßchirurgie in: Neue Techniken in der operativen Medizin. Aachen, Springer-Verlag 79—82
5. Spängler HP (1976) Gewebeklebung und lokale Blutstillung mit Fibronogen, Thrombin und Blutgerinnungsfaktor XIII. Wien Klin Wochenschr 88/49: 1—13
6. Borst HG, Haverich A (1982) Fibrin seal in cardiovascular surgery. Proceedings of a workshop. Thorac Cardiovasc Surg 30: 195—224
7. Köveker G, de Vivie ER, Hellberg KD (1981) Clinical experience with fibrin glue in cardiac surgery. Thorac Cardiovasc Surg 29: 287—289
8. Huth C, Seyboldt-Epting W, Hoffmeister HE (1982) Local hemostasis with fibrin glue (Tissucol) after intracardiac repair of tetralogy of Fallot and transposition of the great arteries (TGA) Thorac Cardiovasc Surg 30/I: 30
9. Haverich A, Walterbusch G, Borst HG (1981) The use of fibrin glue for sealing vascular prostheses of high porosity. Thorac Cardiovasc Surg 29: 252
10. Haverich A, Walterbusch G, Borst HG (1983) Abdichtung poröser Gefäßprothesen unter Teil-Heparinisierung und extrakorporaler Zirkulation. Angio 5: 215—220
11. Walterbusch G, Saathoff M, Haverich AM, Mlasowsky B (1983) Die Abdichtung poröser Gefäßprothesen — Eine Gelegenheit zur lokalen Antibiotikaapplikation? Angio 5: 239—244
12. Lange U, Jenkner J (1983) Erfahrungen bei der Verwendung von Humanfibrinkleber zur Abdichtung von Gefäßprothesen. Angio 5: 221—223
13. Akrami R, Kalmar P, Pokar H, Tilsner V (1978) Abdichtung von Kunststoffprothesen beim Ersatz der Aorta im thorakalen Bereich. Thoraxchirurgie 26: 144—147
14. Ben Sanchar G, Nicoloff DM, Edwards JE Separation of neointima from Dacron graft causing obstruction. J Thorac Cardiovasc Surg 82: 268
15. Guilmet D, Bachet J, Goudot B, Laurian C, Gigou F, Bical O, Barbagelatta M (1979) The use of biological glue in acute aortic dissection. A new surgical technique: Preliminary clinical results. J Thorac Cardiovasc Surg 77: 516—521
16. Stenzl W, Tscheliessnigg KH, Dacar D, Iberer F, Rigler B (1986) The use of fibrin sealant in cardiac surgery. In: Schlag G, Redl H (eds): Fibrin sealant in operative medicine, 5: 181—184
17. Cooley DA, Romagnoli A, Ailam DJ, Bossart AI (1981) A method of preparing woven Dacron aortic grafts to prevent interstitial hemorrhage. Cardiovasc Diseases Bull Texas Heart Inst 8: 48—52
18. Bethea MC, Reemtsma K (1979) Graft hemostasis. An alternative to preclotting. Ann Thorac Surg 27: 374
19. Redl H, Schlag G, Dinges HR, Kuderna H, Seelich T (1982) Background and methods of fibrin sealing biomaterial. In: Winter GD, Gibbons DF, Plenk H (eds.). Chichester, John Wiley & Sons Ltd. 669—676
20. Rousou J, Levitsky S, Gonzalez-Lavin L, Cosgrove D, et al. (1989) Randomized clinical trial of fibrin sealant in patients undergoing resternotomy or reoperation after cardiac operations. J Thorac Cardiovasc Surg 97: 194—203

Author's address:
PD Dr. A. Haverich
Hannover Medical School
Division of Thoracic and Cardiovascular Surgery
Konstanty-Gutschow-Str. 8
3000 Hannover 61, FRG

Retransfusion of Postoperative Drainage Blood

J. von der Emde, F. O. Mahmoud and H. D. Esperer

Chirurgische Klinik mit Poliklinik der Universität Erlangen-Nürnberg, FRG

Introduction

Blood loss and infections were a major problem in all surgical procedures from ancient times up to the early 1950s [1]. Delicate surgical hemostasis was the only tool to prevent a bleeding catastrophe as neither homologous nor autologous blood transfusion was possible. There were many unsuccessfull attempts to overcome the problem of blood loss, but firstly, it was technically difficult to transfuse from one to another and secondly, there was the unknown problem of incompatibility.

It is quite astonishing that blood transfusions were carried out between 1666 and 1775 (Landois) in 347 humans and 129 animals, half of the first group and one-third of the animal group being reported to be successful.

In 1818, Blundell intraoperatively transfused autologous blood for the first time. As he was a gynecologist, he used blood extravasated during delivery for transfusion into a vein. He also used homologous blood from one individual to another in a patient suffering from carcinoma. This was done without knowledge of blood groups, as these were not discovered by Landsteiner until 1901.

One hundred years later, Elmendorf (1917) postoperatively transfused blood from the hemothorax, and Robertson was the first to use a unit of citrated blood.

Early progress was accomplished by the Russians, who founded the first institute of blood transfusion in 1926. Shamow started to use cadaver blood, and this method is still in use in the USSR. The Mayo clinic established the first blood bank in 1936, and it is quite astonishing that the German, Austrian and Swiss Surgical Society recommended blood transfusion only between two individuals.

There was an increasing need to transfuse large amounts of homologous blood in the USA. Four million liters of blood were used in the early 1950s during the Korean Conflict. At the same time the problem of serum hepatitis emerged as a serious major problem.

With the advent of cardiac surgery under extracorporeal circulation there arose an increasing need for an enormous amount of banked blood.

In the Mayo-Gibbon heart-lung machine we used at least 6 liters of blood in every operation in the early 1960s although Cooley favored the hemodilution technique at that time. It was Buckley, however, who did the scientific work on hemodilution techniques published in 1972.

George Noon was the first to publish a simple method of intraoperative auto-transfusion in 1976, but it was Cooley who collected blood from the heart-lung machine and its tubing, and retransfused it.

Finally, Schaff, and at the same time our group in Erlangen used the technique of autotransfusion in the early and late postoperative periods.

Once we had become aware of the drawbacks of bank blood transfusion and become very keen on saving blood, we were able to reduce our blood requirements to 0.3 units per patient in 1980.

Then we were greatly suprised to find that during the following years our blood requirement again increased and has risen to one unit per patient at the present time. We have examined our data to see what the reasons for this increase are.

First of all, I would like to introduce our retransfusion system, which we have been using with minor changes since 1977.

All the drainage blood from the substernal tube and from both pleural spaces, if they are opened during the procedure, is collected in the reservoir already used during extracorporeal circulation. The blood is collected without adding heparin.

Retransfusion is carried out in the following way: after 200 ml of blood has accumulated in the reservoir the blood is intermittently retransfused into a central venous line passing a filter of 40.

For the st 3 years we have been using a special infusion pump, which is no longer driven by a finger or roller pump but a piston-like system. The syringe takes 10 ml out of the reservoir and sends the blood back into the circulation, past a bubble trap.

This console (Fig. 1) is designed so that we can adjust it to a fixed rate per hour (ml/h), and at the same time we are able to set the scale to the amount of blood loss we expect during the next hours. Finally, we have a digital read-out of what was actually transfused during the postoperative period until the reservoir was empty. It is possible to estimate the ml/h, the expected amount of drainage blood per hour. Blood should be retransfused at a slow rate to preclude hemolysis and to prevent air entering into the tubing. If this happens, the air has to be eliminated or the whole tubing system has to be replaced.

If there is only some blood left after 12 h we still collect the blood and suck the remaining blood from all the tubing into a bag in order to transfuse it directly or, if there is too much hemolysis, we prefer to give back only centrifuged erythrocytes.

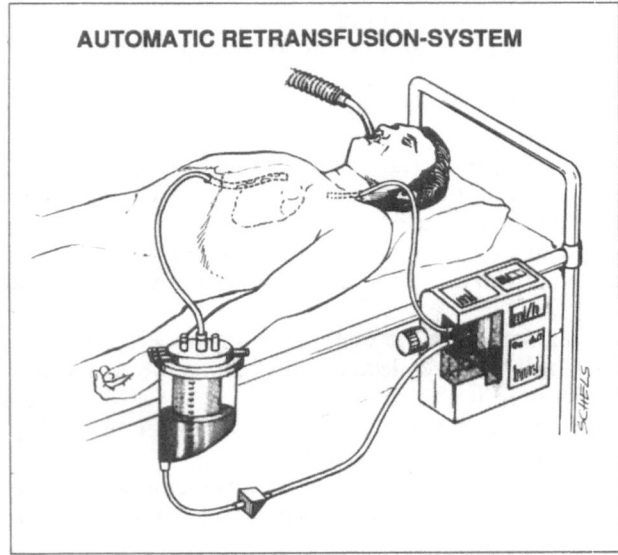

AUTOMATIC RETRANSFUSION-SYSTEM

Fig. 1. Retransfusion system adjustable pump: 1) ml per hour; 2) ml total amount of retransfused blood.

We retransfuse for about 12 h but we have quite liberally done this for 24 h, and observed in this group reactions such as a rise in temperature or even "goose bumps".

The usal amount of drainage blood is between 400 and 600 ml. Just after surgery, hematocrit is about 12—15 % and drops during the first 15 h to 15 % or 4 %. We also transfuse pleural effusion because we think there is a world-wide need to save as much protein as possible.

To present our results, we collected all our data concerning retransfusion during the last 6 months and were especially looking for reasons why our bank blood requirement had increased.

Comparing the data from 1980 with those of the patients from 1989, it was obvious that the latter belonged to a higher age group. 10 % were above 17 years, the average age being 60 years. In women, the bank blood requirement was higher for various reasons. 4 % of our patients suffered from renal insuffiency with a creatine value above 5 mg %, and 2 % of patients were on hemodialysis.

Bypass time has increased because of the increasing number of coronary anastomoses and the use of the internal mammary artery, which requires a higher rate. Total bypass time has increased from 53 to 81 min and ischemic time from 23 to 36 min. 5.6 % of our patients were operated on an emergency basis and were carried from catheter-lab directly into the operating room; they were on catecholamines and nearly 10 % of the patients were having a second operation.

In the transfusion group there were three times as many women, more diabetic people, and significantly more second and emergency cases, and many more renal failures and rethoracotomies. It is not very encouraging and we are not very happy about the fact that only a small amount of drainage blood was retransfused; in primary operations it was only 47 % and in secondary operations 51 %. There was a significant reduction in drainage blood by administering applying aprotinin.

In another combination of our data, 1 unit of blood was given in primary operations and 3.1 in secondary, but if aprotinin was administered perioperatively only 1.7 units had to be given.

The data presented here are all but optimal concerning reduction of bank blood, although the equipment demonstrated might optimise the reduction of bank blood. In addition, in our hospital it was not possible for logistic reasons for our patients to pre-donate blood.

What are our recommendations in spite of this? Surgical hemostasis is the most important factor beside pre-, intra- and postoperative autologous blood collection. Therefore, meticulous retransfusion postoperatively and hemodilution under extracorporeal circulation with hematocrit values between 20 und 25 %, depending on the patient's condition, are helpful. Controlled hypotension and hypothermia will reduce mechanical blood trauma due to pump revolutions.

The use of aprotinin leads to a sginificant reduction of bleeding.

We do not use the cell-saver as do other centers, especially after long bypass times with significant hemolysis. Normalizing physiological coagulation is mandatory.

It is unlikely that artificial blood will reduce bank blood requirements in the near future.

Although we cannot measure it, we would estimate the quantity of unretransfusable blood to be around 1 liter per operation: 1) 300 ml — wall suction; 2) 200 ml — blood absorbed into the swabs; 3) 500 ml blood remaining in all tubing from chest and wound; 4) 100 ml remaining in the tissue forming a hematoma; 5) 200 ml sequestration due to ECC trauma to the erythrocytes which can best be calculated from the degree of hematocrit during the first postoperative days.

In spite of our less than optimal results, we think retransfusion is a good method of reducing bank blood requirements. All efforts should be mode to reserve homologous blood transfusion by the use of predonated blood; in special cases the use a cell — saver for autologous blood retransfusion — and, hopefully, there will be more wide-spread use of pharmacological hemostasis after surgery as we found by the use of aprotinin. Only for special cases will fibrin sealing be useful. Furthermore, it seems worthwhile to use our system of shed blood retransfusion, because blood lost in major bleeding after surgery can be retransfused and rethoracotomy can be postponed until the patient has been rewarmed and coagulation factors have been controlled and substituted; therefore, in some cases a rethoracotomy can even be avoided.

Reference

1. Paravicini D (1986) Intraoperative autotransfusion. Anaesthesiology and Intensive Care Medicine 183: 1—18

Author's address:
Professor Dr. J. von der Emde
Herzchirurgische Abteilung
Chirurgische Universitätsklinik
Maximiliansplatz 1
8520 Erlangen, FRG

Bacteriological Methods to Monitor the Quality of Intraoperative Autotransfusion

H. Ezzedine and P. Baele

Catholic University of Louvain, Saint-Luc Hospital, Brussels, Belgium

Introduction

Intra- and post-operative blood salvage techniques have gained wide acceptance during the last decade [5—7]. The benefits of reduced viral exposure and its long-term immunological advantages are so obvious that the practice developed without reference to specific quality-control standards. In particular, no standard evolved to assess the bacteriological quality of retransfused blood [1, 9]. This paper provides a clinical and experimental comparison of two bacteriological techniques used to monitor the quality of intraoperative retrieved blood.

Material and methods

Patients

Three-hundred-twenty-nine patients undergoing cardiac surgery were included in this study. Patient characteristics are summarized in Table 1.

Table 1. Clinical study: characteristics and number of surgical procedures performed.

Type of surgery	n	Mean duration of surgery (min)	Mean duration of extracorporeal circulation (min)	Quantity of retransfused erythrocytes: (grams) mean and range	Age
Coronary surgery	256	360	169	588 (0—1960)	63 (28—81)
Single valve replacement	27	249	112	525 (240—1020)	64 (8—83)
Complex repair	46	362	181	685 (0—1680)	60 (5—77)
All	329	351	166	597	62 (5—83)

133

Intraoperative blood salvage

The Sorensen Auto Transfusion System (ATS Receptal, Sorensen Research, Salt Lake City, Utah, USA) was used to collect shed blood in the operating room. The anticoagulant solution used was ACD (citric acid trisodium citrate-dextrose). Two grams of cefazolin were added per liter of ACD. Collected blood was brought to a central facility to be centrifuged and washed, using an automated cell processor (IBM-COBE 2991, Lakewood, California, USA). Plasma, leucocytes, platelets, red cell debris, anticoagulant, washing solution, and other drugs were discarded in the process. Centrifugation and washing took 20 min and packed red cells with a hematocrit of 68% were reinfused within 6 h of the start of collection. For all patients antibiotic prophylaxis consisted of 2 g of Cefazolin given iv at induction of anesthesia and subsequently, every 6 h during 48 h [8].

No specific schedule was defined for postoperative bacteriological sampling, the decision for blood cultures or other investigations being left to the attending physicians. Bacteriological data of the patients were followed for at least 3 months after the procedure.

Bacteriological methods

Two methods were compared in this study: a quantitative spread-plate technique and a conventional radiometric blood-culture technique. Autotransfused blood samples were drawn in a sterile fashion from the reinfusion bag just prior to retransfusion to the patients and were immediately processed by the laboratory or kept overnight at 4 °C in case of late surgery. For the quantitative spread-plate technique a total volume of 1 ml of red cells was examined. Aliquots of 0.2 ml were spread on five blood agar plates (10% horse blood) using bent glass rods. Inoculated plates were incubated at 37 °C for 24 to 48 h after which colonies were counted. Results are expressed as the number of colony forming units per ml (CFU/ml).

The radiometric method was performed using Bactec bottles (Becton Dickinson Diagnostic Instrument Systems, Towson, Maryland, USA). Five mls of red cells were injected into the bottles, which were incubated at 37 °C and checked daily for 1 week. Subculture took place whenever bacterial growth was suspected. A threshold of > 30 for the growth index was retained. Vials were also subcultured if a change of > 10 occurred between two consecutive readings.

Experimental control study

In order to evaluate the possibility of growth for small inocula in Bactec bottles, control experimental tests were performed, using a suspension containing a known number of *coagulase negative Staphylococci*. This microorganism was a hospital strain characterized by hemolytic activity on blood agar which distinguished it from accidental contamination. Ten-fold dilutions in the range 10^{-1} to 10^{-8} were prepared from a suspension containing approximately 10^6 CFU/ml. From the last four dilutions, 5 ml were inoculated into a Bactec vial and a total volume of 1 ml spread on five blood agar plates. Sixty-eight tests were thus performed under the same conditions as those mentioned above for blood cultures.

134

Results

Autotransfused blood

The spread-plate technique: Table 2 shows the distribution of positive cultures obtained with this technique. Most colonies could be detected after 24 h of incubation. Thirty-four cultures were positive (10.3%), yielding 1–7 CFU/ml. In the only case with 7 CFU/ml two types of *coagulase negative Staphylococci* were distinguished by antibiotic profile. Table 3 details the positive results obtained with the radiometric technique. Seventeen (5.1%) tests were positive; *coagulase negative Staphylococci* were found in eight cases, *Diphteroids* in six, *Micrococcus* in two, and *Candida albicans* in the last one. Discrepancies (Table 3 and 4) between the two methods were found in 27 tests: the direct plating method was positive in 22 cases, yielding mainly *coagulase negative Staphylococci* (mostly, 1–2 CFU/ml) while Bactec bottles remained negative. Other isolates included *Micrococus* (3 CFU/ml), *Diphteroides sp.* (1 test, 1 CFU/ml). However, five tests were positive by the radiometric technique alone: *Diphteroids* grew in two of them and *Micrococcus, coagulase negative Staphylococcus,* and *Candida albicans* were each found once. Two tests positive by both methods showed discrepancies regarding the type of bacteria: *coagulase negative Staphylococcus* were isolated on Agar plates, while Bactec bottles grew *Diphteroids*.

Postoperative outcome

Two-hundred-one patients had at least one postoperative blood culture. Sixteen (8%) were positive, but the corresponding samples of autotransfused blood remained negative with both methods used. *Coagulase negative Staphylococcus* was isolated in six postoperative blood cultures. However, these were considered as mere contaminants since they were found only once in each case. Gram negative bacilli were involved in bacteremias in eight instances (mainly *E. coli* or *Enterobacter cloacae*).

Table 2. Type and number of microorganisms (CFU/ml) recovered from autotransfused blood by the spreadplate technique (N = 329 patients).

Bacteria	CFU/ml				Total
	1	2	3	7	
Coagulase negative Staphylococci	17	7	1	1	26
Micrococcus sp.	4				4
Diphteroids	3				3
Acinetobacter lwoffii	1				1
Total	25	7	1	1	34

135

Table 3. Positive cultures by the radiometric method and corresponding findings using the agar-plate method.

Bactec		AGAR	
Number of tests	Bacteria	Number of tests	Bacteria
8	ST AL	7	ST AL
		1	negative
6	DI SP	2	DI SP
		2	ST AL
		2	negative
2	MI SP	1	MI SP
		1	negative
1	CA AL	1	negative

Abbreviations: ST AL = coagulase negative Staphylococci
DI SP = Diphteroïds sp.
MI SP = Micrococcus sp.
CA AL = Candida albicans

Table 4. Comparison of results of autotransfused blood cultures by both methods (N = 329 patients).

		Agar		Total
		+	—	
B A C T E C	+	12	5	17
	—	22	290	312
Total		34	295	329

Table 5. Control tests comparing growth of a selected coagulase negative staphyloccus in Bactec bottles (at 24 h and 72 h incubation) and on agar plates.

Number of tests (N = 68)	CFU/ml on agar plates	Radiometric results: Number of tests			
		24 h		72 h	
		+	—	+	—
8	5—8	6	2	8	0
6	3—4	3	3	6	0
26	1—2	6	20	18	8
28	0	0	28	1	27

136

One patient has *Pseudomonas Fluorescens* septicaemia secondary to *homologous* blood transfusion with a culture of the incriminated blood bank unit disclosing the same microorganism.

Eight patients had bacteriologically documented wound, sternum, or mediastinal infection. In one patient, cultures of mediastinal pus remained negative.

No endocarditis was found in this study.

In only one patient did cultures reveal the same microorganism intra- and post-operatively. This 67-year-old male underwent an extensive myocardial revascularization using bilateral mammary artery grafts and a carotid endarterectomy. A severe anaplylactoid reaction complicated the course of the procedure, which lasted 7 h. Autotransfused blood cultures yielded *Candida albicans* by the radiometric method alone. Early graft obstruction required reintervention. The next day the patient was found to be heavily colonized with *Enterobacter cloacae* in his upper respiratory tract and saphenous wound. On day 10, cardiac tamponade prompted a third intervention. In the following days, sternal dehiscence lead to two more operations during which *Candida albicans* was found subcutaneously in the sternum, the mediastinum, and in the wound drainage. The patient was discharged after 3 months of a very difficult recovery.

Experimental tests comparing both systems

Fourteen out of 68 tests showed 3 or more CFU/ml on agar plates after 24 h of incubation. In only nine of these was bacterial growth detected by the radiometric method at the same time (Table 5). Seventy-two-h incubation time was required for radiometric detection of all 14 cases. When a smaller number of test microorganisms (1—2 CFU/ml) were present on agar plates, only 23% of 26 tests detected bacterial growth at 24 h of incubation in Bactec bottles. Furthermore, this latter method failed to detect eight positive tests, despite a prolonged incubation time (> 72 h).

Discussion

This bacteriological survey revealed that only a small fraction of intraoperative blood reinfusates was contaminated. Furthermore, the concentration of microorganisms as determined by the spread-plate technique was low. This confirms the prevailing clinical experience, i.e., that intraoperative autotransfusion of centrifuged and washed retrieved blood carries a minimal bacteriological risk in clean-field surgery, such as cardiac surgery [1, 2, 4, 5].

In only one case did the same microorganism grow both in autotransfused blood and postoperatively in the mediastinum. This patient had undergone a prolonged operation while in a precarious hemodynamic state. The positive Bactec culture indicates that the surgical field was most probably contaminated during the first surgery. The fact that the agar method did not disclose *Candida albicans* may be explained by a too short incubation period in the presence of a small inoculum. Agar plates were incubated for 48 h only, while Bactec bottles were observed for 7 days. Agar plates are now left to incubate 7 days before being discarded.

In both clinical and experimental control studies, positive results were less frequent with the radiometric methods as compared to the plating technique. This is rather surprising because a large volume of blood (5 ml) was inoculated to Bactec bottles, whereas only 1 ml was cultured on agar. This discrepancy may be attributed to a less favorable culture environment. The experimental control tests comparing the two methods showed a slower growth rate and, in some cases, no growth at all with the radiometric technique, especially when small inocula were used. In addition, the radiometric technique requires subcultures to identify detected microorganisms. This adds another delay when compared to the direct-plate count.

In view of these results and since the challenge is to improve the sensitivity of the culture technique in order to detect all viable bacteria present at the time of reinfusing the blood, the spread-plate count seems particularly appealing. The clinical series confirmed the well known pathological importance of *coagulase negative Staphylococcus* [3, 4], and the experimental study showed the high yield of the agar-plate technique in comparison to the radiometric method for this particular microorganism.

Since infection is greatly dependent on the number and virulence of bacteria delivered to the patient, the spread-plate technique is more attractive, regarding rapidity in obtaining quantitative and qualitative results leading, thus, to the institution of adequate antibiotherapy should heavy contamination of autotransfused blood be detected for any patient.

In conclusion, the spread-plate technique proved to be inexpensive and easy to perform. It yielded quantitative, as well as qualitative results in a short time. For all these reasons it has been preferred in our center to monitor intra- and postoperative blood-reinfusion programs.

References

1. Boudreaux PJ, Bornside GH, Cohn I (1983) Emergency autotransfusion: partial cleansing of bacteria-laden blood by cell washing. J Trauma 23: 31—5
2. Chauvaud S, Massonnet-Castel S, Pelissier E, Fabiani JN, Abry B, Carpentier A (1987) Autotransfusion en chirurgie cardiaque: Intérêt du lavage globulaire dans les interventions à haut risque hémorragique. Ann Chir: Chir Thorac Cardio-Vasc, 41: 421—425
3. Dion R, Verhelst R, Goenen M et al. (1988) Endocardites sur prothèses valvulaires intracardiaques. Ann Chir: Chir Thorac Cardio-Vasc, 42: 75—81
4. Kluge RM, Calia FM, McLaughlin JS, Hornick RB (1974) Sources of contamination in Open Heart Surgery. JAMA 230: 1415—1418
5. Orr M (1982) Autotransfusion: Intraoperative Scavenging. In: Stehling LC (ed): International Anesthesiology Clinics. Little, Brown; Boston, pp 97—119
6. Popovsky MA (1988) Intraoperative salvage: equipment and use. In: Autologuous blood transfusion: Current Issues. American Association of Blood Banks, Arlington, Virginia, Maffei L, Thurer RL (eds) pp 33—41
7. Sharp WV, Stark M, Donovan DL (1981) Experience with a washed red cell processing technique. Am J Surg 142: 522—24
8. Scher KS, Jones CW (1985) Which cephalosporin for wound prophylaxis? An experimental comparison of three drugs. Surgery 98: 1: 30—33
9. Schwieger IM, Gallagher CJ, Finlayson DC, Daly WL, Maher KL (1989) Incidence of Cell-Saver Contamination During Cardiopulmonary Bypass. Ann Thorac Surg 48: 51—53

Author's address:
Houda Ezzedine, MD
Department of Microbiology, Hospital Hygiene Section, 1754, Cliniques Saint-Luc,
Catholic University of Louvain (UCL), 10, avenue Hippocrate, 1200 Brussels, Belgium

Blood Salvage in Cardiac Surgery: Comparative Analysis of Three Different Procedures

B. Walpoth, U. Volken, T. Pfäffli, U. Nydegger and U. Althaus

Department of Thoracic and Cardiovascular Surgery, Division of Transfusion Medicine, Inselspital, Berne, Switzerland

Introduction

During the last 10 years, several authors have introduced and propagated various methods of blood salvage in cardiac surgery [2, 4, 5, 7, 11]. Following the reports of transfusion-transmitted infections a marked trend towards autologous blood usage in surgery was noted. Besides viral infections (HIV, hepatitis, CMV, and EBV), a number of bacterial and parasitic infections have been reported [1, 3, 6]. The incidence varies greatly with the geographical and environmental settings, as well as with the blood-donor-recruitment policy (volunteers vs paid blood donors).

Our aim was to significantly reduce the need for homologous blood products during cardiac surgery. We used three different, basic perioperative procedures: 1) washing of the erythrocytes from shed blood (A, Cellsaver), 2) centrifugation of the oxygenator blood (B), 3), retransfusion of shed mediastinal blood (C), and also 4) a combination of the two latter methods(D), and 5) a comparison to patients without any blood salvage procedures (E). In addition, we analyzed prospectively the quality of the three different autologous blood products.

Methods

Patients

Between September 1, 1988, and August 31, 1989, myocardial revascularization was performed in 270 patients (235 men and 35 women with a mean age of 58.9 ± 8.9). Included are five emergencies, six reoperations, and 18 combined cardiac procedures.

Operative methods

In over 80% of the cases, one or two internal mammary grafts were used for myocardial revascularization. Per patient 2.9 ± 1.0 distal anastomoses were performed. Membrane oxygenators were used only during extracorporeal circulation (ECC) with a mean bypass time of 112 ± 21 min.

The average transit time in the intensive care unit was 48 h.

Blood salvage groups

The following modalities or combination thereof were used.

Cell washing (group A): Cellsaver IV, Haemonetics;

Centrifugation of oxygenator blood (group B): At completion of the extracorporeal circulation the remaining blood in the system and in the oxygenator was evacuated through the arterial filter and transferred into a solution-free plastic bag (Jostra Medical), which was subjected to centrifugation for 10 min at 1000 g. The supernatant was discarded, leaving a unit of packed red cells to be retransfused to the patient after surgery in the intensive care unit.

Retransfusion of shed mediastinal blood (group C): Drainage from the chest and mediastinum was collected after surgery in the cardiotomy reservoir (Jostra Medical). Part or all was reinfused intravenously to the patient with an infusion pump (Imed International Corporation, San Diego, USA).

Combination of procedures B and C (group D);

Patients without autologous blood salvage procedures (group E).

Quantitative assessment

The consumption of homologous and autologous blood products was computed for all 270 patients. The following parameters were examined:
— The quantity of retransfused autologous blood.
— The need for homologous blood products (packed red cells = PC, fresh frozen plasma = FFP and fibrinogen).
— Total postoperative mediastinal drainage until removal of chest tubes (as an average, after 36 h).

Qualitative assessment

Five patients in group A and 10 in groups B and C were analyzed prospectively and compared in a randomized fashion to 10 control patients not receiving any autologous blood. The following parameters were analyzed:

Hematology: Hemoglobin concentration and thrombocyte counts (Coulter counter Model S, Coultronics, France).

Hemolysis: Free plasma hemoglobin by the o-Toluidin-method.

Energy rich phosphates of the erythrocytes: Adenosintriphosphate (ATP) and 2,3 diphosphoglycerate (2,3 DPG) (Sigma Diagnostics, St. Louis, USA) to ascertain cellular homeostasis and adequate capacity to deliver oxygen.

Coagulation studies: Activated clotting time (ACT, HemoTec), thrombin times, and fibrinogen (Clauss) were recorded.

Clinical chemistry: Concentration of serum sodium and potassium, as well as of total protein, albumin, and immunoglobulin.

Bacteriology: Samples for both aerobic and anaerobic cultures were examined in group C only; they were considered at risk for infection.

Sampling time

Measurements were carried out preoperatively, after 1 h on ECC, at completion of ECC, and 6 h after completion of ECC.

Statistical analysis

Analysis was performed and is expressed as mean ± 1 standard deviation (SD). Groups were compared with Student's t-test.

Results

Quantitative aspects

Autologous transfusion (Table 1): During the study year the following results were attained. In 189 patients centrifuged oxygenator blood was retransfused, yielding a mean of 509 ± 156 ml/patient. The retransfusion of shed mediastinal blood amounted to 593 ± 430 ml/patient and this procedure was used in 107 cases. In 74 patients a combination of the two procedures was carried out and a total volume of 1144 ± 305 ml/patient was achieved. The cellsaver was set up in 10 patients with a mean amount of 769 ± 194 ml/patient of autologous red cells. In 63 of 270 patients (23%) no autologous blood was used. It should be noted that only 10% of the patients could be operated without homologous blood supply.

Quantitative use of homologous blood (Table 2): Patients without autologous blood salvage procedures (E, n = 63) required 6.0 ± 3.4 units of homologous packed red cells (PC) and 3.4 ± 3.8 units of fresh frozen plasma (FFP). When only centrifugated oxygenator blood was retransfused (B, n = 92), the requirement of homologous blood products was significantly reduced to 3.6 ± 2.3 units PC per patient (p < 0.001) and FFP was reduced to 1.7 ± 2.1 units (p < 0.02). In group D, 74 patients received both oxygenator and shed mediastinal blood, which led to a further reduction of homologous blood products; in fact, patients from group D used only 3.4 ± 1.9 units PC and 2.6 ± 3.0 units FFP.

Table 1. Autologous blood salvage.

Group	n	Quantity of retransfused autologous blood ml/patient
Cellsaver	10	769 ± 194
Centrifugated oxygenator blood	189	509 ± 156 ⎫
Shed mediastinal blood	107	593 ± 430 ⎬
Combination of oxygenator and shed mediastinal blood	74	1144 ± 305 ⎭ *

* p < 0.05

Table 2. Requirement of homologous blood.

Group	n	Units of homologous packed red cells*	
No autologous blood salvage (E)	63	6.0 ± 3.4	⎫
Centrifugated oxygenator blood (B)	92	3.6 ± 2.3	⎬ **
Combination of B and C (D)	74	3.4 ± 1.9	⎭

* 1 unit = 280 ml; ** p < 0.001

The requirement of homologous blood component in the operating room (2.6 ± 2.0 PC and 1.4 ± 1.9 FFP) and in the intensive care unit (ICU; 1.3 ± 2.1 PC and 1.0 ± 2.8 FFP) are represented in Fig. 1.

Drainage: Mean total postoperative drainage amounted to 1801 ± 825 ml in group E (no autologous blood salvage), 1659 ± 767 ml in group B (centrifugated oxygenator blood), and 1905 ± 1057 in group D (combination of autologous blood salvage procedures).

Qualitative aspects

Hematology: The mean hemoglobin concentrations were measured in blood derivatives of all three groups and compared to homologous packed cell units (around 22 g/dl). The mean hemoglobin concentration in the product of the cellsaver was

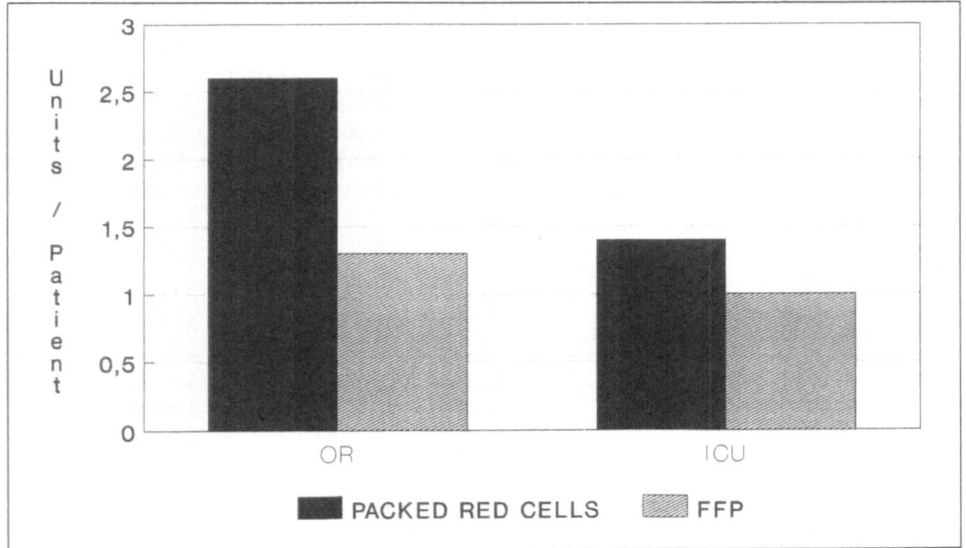

Fig. 1. Mean requirement of homologous blood products in the operating room (OR) and intensive care unit (ICU) per patient. Unit of fresh frozen plasma (FFP) and packed red cells (1 unit = 280 ml).

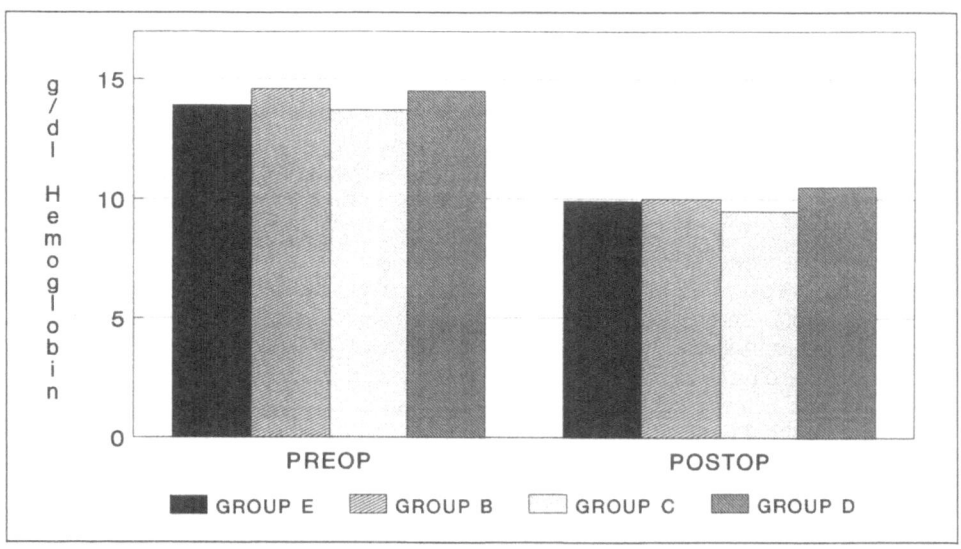

Fig. 2: Mean pre- and postoperative hemoglobin concentration in the patient's venous blood. Groups are: No blood salvage (E), centrifugated oxygenator blood (B), shed mediastinal blood (C), and combined procedures (D).

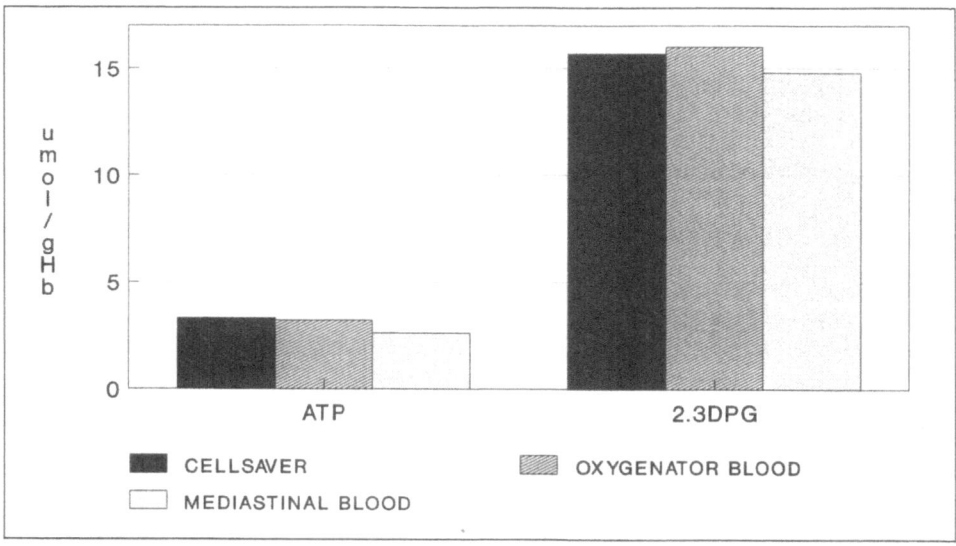

Fig. 3. Energy-rich phosphates of autologous erythrocytes after Cellsaver processing, centrifugation or retransfusion of the shed mediastinal blood. Adenosintriphosphate (ATP) and 2,3 Diphosphoglycerate (2,3DPG).

143

16.3 ± 4.1 g/dl, in group B (centrifugation of oxygenator blood) it was 21.5 ± 1.3 g/dl, and in group C (shed mediastinal blood) it was 9.6 ± 1.5 g/dl. The mean platelet counts in the shed mediastinal blood were $70 \times 10^9/l \pm 37$. Occasional controls in the other blood procedures revealed lower concentrations.

The mean pre- and postoperative (POD 1) hemoglobin concentrations in venipunctured samples from each patient according to the different groups are represented in Fig. 2. Preoperatively, these values range from 13.9 to 14.8 g/dl, and postoperatively, from 9.5 to 10.5 g/dl. The preoperative and postoperative values showed no significant difference between the groups.

Hemolysis: Free plasma hemoglobin was determined in all three autologous blood-product groups. It amounted to 63 ± 7 mg/dl in the cellsaver group (A), 202 ± 57 mg/dl in the centrifugated oxygenator blood (B), and 211 ± 44 mg/dl in the shed mediastinal blood (C). Plasma hemoglobin concentration in the venous blood of the patient (group C) showed the following values: preoperatively 12 ± 15 mg/dl, after 1 h on ECC 34 ± 21 mg/dl, and 35 ± 12 mg/dl 3 h after termination of the ECC. This value decreased to 20 ± 13 mg/dl after retransfusion of the autologous blood products. It is noteworthy that in all groups, regardless of the type and quantity of autologous blood products, no increase of free plasma hemoglobin could be detected in the patient's venous blood. Occasionally, a transient hemoglobinuria was noted.

Energy-rich erythrocyte phosphates (Fig. 3): The ATP-concentration was within the normal range (3.65 — 4.45 μmol/gHb) in group A (cellsaver blood), was reduced by 19 % in group B (centrifugated oxygenator blood), and reduced by 31% in group C (shed mediastinal blood), as compared to the preoperative patient value. The 2,3 DPG concentration was within normal limits in all three autologous blood salvage groups (10.5 — 16.2 μmol/gHb).

Clotting parameters: The activated clotting times (ACT) were prolonged in the samples from all three autologous blood products. In group C the retransfused blood was nearly completely defibrinated (five out of 10 patients showed a fibrinogen value ranging from 0.1 to 0.3 g/l). No patient showed significant prolongations of the ACT and/or thrombin times after retransfusion of autologous blood products. In the 10 patients of group C, ACT values were 112 ± 30 s preoperative, 126 ± 16 s before retransfusion, and 117 ± 15 s after retransfusion of shed mediastinal blood.

Clinical chemistry: Potassium values from samples taken out of the autologous blood products just before retransfusion were: 4.5 ± 0.3 mmol/l for the cellsaver (A), 5.4 ± 0.1 mmol/l in the oxygenator blood (B), and 5.7 ± 0.7 mmol/l in the shed mediastinal blood (C). In addition, albumin, total protein, and immunoglobulin concentrations were comparable with those of the patient's venous blood when studied in products from group B and C.

Bacteriological analysis: In the 10 patients of group C aerobic and anaerobic cultures were sterile up to 7 days. Rarely did patients show transient febrile reactions on POD 2—5. No hypersensitivity reaction was seen.

Discussion

The safety of the blood-salvage procedures under consideration in the present study is documented at various levels: Bacterial cultures were negative in group C throughout. No mix-up between the different blood products occurred, and all patients supported the transfused products without clinical side-effects.

The quality of the autologous blood products was acceptable. As yet, free hemoglobin concentration was elevated, but remained without apparent drawbacks for the patient. Of some concern is the fact that packed cells after 35 days of storage show values of 350 mg/dl free plasma hemoglobin and high levels of serum potassium, up to 80 mmol/l (8, 9). In contrast, our three autologous blood salvage products showed values ranging from 4.5 to 5.7 mmol/l.

The 2,3 DPG values of erythrocytes were all within normal range, indicating that the oxygen delivery is efficient. Conversely, in a previous study homologous erythrocytes after 35 days of storage showed a significant and marked reduction of 2,3 DPG (10). According to some authors (12) the energy-rich phosphates of ex vivo erythrocytes are restored rapidly after transfusion. No overt clotting was found in any of the three autologous blood products. Such absence of clotting is likely due to the remaining heparinization of the centrifuged oxygenator blood and to nearly total defibrination in shed mediastinal blood. In the cellsaver all coagulation factors are removed, causing a need for substitution with FFP.

The efficacy of our procedures indicates that, on average, 2 units of autologous packed cells could be recovered per patient due to the combination of retransfusion of processed oxygenator blood (B) and shed mediastinal blood (C).

The mean hemoglobin concentration in group B blood (21.5 ± 1.3) is not significantly different from the one found in homologous packed red cells, which confers a reasonable transfusion effect to our patients.

The shed mediastinal blood (C) displayed a hemoglobin concentration similar to the one found simultaneously in the patient's venous blood. However, the retransfusion of shed mediastinal blood confers a high concentration of albumin and protein, as well as a relatively high thrombocyte concentration.

The mean homologous blood requirement could be reduced significantly from 6.0 (group E) units of packed red cells per patient to 3.6 (group B) and 3.4 (group D), respectively. In our study, thus far, only 27 patients (10%) could be operated without any homologous blood products. It is noteworthy that since the completion of this study there is an increasing number of cases (28%) operated without homologous blood products (effect of the "learning curve").

Conclusion

In the present study routine use of autologous blood salvage yielded a mean of 2 units of packed red cells per patient. This represents about a 40% reduction of homologous blood use at our institution. Extensive quality assessment of the autologous blood products has shown no substantial difference when compared to homologous blood products. Accordingly, we have now introduced these modalities as routine procedures in all cases of cardiac surgery. We advocate that the cellsaver should be used only in operations where large blood loss is anticipated.

Acknowledgements: The authors would like to express their gratitude for the good collaboration with the staff of the operating room, intensive care unit, chemical and hematological laboratories.

References

1. Bove JR (1987) Transfusion-associated hepatitis and AIDS: what is the risk? New Engl J Med 317: 242—5
2. Carter RF, McArdle B, Morrit GM (1981) Autologous transfusion of mediastinal drainage blood. Anaesthesia 36: 54—59
3. Cohen NA, Muñoz A, Reitz BA, Ness PK, Frazier OH, Yawn DH, Lee H, Blattner W, Donahue JG, Nelson KE, Polk BF (1989) Transmission of Retroviruses by Transfusion of Screened Blood in Patients Undergoing Cardiac Surgery. New Engl J Med 320: 1172—1176
4. Cosgrove DM, Loop FD, Lytle BW (1982) Blood Conservation in Cardiac Surgery. Cardiovasc Clin 12: 165—175
5. Dahmen E, Ohlmeier H, Hoppe I (1978) Eigenblutspende und Eigenbluttransfusion bei kardio-chirurgischen Risikopatienten. Thoraxchirurgie 26: 27—38
6. Frey-Wettstein M, Leder A, Schütze M (1988) HIV-Übertragung durch Bluttransfusionen: eine Studie des Blutspendedienstes SRK. Schweiz med Wschr 118 (5): 149—153
7. Gillot A, Thomas JM (1984) Clinical Investigation Involving the Use of the Haemonetic Cell Saver in Elective and Emergency Vascular Operations. Am Surg 50: 609—612
8. Moroff G, Morse EE, Katz AJ, Kahn RA, Dende D, Swatman L, Staggs SD (1984) Survival and Biochemical Characteristics of Stored Red Cells Preserved with Citrate-Phosphate-Dextrose-Adenine-One and Two and Prepared from Whole Blood Maintained at 20 to 24 °C for Eight Hours Following Phlebotomy. Transfusion 24: 115—119
9. Noble NA, Tanaka KR, Myhre BA, Johnson DE (1982) Red Cell Enzyme Activity during Blood Storage and Reactivation of Phosphofructokinase. Am J of Hem 13: 1—8
10. Rosa J (1989) Recherches sur le 2,3diphosphoglycérate. In Genetet B. und Fauchet R (Hrsg.): La Transfusion Sanguine. Médecine-Sciences Flammarion, Paris pp 115—121
11. Schleinzer W, Mehrkens HH, Weindler M, Wollinsky K, Pohland H (1987) Klinisches Konzept der autologen Transfusion: Hämodilution, maschinelle Autotransfusion, Plasmapherese, Eigen-blutspende. Anästh. Intensivmed. 28: 235—241
12. Valeri CR, Hirsch NM (1969) Restoration in Vivo of Erythrocyte Adenosine Triphosphate, 2,3-Diphosphoglycerate, Potassium Ion, and Sodium Ion Concentrations following the transfusion of Acid-citrate-dextrose-stored Human Red Cells. J Lab Clin Med 73: 822

Author's address:
Dr. B. Walpoth
Department of Thoracic and Cardiovascular Surgery
Inselspital
CH-3010 Bern
Switzerland

Inflammatory Response Due to Cell-Saver in Cardiac Surgery

D. Loisance[1], A. Liou[2], Ph. Deleuze, I. Contremoulin[3], L. Intrator[2], J. P. Cachera[1]

[1] Cardiac Surgery Department, [2] Immunology Department, [3] Anesthesiology Department, C.H.U. Henri Mondor, Créteil, France

Introduction

Various technics have been proposed and evaluated clinically to avoid homologous blood transfusion in cardiac surgery. Transfusion of pre-deposited autologous blood appears quite unrealistic at a time when surgery is frequently performed as an urgent procedure. Reduction of blood loss, given by a precise surgical technique and pharmacological agents such as aprotinin, together with intra-operative autologous transfusion is a more practical approach. Previous reports by Royston [1] and our present prospective double-blind study on coronary patients clearly demonstrate that aprotinin is quite efficient in this attempt to minimize blood loss. Detailed analysis of blood loss during operations performed by different surgeons clearly shows the role of surgery itself. For obvious reasons, this observation is, nevertheless, not presented in the scientific literature. Finally, techniques of intra-operative autologous transfusion are now available. One of the most appealing is given by the red cell-saver (CS) which permits re-infusion of washed red cells, obtained from lost blood. The

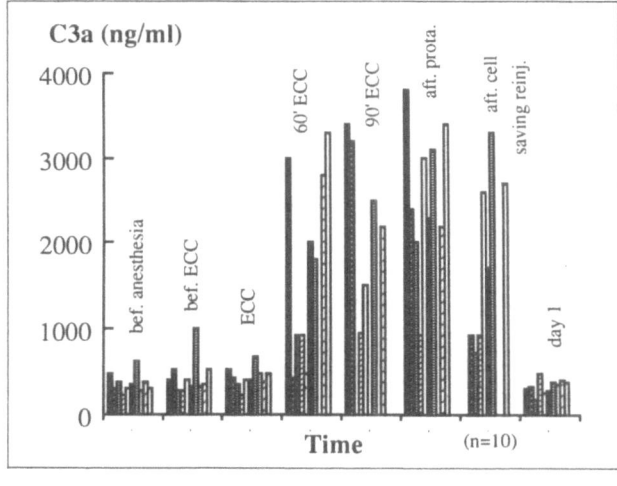

Fig. 1. Individual differences in plasma [C3a] augmentation intra- and post-operatively.

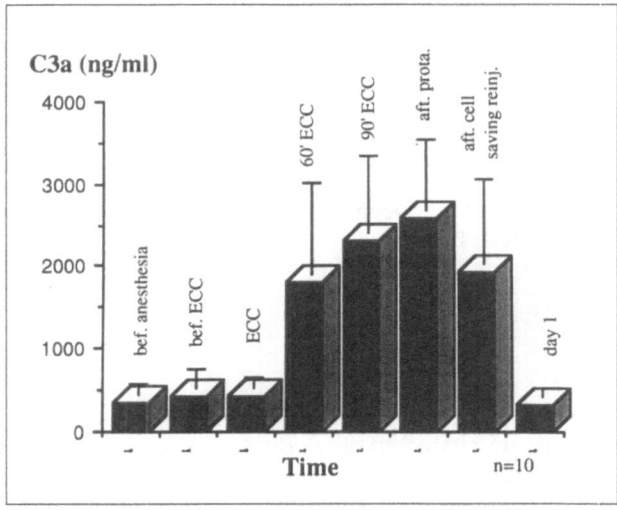

Fig. 2. Plasma [C3a], during and following CPB, in 10 cases (mean ± SEM).

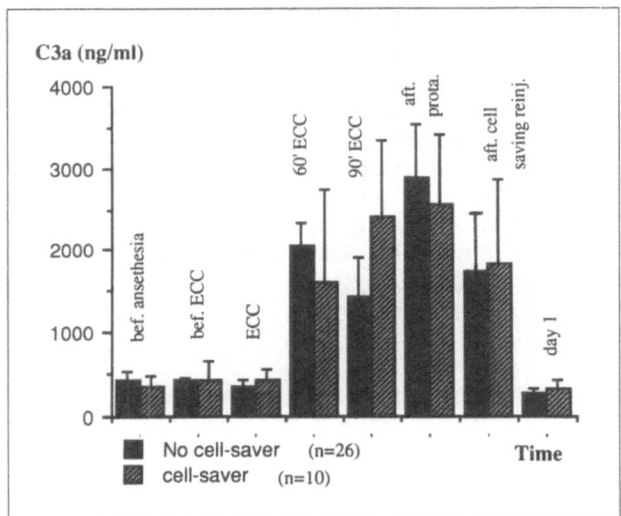

Fig. 3. Plasma [C3a] augmentation in patients (n = 10) receiving cell saver concentrate infusion, and in control group (n = 26).

question of the increased blood trauma and whole-body inflammatory response due to this blood handling has not been addressed precisely. The purpose of the present paper is the study of the C3a generation, used as an index of the inflammatory response in cardiac surgery with red cell re-infusion obtained by a cell-saver.

Method

The study has been carried out on 10 consecutive patients in whom the expected bleeding volume was high — at least higher than the usual 500 ml observed in routine

148

cases. Consequently, the patients to be included were submitted to re-operation. The study was carried out during the first quarter of 1989, with three coronary patients and seven valvular patients (age: 54 ± 15 years, ranging from 31 to 68, body surface area: 1.78 ± .18 m²). Duration of bypass (CPB), using membrane oxygenation and uncontrolled pericardial and intra-cardiac suction was 115 ± 28 min (36–118).

Blood sampling was performed at time of anesthesia, 5 min prior to CPB, at 5, 60, and 90 min after protamine infusion, and 5 min after red cell re-infusion. Volume of red cells injected was 865 ml ± 480. The last blood sample was obtained after 1 day. C3a generation was assessed by [C3a] plasma measurement using Amersham RIA technic.

A clinical score, based on cardiac, pulmonary, renal, and cerebral function (0–2 for each function) was given after the period of post-operative intensive care. This score permitted a gross clinical evaluation of the post operative outcome and an evaluation of the deleterious effects of CPB (wet lung, cerebral dysfunction, renal insufficiency, and myocardial edema).

Data obtained in this group of patients were compared to those obtained from 26 patients, operated for a first elective surgery, without any use of the cell-saver. In this group, age was 57 ± 12 years, BSA 1.75 ± .10 m², time on CPB 110 ± 25 min.

The results are expressed as mean ± SEM. Statistical evaluation used chi-square test for qualitative values and Student's *t*-test for numerical information; significance level was .05.

Results

Figure 1 shows individual values of plasmatic [C3a] at the different times. Figure 2 summarizes the mean and standard error in the 10 patients. The maximal [C3a] is obtained after protamine infusion. No further rise after cell-saver concentrate re-infusion is observed. Figure 3 shows the lack of significant difference between the cell-saver group and the control group.

The clinical score does not show any difference between the two groups: .85 ± .6 in the control group, and 1 ± .1 in the cell-saver group. None of the 10 patients presented a score higher than 3. This suggests that no deleterious effect of the red cell re-infusion may be clinically detected.

Conclusion

This protocol demonstrates the safety of the technique of washed red cell re-infusion in cardiac surgery. No enhanced blood trauma and whole body inflammatory response could be detected when the cell-saver was used. This may be considered surprising when the complex procedure of red cells washing and filtration is considered. This is an important observation when the volume of red cell concentrate is considered.

This protocol suggests that the minimal requirements of autologous blood transfusion can be met by the use of cell-saver. Consequently, the addition of a strict surgical technique, an atraumatic extracorporeal perfusion, and an intra-operative reinfusion of the lost red cells in a patient protected pharmacogically permits cardiac surgery in the safest manner.

Reference

1. Royston D, Bidstrup BP, Taylor KM, Sapsford RN (1987) Effect of aprotinin on need for blood transfusion after repeat open heart surgery. Lancet 1290—1291

Authors' address:
D. Loisance
Cardiac Surgery Department
C. H. U. Henri Mondor
51 Av. du Maréchal De Lattre de Tassigny
94000 Créteil, France

Open-Heart Surgery in Jehovahs Witnesses

V. Schlosser and G. Fraedrich

Department of Cardiovascular Surgery, University of Freiburg, FRG (Head of Department: Prof. Dr. Volker Schlosser)

Introduction

Efforts to reduce blood loss and subsequent donor blood transfusions have gained increasing importance in open-heart surgery over the last few years [1, 2, 4, 8, 16].

Because of the growing awareness about transmission of AIDS, hepatitis, and other malignant disease, as well as the limited availability of adequate quantities of homologous donor blood, the importance of new blood-saving procedures [2—4, 8, 9—11] has been stressed.

Furthermore, financial aspects as well as religious views of some patients — like those of the Jehovahs Witnesses sect — have forced cardiac surgeons to reduce blood loss and subsequent blood transfusions.

Clinical situation

The operative treatment of Jehovah's Witnesses, who refuse all blood transfusions has presented three special problems to the cardiac surgeon: Clinical status, legal implications, religious convictions.

In regards to the *clinical situation* the following prerequisites for any open-heart operation of Jehovah's Witnesses patients have to be fulfilled:
— the urgent need for operation;
— the slightly increased operative risk;
— a plasma hemoglobin level of above 13 g/100 ml

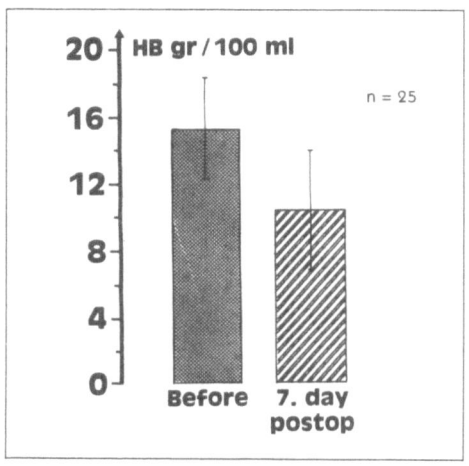

Fig. 1. Hemoglobin mean values.

151

There is no question that the need for urgent operation may cause porblems for the cardiac surgeon if the decision for operation is made by consideration of the slightly increased risk due to religious limitations in this group of patients.

In cases of emergency operations for severe cardiac valve dysfunctions or in patients with unstable coronary artery disease, there is normally a minor problem in making the decision for operation.

Legal situation

The legal situation — referring only to the Federal Republik of Germany — is as follows: In adult patients the most important factor is the confidence of the patient in his doctor, and the unlimited right of self-determination of every patient. The refusal of donor blood transfusions by the patient is part of his unlimited right of self-determination, and has to be fully respected [5, 7, 14, 15, 17, 19, 23, 24]. As an alternative, the surgeon may refuse any further treatment of such patients, but the right of unlimited self-determination by the patient has to be respected as the one basic consideration of the surgeon. Nevertheless, an extensive explanation to the patient with detailed information of all the risks posed by his religious beliefs and the fully informed consent of the patient are the most important prerequisites for any further surgical treatment.

The legal situation is much more difficult with underage children. In the case of underage children, who are aware of their situation and intelligent enough to realize their self-determination, they should be treated as adults, although they are not self-responsible from a legal point of view. In the case of young children the parents are not permitted to make decisions counter to the health of the child. Such a decision by the parents — to refuse blood transfusion during operation — may jeopardize the health of the child, and are, therefore, not legal. In these situations the surgeon may consult the guardianship court, although he is not forced to do so. Naturally, such a course of action by the surgeon could alter the relationship of confidence between the patient and the surgeon [14, 15, 17, 19].

Considering the above, it may be said that, due to the difficult legal situation with underage children, only very urgent operations in life-threatening situations should be done under those conditions.

Referring to preoperative information on the patient, the slightly increased risks due to refused donor blood transfusions, as well as alternative therapeutic steps have to be clearly explained. There has to be an unlimited informed consent signed by the patient or guardion.

Religions situation

Due to the well known religious beliefs of Jehovah's Witnesses any form of blood transfusion is refused. Furthermore, the application of other blood-related substances like fibrin glue, fresh frozen plasma, or coagulating factors are also refused as well as preoperative harvested and stored autologous blood-units. The retransfusion of patient's-own blood is only permitted if the circulation unit is not interrupted. Therefore, it is possible to retransfuse blood from the heart-lung-machine, the hemo-cell-saver, as well as from the mediastinal drainage-system.

The perfusion-system commonly in use in our department consists of a disposable membrane-oxygenator primed with cristalloid fluid, Hartmann's solution, glucose, hydroxyethylated starch, or other (Table 1). The intraoperative suction of blood is done by a cell-saver system and blood prepared by the hemo-cell-separation technique is immediately retransfused. The retransfusion of drained blood starts intraoperatively and is continued up to 10 h postoperatively. Intensive investigations regarding hemoglobin content, blood cell morphology, and incubation rate of retransfused drainage blood, also after 10 h, have been reported by others as well as by our department [4, 25, 26]. In all Jehovah's Witnesses patients we apply high-dose aprotinin in order to limit perioperative blood loss (see the contribution by Fraedrich, p. 221 ff.).

Our own clinical experience, during 1975—1989 is based on the results of the operative treatment of 103 cardiac patients: two patients of the series died in the perioperative period, both after mitral valve replacement (Table 2). One patient suffered a valve-related rupture of the left ventricle, the other died of low-cardiac-output-syndrome due to poor left ventricular function. Neither death was related to blood-transfusion refusal. The mean hemoglobin levels of the patients are shown in Fig. 1. There were several patients with hemoglobin levels between 8 and 10 % at the time of transfer to their hospitals of origin. According to reports of Hagl, there should be intraoperative hemoglobin levels above 10 g/% in patients with coronary artery stenosis and left ventricular hyperplasia, in order to provide adequate oxygen supply to the myocardium at 37 °C [6, 13, 20, 21—22], but today most cardio-surgical centers accept hemoglobin levels of 8 g/100 ml postoperatively without transfusion.

In our own department, 60—70 % of all patients undergoing open-heart surgery — beside the group of Jehovah's Witnesses — are currently operated without any use of donor blood transfusions.

Summary

To summarize the above it may be concluded:

1) The majority of open-heart operations may be done safely without the use of donor blood transfusions or preoperatively harvested blood units.
2) The risk of operation may be slightly increased under these conditions.

Table 1. Perfusion techniques.

Disposable Oxygenator (Harvey)
Priming with cristalloids (Hartmann's solution, glucose, hydroxyethylated starch)
Intraoperative cell-separation (Hemo-cell-saver)
Early postoperative retransfusion of drainage blood
High-dose aprotinin

Table 2. Clinical experiences (1/1975—9/1989, n = 103).

CHD		77
Valve replacement		
MVR	6	
AVR	15	
AVR + MVR	3	
Reoperations		2

3) We think that the blood-saving operations are most useful in adults, but in underaged children we are very restrictive.

4) The preoperative hemoglobin level must be higher than 13 g/100 ml.

5) A detailed and specific written informed-consent by the patient or legal guardian is an important prerequisite.

In cases of urgent cardiac operations in Jehovah's Witnesses, surgery with calculated risk is possible in respect to the above-mentioned prerequisites. Jehovah's Witnesses should not be excluded from cardiac operations, since open-heart surgery without the use of donor blood transfusions is becoming a routine procedure.

References

1. Bailey Ch8, Hirose T, Gollub S, Evertt HB, Folk F (1969) Open heart surgery without blood transfusion. Vasc Dis 5: 179
2. Boldt J, Kling D, Bormann VB, Züge M, Scheld HH, Hempelmann G (1989) Blood conservation in cardiac operations. J Thorac Cardiovasc Surg 97: 832—840
3. Dietrich W, Göß E, Barankay A, Mitto HP, Richter JA (1983) Reduzierung des Fremdblutverbrauchs in der Koronarchirurgie durch Hämoseparation und isovolämische Hämodilution. Anästhesist 32: 427
4. Fraedrich G, Weber C, Bernhard C, Hettwer A, Schlosser V (1989) Reduction of blood transfusion requirement in open heart surgery by administration or high doses of aprotinin. Preliminary results. Thorac Cardiovasc Surgeon 37: 89—92
5. Gombotz H, Metzler H, Hiotakis K, Dacar D (1985) Offene Herzoperation bei Zeugen Jehovas. Wi Kli Wo 12: 525
6. Hagl S, Bornikoel S, Mayr N, Messmer K, Sebening F (1975) Cardiac performance during limited hemodilution. Bibl Haemotologica 41: 152
7. Kamat PV, Baker CB, Wilson JK, Finlayson DC (1977) Open heart surgery in Jehovah's Witnesses: experience in a Canadian hospital. Ann Thorac Surg 23: 367
8. Kaplan J, Canarell Ch, Jones EL, Kutner MH, Hatcher CR,Dunbar RW (1977): Autologous blood transfusion during cardiac surgery. J Thorac Cardiovasc Surg 74: 4—10
9. Kawashima Y, Yamatomoto Z, Manate H (1974) Safe limits of hemodilution in cardiopulmonary bypass. Surgery 76: 391
10. Klövekorn WP, Richter J, Sebening F (1981) Hemodilution in coronary bypass operations. Bibl Haematologica 47: 297
11. Messmer K (1981) Compensatory mechanisms for acute dilutional anemia. Bibl Haematologica 47: 31
12. Oeveren van W, Jansen NJG, Bidstrup BP, Royston D, Westaby S, Wildevuur Ch (1987) Effects of Aprotinin on hemostatic mechanisms during cardiopulmonary bypass. Ann Thorac Surg 44: 640—645
13. Rand PW, Lacombe E, Hunt HE et al. (1964) Viscosity of normal human blood under normothermic and hypothermic conditions. J Appl Physiol 19: 117
14. Rieger HJ (1975) Transfusionsverweigerung aus religiösen Gründen. DMW 100: 639
15. Rieger HJ (1984) Lexikon des Arztrechtes. Walter de Gruyter, Berlin

17. Rüping H (1987) Der Einsatz der Haemodilutionsperfusion bei Zeugen Jehovas aus juristischer Sicht. Pers Mitt
18. Sandiford FM, Chiarello L, Hallman GL, Cooley DA (1974) Aortocoronary bypass in Jehovah's Witnesses. Thorac Cardiovasc Surg 68: 1
19. Schlosser V, Kuttler H, Johannesson T, Schindler M (1987) Herz- und Gefäßchirurgische Operationen ohne Fremdbluttransfusionen. Herz/Kreisl 19: 400—403
20. Sunder-Plassmann L, Klövekorn WP, Messmer K (1976) Präoperative Hämodilution: Grundlagen, Adaptionsmechanismen und Grenzen klinischer Anwendung. Anästhesist 25: 124
21. Urbanyi B, Spillner G, Kameda T, Schlosser V (1983) Autotransfusion with hemodilution in vascular surgery. Int Surg 68: 37
22. Urbanyi B, Spillner G, Santana A, Schlosser V (1986) Klinische Applikation der Hämodilution in der Gefäßchirurgie. Thieme, Stuttgart—New York
23. Weissauer W, Frey R (1978) Ärztliche Haftung für Anästhesiezwischenfälle. DMW 103: 724
24. Weissauer W, Hirsch G (1978) Bluttransfusion und Einwilligung des Patienten. DMW 103: 1770
25. Weninger J, Emde vd J, Schricker Th, Blechschmidt J (1980) Retransfusion von Drainageblut nach herzchirurgischen Eingriffen. Langenbeck's Arch Klin Chir 351
26. Weninger J, Shanahan R (1982) Reduction of bank blood requirements in cardiac surgery. The Thoracic and Cardiovasc Surg 30: 142—146
27. Zaorski JR, Hallmann GL, Cooley DA (1982) Open heart surgery for acquired heart diseases in Jehovah's Witnesses. Am J Cardiol 20: 186

Authors' address:
Prof. Dr. V. Schlosser
Dept. of Cardiovascular surgery
University Clinics
Hugstetterstraße 55
7800 Freiburg, FRG

Autologous Blood Transfusion in Cardiac Surgery — 15-Year Experience

C. Saavedra[1], S. Seidl[1], P. Satter[2], M. Kaltenbach[3], and R. Dudziak[4]

[1] Department of Immunohematology, University of Frankfurt and Red Cross Donor Service, Hessen, FRG
[2] Department of Cardiac Surgery
[3] Department of Cardiology
[4] Department of Anesthesiology, University Hospital, Frankfurt/Main, FRG

Introduction

A major risk of blood transfusion is transmission of infectious diseases. Apart from the screening techniques the most "effective technique" is the utilization of autologous blood which circumvents many associated risks. The term "autologous" includes various procedures such as intra-operative autologous blood transfusion or re-transfusion of autologous blood in the course of hemodilution. Another method is the transfusion of autologous blood donated 3—5 weeks before elective surgery. It has been shown that withdrawal of red cells over several weeks can be performed easily and without harm to the patient.

An autologous pre-deposit (APD) blood program was introduced in Frankfurt in 1974. One of the reasons for this was the reported high incidence of post-transfusion hepatitis (PTH) in cardiac surgery patients, ranging from 2.2% to 20%.

Method

From 1974 to 1988 a total of 9 147 cardiovascular patients underwent open-heart surgery in the University Hospital of Frankfurt; 2 406 patients (26.5%) had been enrolled in the APD-blood program. Most patients donated 2 to 3 units of blood over 3 weeks. The average interval between each donation and between the last donation and the date of surgery was 7 days (5—10 days). The patients received oral iron, beginning 1—2 weeks before the first donation (if possible) and continued through the period of donation. The dose of elemental iron was 3—6 mg/kg/day, with a maximum of 300 mg/day.

Criteria for donor selection

The absolute requirement is that the patient must be able to regenerate red blood cells and should generally not be older than 65 years. The hemoglobin concentration must be 12 g/dl or above in cardiac surgery patients; the blood pressure should not exceed 180 mm Hg syst.

All donations are screened for syphilis (GAST), SGPT, and by EIA for HBsAg and HIV antibodies. Autologous blood is not transfused if HBsAg and/or HIV-antibody positive in order to protect the staff.

156

Blood was stored as whole blood, but this procedure was recently changed and plasma is now separated and stored separately at −20 °C to maintain coagulation factor activity.

Results

Table 1 shows the number of patients per year undergoing cardiovascular surgery (1986—1988) along with the actual number of patients who were selected for the APD-blood program. We have chosen these years because remarkable changes were observed in the average percentage. In the years between 1975 and 1982 approximately 30% of patients were included, thereafter this percentage decreased to 11.8% (1984). In recent years the number of patients increased again, reaching a maximum of 42.4% in 1987. This may, at least in part, be attributed to the AIDS epidemic which was first recognized in the FRG in 1985—1986.

The total number of patients undergoing open-heart surgery remains more or less constant (824, 885, 880). This also holds true for the number of patients who were found to be suitable candidates by the cardiologist (630, 618, 607). However, the number of patients who elected surgery is much higher in 1987 and 1988 (73.3% and 60.7%, respectively) as compared to 1986 (34.6%). Furthermore, in 1987 and 1988 there was also a remarkable increase in the number of patients included in the APD-blood program (83% or 77% vs 55%).

Table 2 shows the number of patients and the reasons why these patients were *not* included in the APD-program by decision of the blood bank physician. The great distance between the blood bank and the home of the patient accounted for only a few rejections patients. Approximately one-fourth of the patients was not accepted because of their high blood pressure, whereas a rather high percentage demonstrated a low hemoglobin level ($>$ 12.0 g%). Surprisingly, there was a remarkable increase in 1987 and 1988 (33.8% and 44.2% vs 15.4%). Several patients suffered from severe complications such as angina pectoris or arrythmia, or refused blood donation because of fear, although these percentages decreased in the last 2 years from 23.8% (1986) to 9.0% (1987) and 12.8% (1988), respectively.

With advanced surgical techniques the number of patients who were treated exclusively with autologous blood increased significantly. Among 447 cardiac surgery patients (Table 3) 215 were included in the APD-program during a 6-month period (June 1—November 30, 1988). 157 patients (35.1%) received only autologous blood, whereas 58 (12.9%) were transfused with both autologous and homologous blood.

Table 1. Autologous Pre-Deposit Program (1986—1988).

	1986	1987	1988
Cardiac surgery	824	885	880
Pts. suitable for APD-program (by cardiologist)	630	618	607
Pts. who donated blood	218 (34.6%)	453 (73.3%)	369 (60.7%)
Pts. incl. in APD-program	120 (55%)	376 (83%)	283 (77%)
Pts. deferred (by blood bank physician)	98 (45%)	77 (17%)	86 (23%)

Table 2. Autologous pre-deposit program. Patients found not suitable for inclusion in the APD-Program (1986—1988).

	1986	1987	1988
Reabons for non-inclusion:			
— Distance between blood bank and home	5 5.1%	8 10.3%	3 3.5%
— Hb < 12.0 g dl	15 15.4%	26 33.8%	38 44.2%
— High blood pressure ≥ 180 mm Hg syst.	26 26.6%	20 26.0%	18 21.0%
— Psychological reasons (fears, etc.)	21 21.4%	10 13.1%	12 14.0%
— Cardiovascular complications (Angina pectoris, arrhythmia)	23 23.4%	7 9.0%	11 12.8%
— Miscellaneous (diabetes, fever, etc.)	8 8.1%	6 7.8%	4 4.5%
	98 100%	77 100%	86 100%

Table 3. Autologous pre-deposit program (June 1—November 30, 1988).

Cardiac surgery		447
Pts. without autologous or homologous blood	46	10.5%
Pts. only with autolog.blood (1—3 units)	157	35.1%
Pts. with autolog. and homologous blood 1—3 units 25 (5.5%) > 3 units 33 (7.4%)	58	12.9%
Pts. without autolog.blood (1—3 units used)	130	29.0%
Pts. without autolog.blood (> 3 units used)	56	12.5%

In 10.5% (46 patients) no blood transfusion was necessary. Out of the transfused patients the majority received 1 to 3 units, i.e., the number of blood units which can be easily collected by the APD-program.

Adverse Reactions

By careful medical examination only two severe side-effects occurred during the previous 15 years. In both cases, the patients lost consciousness, with signs of a severe cardiovascular reaction. Under appropriate treatment both patients recovered after 5—10 min and a few weeks later underwent cardiac surgery without complication.

Conclusion

An APD-blood program for patients undergoing open-heart surgery was introduced in 1974. Since that time, out of 8 670 patients, 2 276 (26.5%) were included in this program.

Clinical experiences has shown, that this APD-program can be considered a safe procedure that prevents the transmission of infectious diseases.

Authors' address:
C. Saavedra, M. D.
Department of Immunhematology
University of Frankfurt
Sandhofstr. 7
6000 Frankfurt, FRG

Preoperative Autologous Blood Donation to Minimize Homologous Blood Transfusions

H. Sons, H. D. Schulte, W. Bircks

Chirurgische Klinik und Poliklinik, Abteilung für Thorax- und Kardiovaskuläre Chirurgie, Heinrich Heine Universität, Düsseldorf, FRG

Introduction

The transfusion of homologous blood and its derivates is still associated with a certain risk [2, 5, 7, 10] in spite of all improvements in donor selection [1, 9]. Therefore, since 1982 it is a standard procedure in our institution to collect autologous blood before operations performed with extracorporeal circulation. The advantages of the retransfusion to the donor-recipient are obvious: there is no risk of disease transmission or incompatibility. Acute normovolemic hemodilution combined with retransfusion [3, 6] reduces the need for homologous blood and/or its derivates [4, 8, 11].

Patients and methods

The standard regimen for adult patients is as follows: Two and three days before the scheduled operation two bags (each 450 ml) of autologous whole blood are collected. The bags are provided with ACD buffer solution and are stored in the blood bank. The donor drinks mineral water to substitute the blood volume. Retransfusion is usually performed after cardiopulmonary bypass and/or after retransfusion of the blood from the extracorporeal circuit. Additional volume requirements in the peri/postoperative course can be met by infusions of Ringer's lactate solution; tolerating Hb values = > 8 g/dl presume an uneventful postoperative course.

Contraindications for the autologous blood donation are poor clinical condition, emergency cases, Hb levels < 12 g/dl, clotting and/or coagulation disturbances, and infancy. Relative contraindications are age, hypovolemia, congestive heart failure, and decreased pulmonary function.

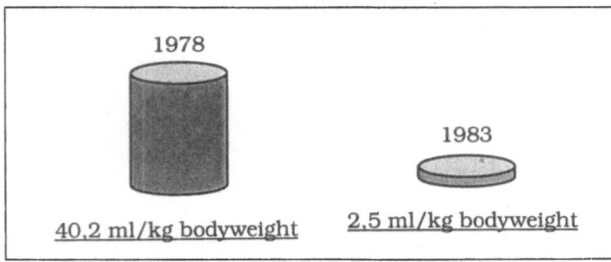

Fig. 1. Homologous blood transfusion before (1978) and after (1983) introduction of the preoperative autologous blood donation in n = 161 (1978) and n = 265 (1983) comparable patients with aorto-coronary bypass grafting procedures. Mean value of transfused homologous blood volume.

Using Ringer's lactate solution for priming of the extracorporeal circuit extended hemodilution is achieved down to a Hb-value = > 7 g/dl.

Patient groups

We calculated the amount of transfused homologous blood and/or blood derivates in 409 patients before (1978) and 509 patients after introduction of the preoperative autologous blood donation. To support these retrospective data we analyzed the data of 518 consecutive patients from 1983, with and without autologous blood donation. The exposition to donors was calculated from the 1986 data of 99 patients with (50) and without (49) preoperative blood donation, assessing comparable variables including age, gender, diagnosis, NYHA class, and LV function.

Results

After the introduction of preoperative blood donation the mean per- patient homologous blood transfusion volume could be reduced from 40.2 ml to 2.5 ml/kg bodyweight in aorto-coronary grafting procedures (Fig. 1), respectively, from 52.8 ml to 7.7 ml/kg bodyweight in aortic/mitral valve replacement or repair (Fig. 2).

In 1983, 518 operations were performed that did not require homologous blood and/or derivates. Autologous blood donation increases the percentage of the procedures without need of foreign blood in patients undergoing elective CABG, valve replacement/repair, and transaortic myectomy (Fig. 3).

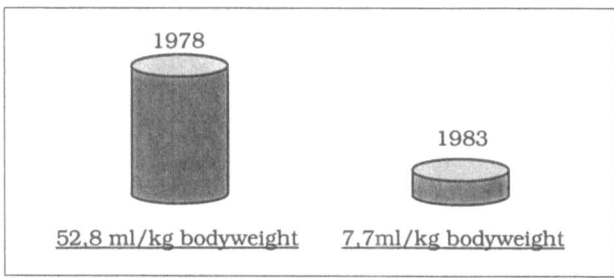

Fig. 2. Homologous blood transfusion before (1978) and after (1983) introduction of the preoperative autologous blood donation in n = 248 (1978) and n = 244 (1983) comparable patients with valve replacement/repair procedures. Mean value of transfused homologous blood volume.

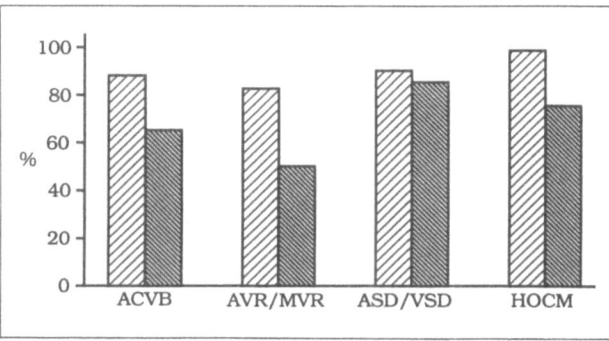

Fig. 3. Procedures performed without homologous blood and/or derivates in n = 518 patients (1983) with and without preoperative autologous blood donation.
▨ with autologous blood donation,
▩ without autologous blood donation.

The autologous blood donation is a main determinant for a reduced exposition to donors derived from the units of transfused blood or plasma, as illustrated in Fig. 4.

Summarizing the data of 524 (1978), 518 (1983), and 549 (1986) patients with comparable elective procedures there is a considerable decrease in operative procedures requiring homologous blood transfusions (Fig. 5).

Discussion

Our results demonstrate that preoperative autologous blood donation may be helpful in reducing the need for homologous blood transfusions. This should be emphasized against the background of risks related to homologous blood transfusion [1, 2, 5, 9, 10] and of the benefits of blood viscosity [3]. Preoperative hemodilution combined with a guideline for priming the extracorporeal circulation using Ringer's lactate solution is suggested to result in an uneventful postoperative course, as shown by us [11] and others [3]. In conclusion, preoperative autologous blood donation is a simple and economical step in avoidance of the use of foreign blood.

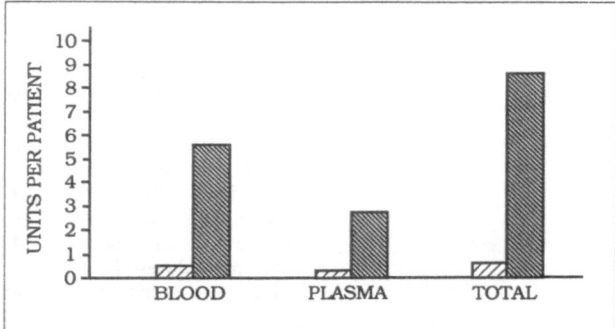

Fig. 4. Exposition to donors in n = 50 patients with and in n = 49 patients without preoperative autologous blood donation (1986).
▨ with autologous blood donation,
▩ without autologous blood donation.

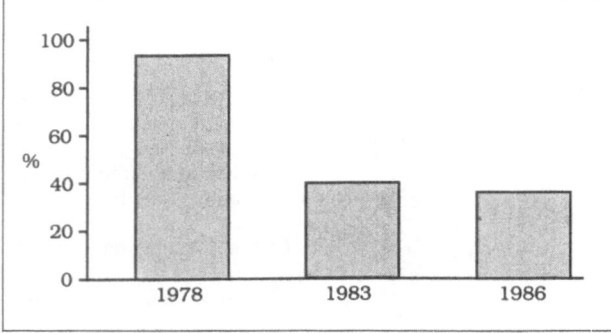

Fig. 5. Operative procedures requiring homologous blood transfusions in n = 524 patients (1978), in n = 518 patients (1983), and in n = 549 patients (1986).

References

1. Alter HJ (1985) Posttransusion hepatitis. Clinical features, risk and donor testing. Progr clin biol Res 182: 47—51
2. Blumberg N, Agarwal MM, Chuang C (1985) Relation between recurrence of cancer of the colon and blood transfusion. Brit med J 290: 1037—1042
3. Bormann v R, Boldt J, Kling D, Weidler B, Scheld HH, Hempelmann G (1987) Kombinierte Autotransfusion in der Herzchirurgie. Dtsch med Wschr 112: 1887—1892
4. Cali RF, O'Hara PJ, Hertzer NR, Diehl JT, Beven EG (1983) The influence of autotransfusion in homologous blood requirements during aortic reconstruction. Cleve Clin Q 51: 143—148
5. Brubaker DB (1983) Human posttransfusion graft versus host-disease. Vox Sang 45: 401—406
6. Dietrich W, Göb E, Barankay A, Mitto HP, Richter JA (1983) Reduzierung des Fremdblutverbrauchs in der Koronarchirurgie durch Hämoseparation und isovolämische Hämodilution. Anaesthesist 32: 427—432
7. Editorial (1984) Transfusion associated A.I.D.S. — a cause for concern. New Engl J Med 310: 115—116
8. Groschopp C, Schulte HD, Körfer R, Thum G (1985) Volumenbedarf während Herzoperationen in den Jahren 1978 und 1983 — Bedeutung von Hämodilution und Eigenblutspende. Kardiotechnik 8: 24—26
9. Kretschmer V (1987) Blut und Blutderivate. Anästh Intensivmed 28: 337—342
10. Robinson NB, Heimbach DM, Reynolds LO (1982) Ventilation and perfusion alterations following homologous blood transfusions. Surgery 92: 183—187
11. Sons H, Güttler J. Kielgas S, Schulte HD (1988) Preoperative autologous blood donations to minimize homologous blood transfusions. Thorac cardiovasc Surgeon 36 (Supp I): 29

Author's address:
Hermann Sons, MD
Chirurgische Klinik und Poliklinik
Abt. f. Thorax- und Kardiovaskuläre Chirurgie
Heinrich Heine Universität
Moorenstraße 5
D-4000 Düsseldorf, FRG

Use of Predonated Autologous Blood in Cardiac Surgery

E. Donauer[1], B. Babik[2], E. Mészáros[3], G. Gál[3], G. Kovács[1]

[1] Department of Cardiac Surgery,
[2] Department of Anaesthesiology,
[3] Blood Transfusion Center of Albert Szent-Györgyi Medical University, Szeged, Hungary

Introduction

Owing to increasing demands [6, 15] and risks of homologous blood transfusion, a program was started for the more extensive application of various blood conservation techniques [7, 9, 10, 15]. These included total hemodilution [15] and the use of cryopreserved predonated autologous blood [6, 7].

Patients and methods

Group I and Group II consisted of consecutively operated adult patients during the first and second half of the year 1987, respectively. In Group III selected patients were included, who agreed to take part in the predonation program in 1988 and 1989, (Table 1).

In all three Groups one or two units (average 405 ml in Group I, 380 ml in Group II, and 370 ml in Group III) of autologous blood were drawn 5—10 days prior to surgery using citrate-phosphate-dextrose (CPD) as anticoagulant (from patients with a hematocrit above 0.38); and this was stored under refrigeration for intra- and/or

Table 1. Demographic profile of study population. Group I: moderate hemodilution (35 ml/kg Ringer's lactate); Group II: total hemodilution; Group III: predonated autologous blood. AVR = aortic valve replacement. DVR = aortic + mitral valve replacement. MVR = mitral valve replacement. CABG = coronary artery bypass grafting.

	Group I	Group II	Group III
No.	90	92	53
Age	51 (34—67)	50,6 (19—68)	48,8 (19—71)
Female/male	40/50	33/59	26/27
AVR or DVR	24	30	31
MVR	30	15	16
CABG	31	38	—
Congenital heart disease	5	9	6

postoperative use. During the operation, before start of bypass and the administration of heparin, another one or two units (average 635 ml in Group I, 650 ml in Group II, and 627 ml in Group III) of autologous blood were withdrawn into CPD from all patients, irrespective of the hematocrit; this was given back following bypass and the administration of protamine in order to enhance normalization of hemostasis. Thrombocyte suspension was not used throughout the study. Anaesthesiological, surgical and perfusion techniques were the same in the three Groups. Except for two cases, Dideco HIFLEX D 700 S oxygenator (Dideco, Mirandola, Italy) was used throughout. Deep systemic hypothermia (20 °C) was applied in each case, with additional local cooling of the heart with ice slush. Myocardial preservation was done with repeated retrograde cardioplegia through the coronary sinus, with a modified St. Thomas's solution. Average perfusion times were 161 min in Group I, 153 min in Group II, and 161 min in Group III.

In Group I *moderate hemodilution* was applied; the oxygenator was primed with a mixture of homologous blood and 35 ml/kg body weight of Ringer's lactate solution. During perfusion autologous blood taken several days before surgery and/or homologous blood was used for volume replacement; no further clear fluid was used in this Group.

In Group II *total hemodilution* consisted of priming the oxygenator with Ringer's lactate only, and using the same fluid for volume replacement during perfusion; autologous and/or homologous blood was used for replacement only when the hematocrit dropped below 0.20.

All 53 patients participating in the predonation program (Group III) had a hematocrit over 0.37, and only patients waiting for valve replacement or correction of congenital lesions were selected. One unit of blood (420 ml each) was drawn into bottles containing CPD every 3 weeks during a 6-month period. Half of the patients received oral iron supplements (500 mg/day ferrous sulfate; Tardyferon, Egis, Budapest); and the other half did not. Within few hours of blood collection, red cells were separated by centrifugation, resuspended in glycerol solution and deep frozen to −30 °C; buffy coat was discarded. Plasma was deep frozen and both plasma and red cells were kept in the deep freezer until the day of operation [10]. On the evening before operation the red cells were thawed, deglycerolized, and resuspended in CPD solution (Group III/B). Frozen plasma was thawed in the morning of the operation (Group III/B).

In 22 patients (Group III/A) autologous whole blood was prepared by resuspending deglycerolized red cells in autologous thawed plasma. In Group III/A the oxygenator was primed with a mixture of reconditioned autologous blood and 35 ml/kg Ringer's lactate, as in Group I; and autologous or homologous blood was used for further volume replacement.

In Group III/B the oxygenator was primed with thawed autologous plasma with added Ringer's lactate; and during perfusion Ringer's lactate was used for volume replacement, with the addition of thawed autologous red cells, or autologous blood (taken days before surgery) when the hematocrit dropped below 0.20.

Reconditioned autologous red blood cells not used during the operation, were routinely reinfused on the first postoperative day even without signs of anemia or hypovolemia, since their use was limited to 48 h. Cell-saving techniques were not used throughout the study. Postoperative blood loss was collected in suction bottles and measured in the first postoperative 48 h.

Results

Six to ten units of blood were predonated by each patient. There were two episodes of fainting out of over 400 occasions of blood withdrawal: both occurred in patients waiting for aortic valve replacement, and both recovered fully within 20 s. No other complication was observed. Patients without oral iron supplements had a slightly lower hematocrit (Table 2), but the differences were not significant. Hematological control before each withdrawal did not contraindicate donation of blood in any case. There were no transfusion reactions at the administration of autologous blood. Approximately 20% of the erythrocytes were lost during the technical procedures.

Table 2. Changes in hematocrit in patients receiving predonated blood (Group III).

	without iron supplement	with iron supplement
Before start of predonation program	0,43	0,42
At admission for operation	0,40	0,43
First postoperative day	0,36	0,39
At discharge	0,36	0,37

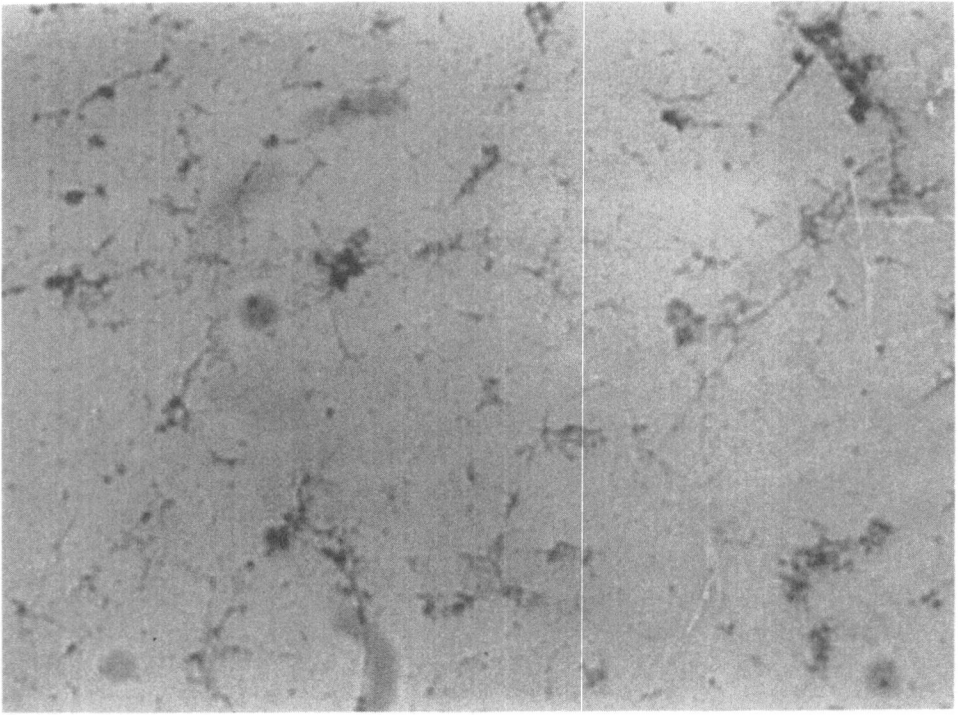

Fig. 1. Microscopic picture of thawed autologous plasma without filtration; magnification 480 x.

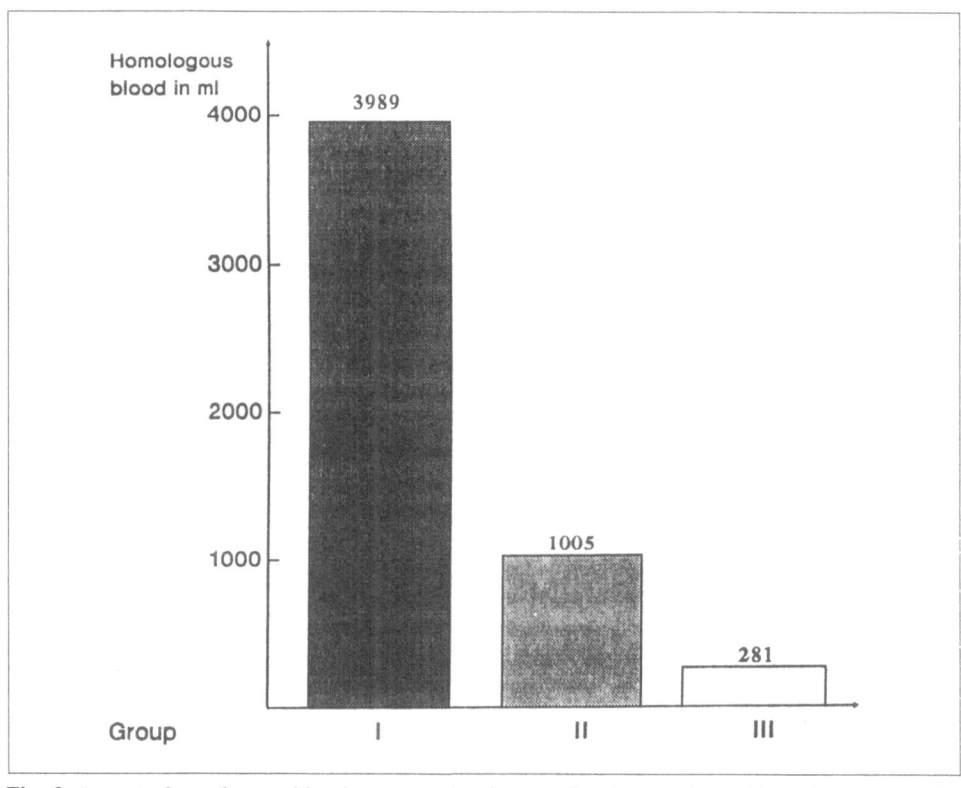

Fig. 2. Average homologous blood consumption in open heart operations: Group I: moderate hemodilution (35 ml/kg Ringer's lactate); Group II: total hemodilution; Group III: predonated autologous blood.

Thawed plasma contained vast amounts of relatively large particles (Fig. 1). In Group III/B a Polystan Venotherm bubble-oxygenator was primed with thawed autologous plasma, without filtration. The arterial filter of the oxygenator became clogged shortly after start of the bypass with a resulting obstruction of blood flow through the oxygenator. This necessitated urgent change of the oxygenator during bypass, which was followed by an uneventful perfusion and recovery of the patient. In the rest of the cases the oxygenator was primed via the cardiotomy reservoir with filtered plasma (using a 30 μ filter); no such problem occurred in the following 30 cases.

On the institution of total hemodilution (Group II) the need for homologous blood could be reduced by 75% (Fig. 2), with 24% of all patients being operated without the use of foreign blood (Table 3). With the use of predonated blood (Group III) a further 75% reduction of homologous blood consumption could be achieved, with 77% of the patients being operated without foreign blood or plasma administration (Table 3). Homologous blood consumption was slightly higher in Group III/A patients, however, in this subgroup four cases had to be reoperated because of bleeding, whereas in Group III/B there was no reoperation (Table 4). Hospital mortality was

167

0.9% in Group I, and 0.9% in Group II; in Group III there was no hospital mortality. However, no death could be attributed to the dilution technique. Postoperative renal failure did not occur in any patients of the study.

Comment

Complications of homologous blood transfusions are well documented [1, 11, 12, 13], some of them being lethal (AIDS [12], hepatitis [1], etc.). Since the risk of homologous blood administration is increasing with the number of donors, its less wasteful use was urged, and several blood conservation techniques were more frequently applied in the last decade. They include use of extensive hemodilution [8], return of intra- [2, 16] and postoperatively [2, 4, 14] lost blood by cell-saving techniques, and better control of blood coagulation by surgical, pharmacological, and physiological means. Although the average foreign blood consumption per operation

Table 3. Homologous blood consumption in patients operated with moderate (Group I), and total hemodilution (Group II), and in patients receiving predonated autologous blood (Group III).

	Group I	Group II	Group III
No.	90	92	53
Reoperation for bleeding	6 (6,7 %)	0 (0 %)	4 (7,5 %)
No of patients operated without use of homologous blood	0 (0 %)	22 (24 %)	41 (77 %)
Average homologous blood consumption in ml	3989	1005	281
Average postoperative blood loss in ml (first 48 h)	780	715	678
Haematocrit at discharge	0,39	0,36	0,36

Table 4. Homologous blood transfusion in patients operated with the use of predonated autologous blood (Group III). Group III/A: oxygenator primed partly with reconditioned autologous full blood (erythrocytes + plasma). Group III/B: oxygenator primed with reconditioned autologous plasma.

	Group III	Group III/A	Group III/B
No.	53	22	31
No. of patients receiving homologous blood transfusion	12 (22.6 %)	6 (27,3 %)	6 (19,3 %)
Sum of homologous blood in ml	14 900	8 700*	6 200**
Average homologous blood consumption in ml	281	395	200
Average postoperative blood loss in ml	678	761	595

* 7500 ml homologous blood was given to four patients who were reoperated for postoperative bleeding.
** 4350 ml homologous blood was given to two adult patients with Fallot's tetralogy.

168

could be greatly reduced in this way, complete elimination of the use of homologous blood transfusion could not be achieved.

Institution of predonation of autologous blood — which can be well applied in all sorts of elective surgery with high blood requirements — can result in further substantial reduction of foreign blood consumption [3, 5, 6, 7]. The patients taking part in the present study well tolerated withdrawal of 3.0—4.5 liters of autologous blood at 3-week interval. According to other studies this interval can be further reduced to 1 week without increasing risk [3, 6].

The combined use of autologous blood predonation, total hemodilution and other blood conservation techniques can reduce homologous blood requirements in open heart surgery to a minimal amount.

Conclusions

1. Homologous blood requirement in open heart surgery can be reduced by 75% by the application of total hemodilution.
2. Use of cryopreserved predonated autologous blood will almost eliminate the need for foreign blood.
3. Repeated withdrawal of blood in 3-week periods is well tolerated by the patients.
4. Thawed autologous plasma must be filtered before use.

References

1. Aach RD, Kahn RA (1980) Post-transfusion hepatitis: current perspectives. Ann Intern Med 92: 539—546
2. Breyer RH, Engelman RM, Rousou JA, Lemeshow S (1987) Blood conservation for myocardial revascularisation. J Thorac Cardiovasc Surg 93: 512—522
3. Britton LW, Eastlung DT, Dziuban SW, Forster ED, McIlduff JB, Canavan TE, Older TM (1989) Predonated autologous blood use in elective cardiac surgery. Ann Thorac Surg 47: 529—532
4. Cosgrove DM (1985) An improved technique for autotransfusion of shed mediastinal blood. Ann Thorac Surg 40: 519—520
5. Giordano GF, Goldman DS, Mammana RB, Marco JD, Nestor JD, Raczkowski AR, Rivers SL, Sanderson RG, Strug BS, Sandler SG (1988) Intraoperative autotransfusion in cardiac operations. Effect on intraoperative and postoperative transfusion requirements. J Thorac Cardiovasc Surg 96: 382—386
6. Haugen RK, Hill GE (1987) A large-scale autologous blood program in a community hospital. JAMA 257: 1211—1214
7. Kay LA (1987) The need for autologous blood transfusion. British Medical Journal 294: 137—139
8. Lilleaasen P, Stokke O (1978) Moderate and extreme haemodilution in open-heart surgery: fluid balance and acid-base studies. Ann Thorac Surg 25: 127—133
9. Mann M, Sachs HJ, Goldfinger D (1983) Safety of autologous blood donation prior to elective surgery for a variety of potentially "high-risk" patients. Transfusion 23: 229—232
10. Meryman HT, Hornblower M (1972) A method of freezing and washing red blood cells, using a high glycerol concentration. Transfusion 12: 145—156
11. Myhre BA (1985) Bacterial contamination is still a hazard of blood transfusion. Arch Pathol Lab Med 109: 982—983
12. Peterman TA, Jaffe HW, Feroino PN, et al. (1985) Transfusion associated acquired immunodeficiency syndrome in the United States. JAMA 254: 2913—2916
13. Popovsky MA, Abel MD, Moore SB (1983) Transfusion related acut lung injury associated with passive transfer of antileukocyte antibodies. Am Rev Respir Dis 128: 185—189

14. Shaff HV, Hauer JM, Bell WR, et al. (1978) Autotransfusion of shed mediastinal blood after cardiac surgery: a postoperative study. J Thorac Cardiovasc Surg 75: 632—641
15. Utley JR, Moores WY, Stephens DB (1981) Blood conservation techniques. Ann Thorac Surg 31: 482—490
16. Winton TL, Charette EJP, Salerno TA (1982) The cell saver during cardiac surgery. Does it save? Ann Thorac Surg 33: 379—381

Author's address:
Elemér Donauer
Department of Cardiac Surgery
Albert-Szent-Györgyi Medical University
Szeged
Hungary

Blood Use Reduction by Predonation — How Effective is It?

H. Achenbach, A. Tanzeem, W. Saggau, S. Hagl

Department of Heart Surgery, University of Heidelberg, Germany

Methods

We studied the efficacy of predonated autologous blood in decreasing homologous transfusion in two matched groups of 42 patients each.

Patients with acute infection, emergency cases, aortic stenosis, unstable angina pectoris, and those being 3 months or more after myocardial infarction were excluded in both groups.

The patients were matched for age, sex, procedure performed (aorto-coronary bypass only), length of cardiopulmonary bypass, and history of previous cardiac operation.

Group 1 received homologous blood perioperatively. Group 2 was transfused with predonated autologous blood.

Group 2 patients donated 1 to 4 autologous blood units 1 to 3 weeks preoperatively. Blood collection was performed in the hospital blood bank under physician supervision. Nearly each 500-ml volume of donor blood was separated into red packed cells and fresh frozen plasma.

Table 1. Perioperative transfusion requirements and volume of mediastinal drainage.

	Group 1 (N = 42)	Group 2 (N = 42)
Total units transfused	2.45	2.75
Autologous units	—	2.0
Homologous units	2.45*	0.75*
FFP units	3.6*	2.44*
Autologous FFP	—	2.38
Homologous FFP	3.6	0.06
Mediastinal Drainage (ml)	485	469

Data shown as he mean, * $p < 0.01$

Table 2. Type of blood transfusion required.

	Group 1 (N = 42)	Group 2 (N = 42)
No Transfusion	7.3 %	0
Autologous Transfusion only	–	72.7 %
Homologous Transfusion	92.7 %	27.3 %

Data shown as percents

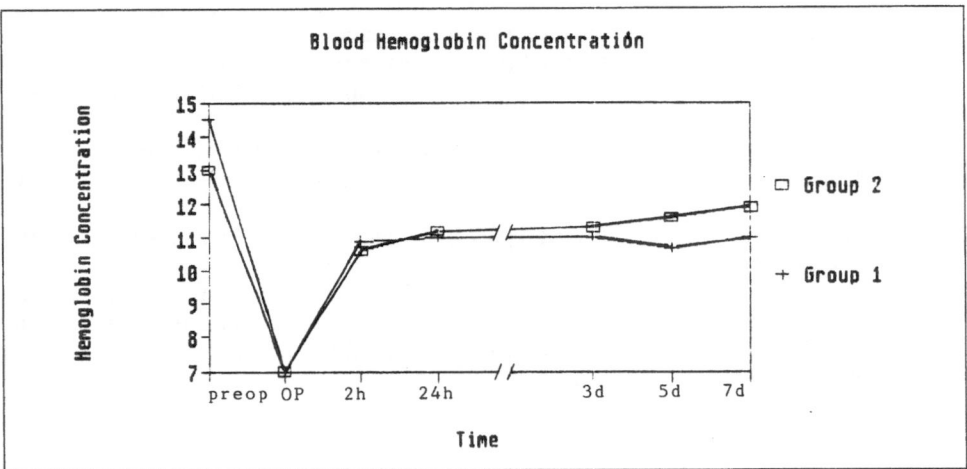

Fig. 1. Blood hemoglobin concentration (mg/100 ml) preoperatively to 7 days postoperatively.

Results

An average of 2.49 (± 0.9) units of blood was predonated by Group 2 patients for 18 days.

This predonation significantly reduced the preoperative hematocrit and hemoglobin in Group 2 (Table 3). There was no morbidity associated with the predonation process itself, and its effects on the preoperative blood determinations were not clinically important.

Table 1 and 2 shows the perioperative transfusion requirements: The mean number of units of blood transfused per patient in Group 2 was 2.75 compared with 2.45 units in Group 1. The mean volume of autologous blood transfused in Group 2 was 2.0 units. The mean number of homologous units transfused in Group 2 was 0.75, however, compared with 2.45 units in Group 1 (p < 0.01). Therefore 72.7% of the patients in Group 2 had no homologous blood requirement.

The total FFP usage was lower in Group 2: 2.44 units of FFP per patient in comparison to 3.6 units in Group 1 (p < 0.01); 97.5% Group 2 patients received homologous plasma.

Conclusion

We conclude from our experience, that safe implementation of an autologous blood predonation program for patients undergoing elective cardiac procedure provides significant reduction in both homologous red blood cells and FFP requirements and their inherent risks; it presents remarkable high patient acceptability, low risk, and few additional costs.

Author's address:
Dr. H. Achenbach
Abt. Herzchirurgie
Chirurgische Klinik
Universität Heidelberg
Im Neuenheimer Feld 110
6900 Heidelberg 1

Autologous Blood Transfusion in Cardiac Surgery

L. Castro, T. Araújo, R. C. Ferreira, J. Q. Melo

Instituto do Coraçao, Lisboa, Portugal

Introduction

The safest transfusion for a patient is with his own blood, a procedure known as autologous transfusion [1]. The most important benefit of autologous transfusion is the prevention of alloimmunization and transfusion-transmitted diseases [1, 3]. There are several methods of autologous transfusion: predeposit; preoperative hemodilution; intraoperative blood salvage; and postoperative mediastinic drainage reinfusion [2]. One of the major indications for predeposit autologous blood is presurgical donation for elective surgery. There are several reports on experience with its utilization in patients undergoing cardiac surgery [4—6]. We report our experience with the first selected 20 patients for this program of predeposit autologous transfusion.

Material and methods

All patients participating in this program were selected by the cardio-thoracic surgeon, who excluded those with: unstable angina, or clinical symptoms of heart failure.

The 20 (14 male, 6 female) patients had: coronary disease (11 patients), valvular heart disease (seven patients), congenital heart disease (one patient), and mediastinic tumour (one patient).

Their mean age was 51 (range 18—69).

At the time of first donation the mean weight (kg) was 68.7 (range 46.6—93).

The criteria for donation were [1]:

— Hb $\geqslant$ 11 g/dl and/or Ht $\geqslant$ 34%;

— Patients weighing less than 50 kg; drawn blood amount was 7 ml for every kg bw;

— Last phlebotomy should have been at least 72 h before surgery. The minimal interval between phlebotomies was 4 days.

Iron supplementation to all patients was by ferrous sulfate 525 mg daily, started 1 week before first donation and continued after surgery, according to the levels of hemoglobin and hematocrit.

The advantages, risks involved, and the possibility of complications were explained to each patient. Written consent from each patient was obtained prior to phlebotomy [5].

The units of blood were collected in CPD-A anticoagulant and stored as red cells and fresh frozen plasma.

Results

The total number of units donated was 73, and the mean number 3.6 (range 1—5). Three patients donated 1 unit; one patient donated 2 units; two patients donated 3 units; eight patients donated 4 units; and six patients donated 5 units.

Three patients had to interrupt donation due to low levels of hemoglobin and hematocrit. The number of donations of the remaining patients depended on the available time until surgery. The longest delay between first donation and surgery was 30 days.

Clinical tolerance to phlebotomy was good, and no adverse reaction or complication was observed.

The mean levels of hemoglobin before each donation are shown in Fig. 1.

A decrease of 0.6 g/dl in mean hemoglobin levels was between the first and second donations and also between the second and third donations. The decrease of mean hemoglobin levels between the third and fifth donations was 0.4 g/dl. The mean hemoglobin level stabilized since the fourth donation.

In a total of 73 units donated, 66 were administered as autologous blood, 3 were discarded, and 4 were used as homologous blood, since the patients fulfilled donor criteria.

Only five patients were transfused with additional homologous blood. One of them required 5 units of homologous blood because of massive surgical bleeding that occurred in the imediate postoperative period (Tables 1 and 2).

Discussion

Our experience, although of only a small subject group, shows that there is a good clinical tolerance to phlebotomy, and this method is well accepted by the patients. However, there should be adequate medical support in the event of any adverse reaction. Previous experiences reveal that these are not superior to those of normal donors [6].

The cause for suspending the donations was anemia in three patients.

The mean units donated by each patient was 3.6 units, with a total of 73 units for 20 patients.

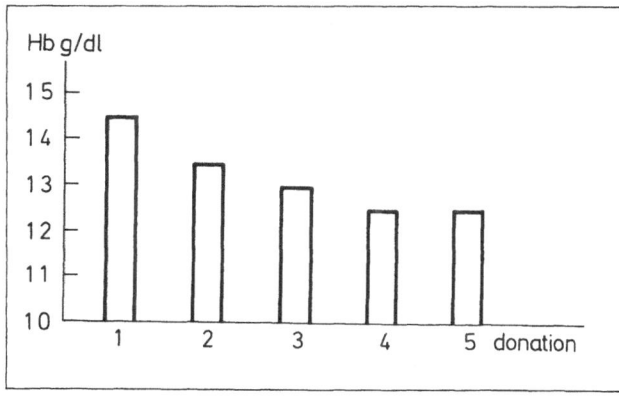

Fig. 1. Mean hemoglobin levels.

175

Table 1. Autologous blood transfused.

No. of Patients	Autologous blood No. of units
2	5
9	4
5	3
1	2
3	1
Total 20	

Table 2. Homologous blood transfused.

No. of Patients	Homologous blood No. of units
1	5
0	4
1	3
1	2
2	1
Total 5	

The decrease of hemoglobin level between the first and the fifth donations was of 1.6 g/dl.

The decrease in the hemathological patterns is compensated by the rheological advantages, since the decrease in blood viscosity allows a better tissue oxigenation [6].

The number of autologous blood units transfused was 66, and only 11 units of homologous blood were needed. This enhances the autologous blood program efficacy which is easily appliable and, therefore, should be implemented in order to decrease the need of homologous blood and the associated risks.

References

1. American Association of Blood Banks (1985). The technical manual of the American Association of Blood Banks, 9th Ed. Philadelphia: JB Lippincott; 359—368
2. Popovsky MA, Devine PA, Taswell HF (1985) Subject Review — Intraoperative Autologous Transfusion. Mayo Clin Proc 60: 125—134
3. Cona J (1977) Autotransfusion: current status. Medical Instrumentation 11: 6: Nov—Dec
4. Goldfinger D (1976) Use of Autologous Transfusion in Elective Surgery. In: Dawson RB (ed). Autologous Transfusion. Washington: American Association of Blood Banks, pp 115—120
5. Mann M, Sacks HJ, Goldfinger D (1983) Safety of autologous blood donation prior to elective surgery for a variety of potentially "high-risk" patients. Transfusion 23: 229—239

176

6. Fruchart MF, Weiss P, Boulat C, Simonneau M, Delorme G, Varin J, Dubourg O, Bardet J, Bourdarias JP (1989) Prélèvements programmés en vue de transfusion autologue lors de la chirurgie cardiaque. Rev. Fr. Transf. Hemobiol. 32: 169—178

Author's address:
L. Castro, M. D.
Instituto do Coraçao
Rua Prof. Reynaldo dos Santos, no 27
Carnaxide
2795 Linda-A-Velha
Portugal

Intraoperative Blood Conservation Using Cell-Saver

S. K. Bhattacharya, G. P. Sharma, P. I. Polimeni, L. Dyck, M. Roy

University of Manitoba Department of Surgery, St. Boniface General Hospital, Winnipeg, Manitoba, Canada

Introduction

Despite meticulous surgical technique a significant blood loss still occurs in routine cardiac surgery. In the past this was routinely replaced with a "banked" blood transfusion. Concerns about the well known complications of the bank blood transfusion, including those of transmitted disease recognized recently, have led to the development of various perioperative blood conservation techniques. Our initial experience in 225 selected patients using Hemanetics-cell-saver equipment has been reported previously [2]. Since 1987, this method of intraoperative blood conservation has been used routinely in all of the approximately 900 cardiac surgery procedures performed in our service. The present study details our most recent experience with this technique in 100 consecutive and unselected cardiac surgical procedures performed by several surgeons.

Materials and methods

Medical records of 100 consecutive patients who underwent cardiac surgical procedures in our service, April—June 1989, were examined in retrospect. The following operative procedures were performed: 79 aorto-coronary bypasses (double, 11; triple, 36; quadruple, 25; five or more, 7), six aortic valve replacements, seven mitral valve repair, one combined aortic and mitral valve replacement, four repairs for congenital heart disease, and three others. The general demographic data, operative data including intraoperative blood salvage, blood loss in the first 24 h postoperatively, and other hematological data such as pre- and postoperative hematocrit, prothrombin time (PT), partial thromboplastin time (PTT), and platelet count were noted.

Median sternotomy approach was used in all patients who underwent a standard cardiopulmonary bypass (CPB). Systemic hypothermia (25—28 °C) along with an intermittent hypothermic potassium blood cardioplegia supplemented with topical cooling (Pericardial Irrigation) were employed in all cases. Hollow fibre oxygenators were used in 97 patients (Turino, 92; Medtronic, 5). A Bentley bubble oxygenator was used in the remaining three patients. Moderate hemodilution employing a non-blood prime and standard dosage of heparin was used in all cases. On termination of the CPB heparin was neutralized with a calculated dose (1.5 times dose of heparin) of protamine sulphate.

The cell-saver discard suction apparatus was used in each case throughout the entire procedure, including the CPB, in order to salvage most of the shed blood in the operative field, keeping use of sponges to the very minimum. The recovered blood thus collected in the cell-saver reservoir was washed, concentrated, and transfused back to the patient. The residual blood in the oxygenator, left over after heparin neutralization, was also processed through the cell-saver system and retransfused back to the patient.

Results

The mean age of the patients was 61.7 ± 11.5 years with a male/female ratio of 2 : 1. Within the isolated coronary bypass group the average number of grafts per patient was 3.4. Ninety-one % of these patients had at least one internal mammary artery as a conduit for pypass. Three patients had a "redo" operation in the entire series. The mean CPB time was 149 ± 53.9 min with the aortic cross-clamp time of 75.7 ± 50.9 min. Four patients donated their own blood preoperatively (3 units each) over 3 weeks; this was then transfused back to each of them during the perioperative periods. Only one patient in this group required transfusion of 2 additional units of homologous blood.

The mean washed red blood cell yield was 2.0 units with a hematocrit of 0.550. The pre- and postoperative hematocrits, PT, PTT, and platelet counts are shown in Table 1. The mean postoperative blood loss was 775 ± 649 ml (range: 145–5941). Two patients required reoperation for the control of bleeding. The requirement for bank blood transfusion during the entire hospital course was a mean of 2.75 ± 2.99 units. Nineteen patients received no bank blood transfusion.

Discussion

Following Cosgrove et al. [2], we started using the cell-saver system for intraoperative blood conservation in 1980, initially using it only in selected cases, such as "redo" operations, thoracic aortic surgery, etc.. This was later gradually extended to all routine cardiac procedures. In the last few years, confronted with an increased risk of various infectious diseases transmitted through bank blood transfusion, further efforts were made to reduce the amount of homologous blood transfusions. Various authors have reported contradictory views on the value and effectiveness of these techniques [1, 3—5]. The present study indicates that considerable salvage of shed blood could be achieved with intraoperative blood conservation alone. This has resulted in significant reduction of the amount of bank blood transfused in our practice.

Table 1. Hematological studies.

Parameter	Preoperative	Postoperative
Hematocrit	0.412 ± 0.045	0.310 ± 0.039
PT	11.0 ± 0.7	15.2 ± 1.5
PTT	34.3 ± 13.3	46.4 ± 7.7
Platelets	291 ± 89	149 ± 53

In our experience, intraoperative blood conservation techniques are worthwhile and are a useful adjunct to modern cardiac surgery. There are certain areas in the application of the cell-saver system, especially with respect to loss of clotting factors, which are reasons for concern. Important coagulation factors and platelets are lost because only the washed red blood cells are returned back to the patient. In patients with significant blood loss processed through the cell-saver, this technique may actually exacerbate the underling coagulopathy (Table 1). We have now undertaken evaluation of other forms of blood salvage, where the shed blood is returned after ultrafiltration or simple filtration. With the introduction of additional new techniques to salvage postoperative mediastinal shed blood, perhaps a majority of the patients could undergo routine cardiac operations with a significantly reduced need for bank blood transfusions.

References

1. Bayer RH, Engelman RM, Rousou JA et al. (1987) Blood conservation for myocardial revascularization. Is it cost effective? J Thorac Cardiovasc Surg 93: 512—522
2. Bhattacharya SK (1982) Intraoperative blood conservation and autotransfusion in cardiovascular operations. Ann RCPSC 15: 279
3. Cosgrove DM, Thurer RL, Lyttle BW et al. (1979) Blood conservation during myocardial revascularization. Ann Thorac Surg 28: 181—189
4. Keeling MM, Lamen AG, Brink MA et al. (1983) Intraoperative autotransfusion. Ann Surg 197: 536—540
5. Winton TL, Charette EJP, Solerno TA (1982) The Cell Saver during cardiac surgery: Does it save? Ann Thorac Surg 33: 379—381

Author's address:
S. K. Bhattacharya, M. D.
Department of Surgery
St. Boniface General Hospital
Winnipeg, Manitoba R2H 2A6

Intraoperative Autotransfusion

L. Claeys, M. Horsch, G. Hanisch, S. Horsch

Department of General and Vascular Surgery, Academic Hospital Cologne-Porz, Cologne, FRG

Introduction

The potential problems associated with homologous blood-transfusions, for instance, transmission of infectious diseases, and the rising number of major operations with a continuous increase in the demand for blood have caused an increased interest in autotransfusion [1].

There are four different methods of autotransfusion. The first is the preoperative elective collection of blood. The second is the acute hemodilution immediately preoperative [4, 5]. The third method consists of the intraoperative transfusion. The fourth type is the postoperative collection of blood for autotransfusion.

Indications and contraindications

Intraoperative autotransfusion (IAT) has two main indications: as a life-saving procedure in acute severe hemorrhage and as part of an autotransfusion program to minimize homologous blood transfusion. We consider vascular surgery, especially venous thrombectomy, elective or ruptured aortic aneurysm surgery and aortic bypass surgery as being the prime indication for intraoperative autotransfusion [2]. Absolute contraindications are surgery for malignant tumors or surgery in septic or infected surroundings. The transfusion of blood contaminated with intestinal matter is also contraindicated.

Materials and methods

Within a period of 45 months we used a small, simple, disposable set for IAT [3, 6]. It requires no additional equipment and enables a fast autotransfusion. The system consists of a semi-rigid flask with a compressible flexible interior plastic bag with a capacity of 500 ml. The bag and suction tube ($\pm$ 12 inches) are made of polyvinylchloride. Into this bag a red and yellow dual tube connection is integrated. At the red connection the extension tube is adapted to the aspirator. At the yellow connection the vacuum tube for aspiration of the blood, the blood filter, and the transfusion set for retransfusion are attached. Blood can be collected after aspiration of 30 ml of citratephosphate-dextrine (CPD). If the patient is fully heparinized no anticoagulant is necessary. The subatmospheric pressure during aspiration should not exceed 80—100 mmHg in order to avoid mechanical damage to the red blood cells. The vacuum tube should be submerged in the blood pool in order to avoid aspiration of air, and to prevent foaming and hemolysis. The flask should be shaken slightly during collection to achieve a good mixing of the blood with the anticoagulant. When the interior bag is filled, it should be closed and the vacuum disconnected. The blood is immediately reinfused via a micropore filter (40-micron filter), eventually under pressure.

Results

In the period from February 1986 to November 1989 we used this system in 483 patients; 89 of them underwent venous thrombectomy, 394 an aortic bifurcation bypass operation. We autotransfused 603 liters and transfused 412 units of homologous blood. In 62 % of our patients transfusion of homologous blood was not necessary; 21 of the 89 patients undergoing venous thrombectomy required banked blood during or after the operation (average 2,6 units/patient); 163 of the 394 patients undergoing aortic bypass operation required homologous blood (average 2.2 units/patient) (Table 1).

To control the quality of the autotransfused blood we studied the following parameters in the patients who did not recieve a homologous transfusion: hemoglobin, hematocrit, WBC, RBC, platelet count, fibrinogen, and haptoglobin preoperatively, immediately postoperative, and on the first, second, and third postoperative days. We checked also bilirubin, amylase, and creatinine (Fig. 1a—e).

To investigate an eventual influence of autotransfusion on the hematologic system we created two groups of patients. The fist group (69 patients) received a volume of maximum 500 cc and the second (127 ptients) received between 500 cc and a maximum of 2500 cc (average 1200 cc). Of all the parameters tested no statistically significant changes were observed after autotransfusion; also no significant electrolyte disorders could be observed. The coagulation-function tests, viz. prothrombintime and thromboplastin-time stayed within normal range. There was no evidence of increased bleeding, consumption coagulopathy or renal failures, etc. Our experience shows that this autotransfusion set is well suited for IAT in major vascular surgery.

Table 1. Personal experience with intraoperative autotransfusion.

Operation	Number of patients	Number of systems used	Volumes transfused	
			Autologous blood (liter)	Homologous blood (units)
Venous thrombectomy	89	338	170	54
Aortic surgery	394	866	433	358
Total	483	1204	603	412

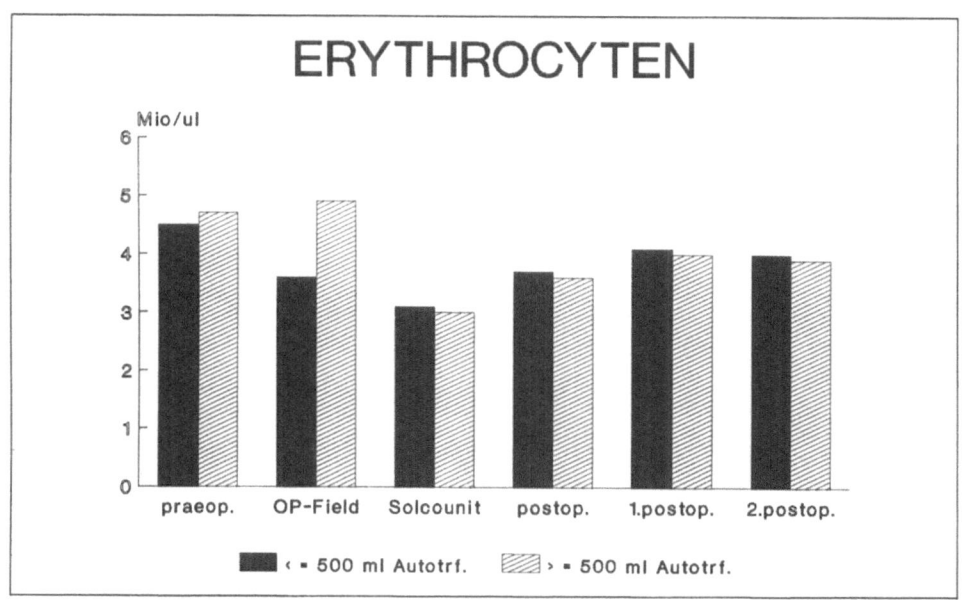

Fig. 1 a

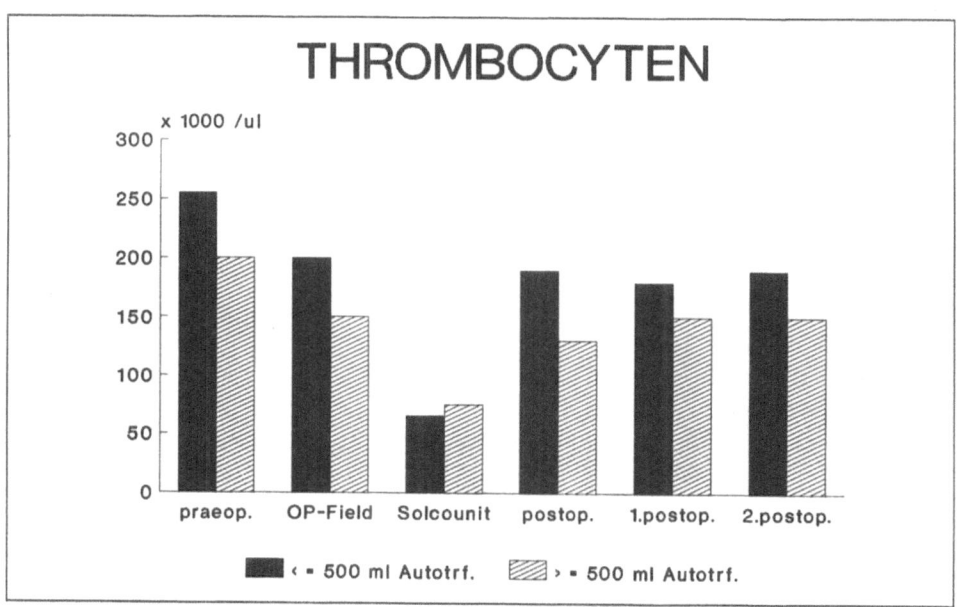

Fig. 1 b

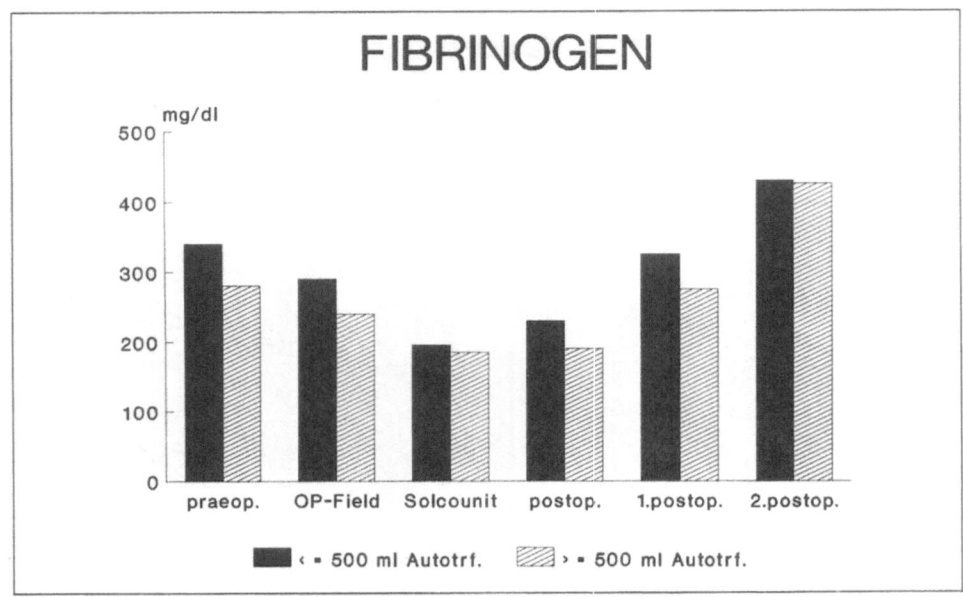

Fig. 1 c

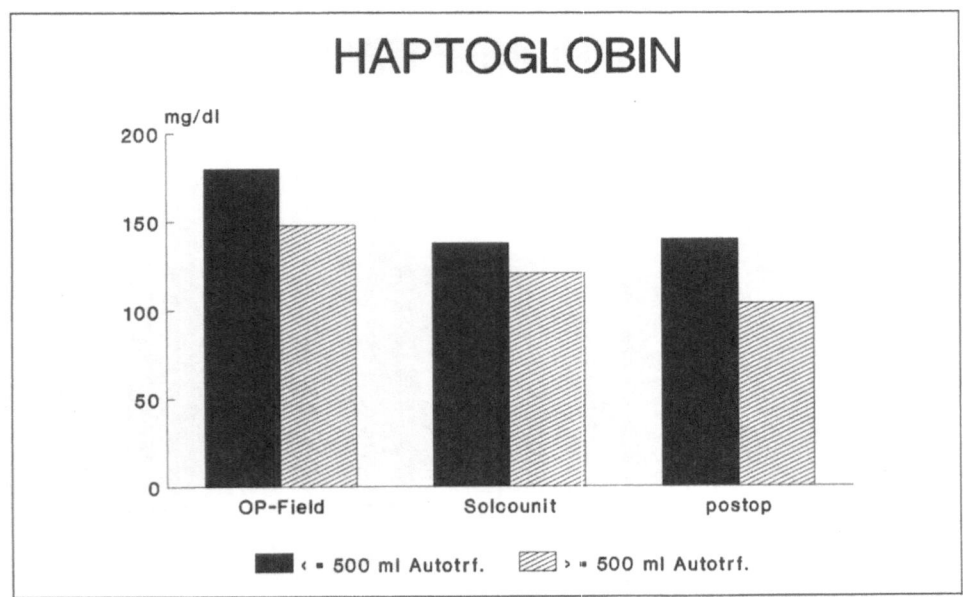

Fig. 1 d

184

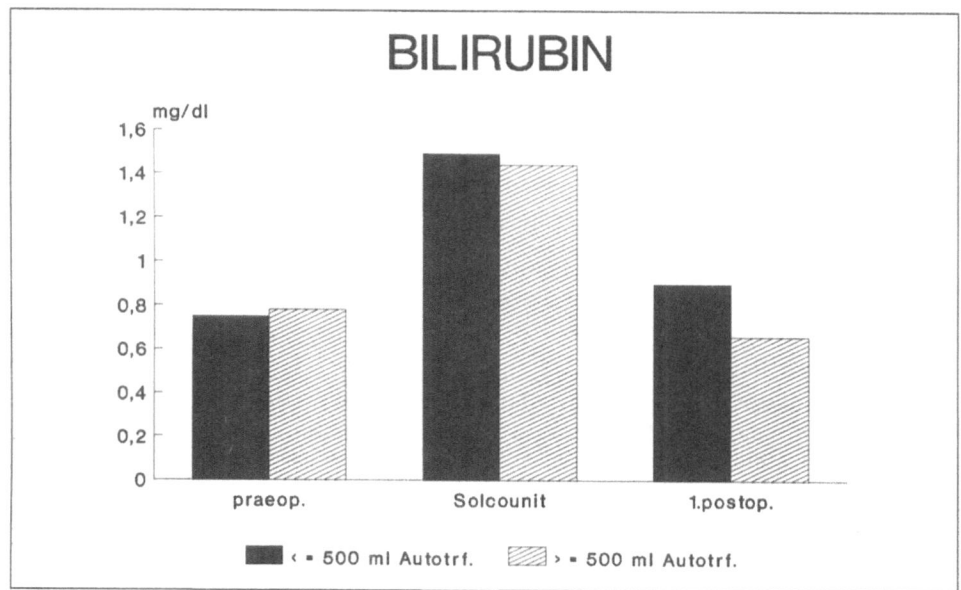

Fig. 1 e

Fig. 1 a—e. Mean plasma value of biological parameters: preoperatively, in the shed blood, in the Solco-unit, immediately postoperative on the first and on the second postoperative day in 196 patients (69 patients < 500 ml autotransfusion and 127 patients > 500 ml autotransfusion).

References

1. Blumenberg B (1982) Spezifische Probleme der Autotransfusions-Gerinnung und Infektion. Vortrag beim Symposium über Plasmaaustausch und Autotransfusion, Berlin 1982
2. Brewster CD, Ambrosino JJ, Darling RC (1979) Intraoperative autotransfusion in major vascular surgery. Am J Surg 137: 507—513
3. Horsch S, Schmidt R, Imhoff M, Pichlmaier H (1983) Ein neues Verfahren zur intraoperativen Autotransfusion. Infusionstherapie 10: 71—73
4. Klövekorn WP, Pichlmaier H, Ott E, Bauer H, Sunder-Plassmann L, Messmer K (1974) Akute präoperative Hämodilution - eine Möglichkeit zur autologen Bluttransfusion. Chirurg 45: 452—458
5. Pichlmayr I (1976) Hämodilution. Anästhesiol. und intensiv-med. Praxis, Heft 1, Hans Marseille Verlag München
6. Schmidt R, Horsch S, Imhoff M (1983) Eine neue Methode zur intraoperativen Autotransfusion. Angio 5: 31—34

Authors' address:
Prof. Dr. med. S. Horsch
Department of General and Vascular Surgery
Academic Hospital Cologne-Porz
Urbacher Weg 19
5000 Cologne 90 (Porz) FRG

Cardiac Surgery in Jehovah's Witnesses: An Experience of 62 Cases

B. Rigler, H. Gombotz*, H. Mächler, D. Dacar, Ch. Matzer*,
K. H. Tscheliessnig, H. Metzler*

Departments of Surgery and Anaesthesiology*, University of Graz, Austria

Introduction

Jehovahs' witnesses (JW) are rejected for closed and open-heart surgery at most European heart centers as they impose serious moral and ethical problems to surgeons and anaesthetists. Members of JW refuse to accept transfusions of blood and blood products under any circumstances, even in view of the lethal risk of major hemorrhage [5, 9]. In addition, predonation of autologous blood which is one important principle of current techniques of blood saving methods [1, 3, 4], is also not accepted. Despite this, open and closed repair of various congenital and acquired heart defects has been reported by a few centers [2, 5, 6, 10]. We describe our experience with 62 patients who underwent cardiac operation at our institution over the past 10 years.

Patients and methods

From 1979 to 1989 bloodless cardiac procedures were performed in 62 (82%) of 73 JW scheduled for heart surgery at our department. Eleven patients were excluded from surgery mainly because of low weight (< 10 kg), low hematocrit (< 35), advanced age (> 70 years), concomitant diabetes, increased pulmonary vascular resistance (> 8 units), unstable angina, critical aortic stenosis and/or impaired left ventricular function. Mean age of the surgically managed patients was 33.1 years (14 days—70 years), mean weight 51 kg (700 g—95.5 kg). No special blood-saving methods were applied during non-bypass operations. Normovolemic hemodilution, bloodless prime and moderate hypothermia were used in cardio-pulmonary bypass procedures, while cell-separation and retransfusion were feasible in only 10 cases. Hemodilution was induced prior to extracorporeal circulation (ECC) by drawing 15—20 ml/kg of blood into communicating CPD-bloodbags containing 200 000 units of aprotinin. Retransfusion of the autologous blood was started immediately after at a very low rate, thus creating a temporary circuit throughout the period of cardiopulmonary bypass with most of the collected blood volume available at the time of discontinuation of ECC.

Results

Thirty-three patients with congenital anomalies underwent 23 bypass and 10 non-bypass operations (Table 1). Surgery included repair of the aorto-pulmonary window, tetralogy of Fallot, simple transposition (D-TGA), as well as Rastelli-type repair of complicated D-TGA/VSD/PS. 21 (34%) were less than 15 years old and two had undergone previous cardiac surgery. In this group there were two deaths due to elevated pulmonary vascular resistance (D-TGA/IVS-Senning, VSD/pulmonary artery banding). One adult with anomalous course of coronary artery branches died from right-heart infarction after resection of infundibular pulmonic stenosis. Twenty-nine patients were operated for elective myocardial revascularization (mean number of vein grafts 2.4) or prosthetic valve replacement. Two patients required concomitant repair of associated lesions (perforated aneurysm of sinus of valsalva, unilateral carotid artery stenosis). One of four patients with previous cardiac surgery developed a left main coronary-artery stenosis following aortic-valve replacement and was successfully reoperated. Three deaths occurred after coronary artery bypass-grafting. Only one was related to blood-loss or anemia (mediastinal sepsis/multiorgan failure). The distribution of the body weight of ECC-patients, their hematocrit values — on ECC and during the entire perioperative period — are illustrated in Fig. 1 together with a diagrammatic representation of the applied hemodilution technique.

Conclusion

The controversial issue of blood transfusions in JW should not be solved by excluding these patients from open-heart surgery. One of the largest series of cardiac operations of JW describes 362 cases with an early mortality of 10.7% [10].

Table 1. Synopsis of heart defects, cardiac operations, refused patients, and hospital deaths in members of Jehovah's Witnesses.

	Rejected	With ECC	Without ECC	Hospital Deaths
CABG	4	14	—	3
AVR	2	6	—	—
MVR	2	8	—	—
DVR	—	1	—	—
ASD	—	5	—	—
VSD	—	3	2	1
PS	—	3	—	1
PA/VSD	—	—	2	—
TOF	—	5	—	—
TGA	1	4*	—	1
CAVC	—	1	1	—
APW**	—	1	—	—
COA	—	1	3	—
PDA	—	—	2	—
Total (<15 years)	9 (2)	52 (11)	10 (10)	6 (2)

* Two patients with hypothermic circulatory arrest.
** Aortopulmonary window.

187

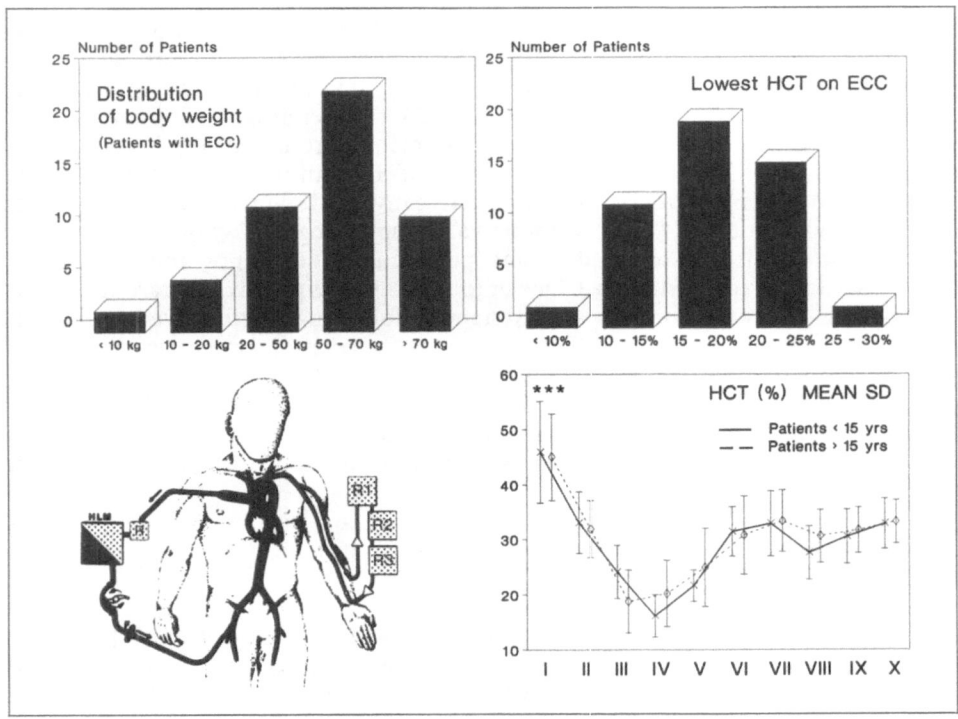

Fig. 1. Distribution of body weight, lowest hematocrit (HCT) levels on ECC; impression of the applied modification of hemodilution technique, as well as the perioperative hematocrit values summarized in patients with ECC. (I preop, II after hemodilution, III and IV during ECC, V after ECC, VI postop, VII day 1, VIII day 3, IX day 6, X day 12 postoperative).

Our study, again, demonstrates the feasibility of bloodless cardiac surgery with and without cardiopulmonary bypass, despite an increased risk — even in patients with redo-surgery or complex cardiac anomalies. In our series no patient died as a consequence of acute hemorrhage, whereas one or two deaths may be attributable to bloodloss or anemia. Hospital mortality was less than 10% (9.6% with bypass-procedures), which is within the range of 5—19%, as reported in the literature [5—8]. However, with predonation of autologous blood not accepted and modified hemodilution technique as the basic principle of open-heart surgery, proper selection of the surgical candidates may be of major importance.

References

1. Breyer RH, Engelmann RM, Rousou JA, Lemeshow S (1987) Blood conservation for myocardial revascularization. J Thorac Cardiovasc Surg 93: 512—522
2. Corno AF, Laks H, Stevenson LW, Clark S, Drinkwater DC (1986) Heart transplantation in a Jehovah's witness. J Heart Transplant 5: 175—178

3. Dietrich W, Göb E, Barankay A, Mitto HP, Richter JA (1983) Reduzierung des Fremdblutverbrauches in der Koronarchirurgie durch Haemoseparation und isovolaemische Haemodilution. Anaesthesist 32: 427—432
4. Fraedrich G, Engler H, Possmann A, Kanz L, Hettwer A, Bernard C, Schlosser V (1989) Fremdbluteinsparung in der offenen Herzchirurgie durch hochdosierte Aprotiningabe. 18. Jahrestagung der Deutschen Gesellschaft für Thorax-, Herz- und Gefäßchirurgie München
5. Gombotz H, Rigler B, Matzer CH, Metzler H, Winkler G, Tscheliessnig KH (1989) 10 Jahre Herzoperationen bei Zeugen Jehovahs. Anaesthesist 38: 385—390
6. Henderson AM, Maryniak JK, Simpson JC (1986) Cardiac surgery in Jehovah's witnesses. A review of 36 cases. Anaesthesia 41: 748
7. Henling CE, Carmichael MJ, Keats AS, Cooley DA (1985) Cardiac operations for congenital heart disease in children of Jehovahs witnesses. Thorac Cardiovasc Surg 89: 914—920
8. Kawaguchi A, Bergsland J, Subramanian S (1984) Total bloodless open heart surgery in the pediatric age group. Circulation 70: 1—30—37
9. Riegler R (1985) Probleme bei Verweigerung von Bluttransfusionen. Anaesthesist 34: 55—61
10. Ott DA, Cooley DA (1977) Cardiovascular Surgery in Jehovah's witnesses. Journal of the Amer Med Assoc 238: 1256—1258

Author's address:
Univ. Prof. Dr. B. Rigler
Univ. Klinik f. Chirurgie
Landeskrankenhaus Graz
Auenbruggerplatz
A-8036 Graz, Austria

Reduction of Homologous Blood Requirement During Myocardial Revascularization — Comparison of Four Different Techniques

H. P. Mitto, W. Dietrich, A. Barankay, J. A. Richter

Institute for Anesthesiology, German Heart Center, Munich, FRG

Introduction

The risks associated with blood transfusion force us to reduce homologous blood transfusions. Different methods have been described which permit the reduction of blood requirement in open-heart surgery. Because of the inhomogenity of patient groups investigated by others, it is difficult to compare these techniques and to judge their quantitative saving effect. We, therefore, investigated the effect of combined application of different methods on homologous blood requirement in selected homogenous patient groups.

Methods

In a prospective randomized study 100 male patients with good LV-function (EF > 50%) and preoperative hemoglobin (HGB) > 140 g/L were investigated. Patients scheduled for myocardial revascularization were assigned to four groups (25 in each). Patients with internal mammary artery grafts and extracorporeal circulation with a duration less than 45 min or more than 90 min were excluded.
Group   I: retransfusion of unprocessed oxygenator blood;
Group   II: cell saving (CS) of remaining oxygenator blood;
Group III: preoperative isovolemic hemodilution (HD) (10 ml/kg) + CS;
Group IV: HD + CS + shed mediastinal blood retransfusion.

Anesthetic, surgical, and perfusion techniques were comparable in all groups. Intra- and postoperative blood and fluid requirements and postoperative blood loss were recorded. HGB values were measured at nine predetermined times intra- and postoperatively.

ANOVA was used for statistics. Differences between groups were analyzed by the Bonferroni adjusted t-test. (* $p < 0.05$ vs group I; + $p < 0.05$ vs group II)

Results

Age, weight, preoperative HGB, duration of extracorporeal circulation and surgery, and number of coronary anastomoses were comparable in all groups. Blood loss was 647 ± 183 ml in group I, 657 ± 253 ml in group II, 890 ± 359 ml in group III (*+), and 698 ± 242 ml in group IV.

190

Blood requirement during hospitalization was 2066 ± 756 ml in group I, 1391 ± 964 ml in group II (*), 833 ± 599 ml in group III (*) and 409 ± 559 ml in group IV (* +). The use of blood-conservation techniques resulted in reductions of homologous blood requirements of 34%, 60%, and 80%, respectively, in groups II to IV, as compared with the requirement in group I.

During the hospital stay the following percentage of patients did not receive homologous blood or blood derivates: group I: 0%, group II: 8%, group III: 20% and group IV: 40%.

Values of HGB in the four groups showed no significant differences on discharge from ICU. Complications related to blood-saving methods were not observed.

Discussion

With retransfusion of autologous packed cells after extracorporeal circulation a rapid increase of hematocrit (HCT) and, therefore, a reduction of homologous blood requirement may be achieved. This is of clinical importance since low HCT and diminished oxygen transport capacity of blood may jeopardize myocardial oxygen supply [2, 3]. Preoperative HD and retransfusion of shed mediastinal blood make volume substitution with autologous blood possible. Diminished coagulation properties and low HCT play a secondary role in this context [1]. The question still remains as to what extent HCT may fall in the postoperative phase without deleterious effect on the patient's recovery.

Conclusion

Combined application of blood-saving methods leads to a marked reduction of homologous blood requirement during and after myocardial revascularization.

References

1. Dietrich W, Barankay A, Dilthey G, Mitto HP, Richter JA (1989) Reduction of blood utilization during myocardial revascularization. J Thorac Cardiovasc Surg 97: 213—219
2. Hagl S, Heimisch W, Meisner H, Mendler N (1977) The effect of hemodilution on regional myocardial function in the presence of coronary stenosis. Basic Res Cardiol 72: 344—364
3. Weisel RD, Charlesworth DC, Mickleborough LL, et al. (1984) Limitations of blood conservation. J Thorac Cardiovasc Surg 88: 26—38

Authors' address:
H. P. Mitto, M. D.
Institute for Anesthesiology
German Heart Center
Lothstraße 11
8000 München 2, FRG

IV. Pharmacological Methods for the Reduction of Blood Use in Cardiac Surgery

Platelet Dysfunction after Coronary Artery Bypass Surgery

K. H. Teoh, R. D. Weisel, J. Ivanov, S. J. Teasdale and M. F. X. Glynn

Divisions of Cardiovascular Surgery, Cardiac Anesthesia and Hematology of the Toronto Hospital, the University of Toronto and the Center for Cardiovascular Research

Summary:

Cardiopulmonary bypass induces platelet activation and dysfunction, resulting in platelet deposition and depletion. Reduced platelet numbers and abnormal function may contribute to postoperative bleeding. In addition, myocardial deposition of activated platelets may contribute to perioperative ischemic injury and early postoperative bypass graft occlusion. Dipyridamole (DIP) reduces platelet activation and may decrease postoperative bleeding, myocardial platelet depostion and perioperative ischemic injury.

A randomized trial was conducted in 58 patients (pts) undergoing coronary bypass surgery (CABG) to compare the effects of oral (n = 19) and intravenous (n = 21) dipyridamole to the results obtained in a control group (n = 18) which received no dipyridamole. Preoperative oral administration of dipyridamole resulted in lower plasma drug concentrations in the early postoperative period than whith perioperative intravenous administration (Oral 0.4 ± 0.2 µg/mL, IV 1.0 ± 0.2 µg/mL, p < 0.05). Postoperative platelet counts were highest in the patients receiving intravenous dipyridamole ($140 \pm 20 \times 10^9$/L), intermediate in those receiving oral dipyridamole ($120 \pm 15 \times 10^9$/L) and lowest in the control group ($100 \pm 25 \times 10^9$/L, p < 0.03). Postoperative blood loss was significantly reduced with both oral and intravenous dipyridamole (control 1.6 ± 0.3 L, oral 0.8 ± 0.2 L, IV 0.9 ± 0.2 L, p < 0.04).

A second randomized trial was conducted in an additional 40 pts undergoing CABG to evaluate the effects of dipyridamole on myocardial platelet and leukocyte deposition and the cardiac release of thromboxane. Twenty patients received dipyridamole perioperatively (0.24 mg/kg/hr IV). Autologous platelets and leukocytes were labeled with ^{111}In and ^{99}Tc respectively and were infused before release of the crossclamp. Myocardial biopsies were obtained after aortic declamping and indicated that platelets and leukocytes were deposited in the myocardium during reperfusion. Dipyridamole reduced both platelet (DIP $1,540 \pm 2100$ cells/mg, No DIP $14,500 \pm 33,000$ cells/mg) and leukocyte deposition (DIP 16 ± 32 cells/mg, No DIP 63 ± 110 cells/mg, p < 0.05). Cardiac release of thromboxane B_2 occurred in the early postoperative period and was reduced by dipyridamole (DIP 0.039 ± 0.16 µg/L, No DIP 0.27 ± 0.18 µg/L, p < 0.05).

In conclusion, dipyridamole preserved platelets and reduced postoperative bleeding and blood product transfusions in patients undergoing CABG Dipyridamole also reduced cardiac platelet deposition and thromboxane release and may reduce perioperative ischemic injury.

* Supported by the Heart and Stroke Foundation of Ontario (Grant AN 1553).

Platelets, leukocytes and reperfusion injury

Cardiac surgery and cardiopulmonary bypass provide a potent stimulus for platelet activation. Exposure of blood to the synthetic surfaces of the bypass circuit and blood-gas-interfaces injured endothelial surfaces induces platelet activation [1—4]. Activated platelets release their granular contents [4], increase thromboxane generation [2, 4], and produce intravascular aggregates [5] which may deposit in the microcirculation [6] or on foreign surfaces [3]. Platelet factors released during activation include platelet factor 4 (PF_4), beta thromboglobulin (B-TBG), fibrinopeptide A (FPA) and thromboxane A_2. Both PF_4 and B-BTG are markers of platelet activation and were released by the heart in patients with coronary artery disease when ischemia was induced [7—9]. Fibrinopeptide A is a vasoconstrictor which, in experimental studies, was shown to affect both the pulmonary and coronary circulation, affecting heart rate stroke volume [10] and vascular permeability [11]. FPA has also been implicated as a cause of ischemia during cardiopulmonary bypass [4]. Thromboxane A_2 is a product of arachidonic acid metabolism which increases platelet aggregability [12] and can produce profound coronary vasoconstriction leading to ischemic injury [13, 14]. Feinberg and colleagues have demonstrated platelet deposition in the canine myocardium after ischemic arrest [15] and after cardioplegia [16]. We have recently documented thromboxane-A_2 release from myocardium of coronary bypass patients after aorticcrossclamp release [17].

Many studies have demonstrated complement activation during cardiopulmonary bypass [18—20]. Complement components activate both platelets [21, 22] and white cells [23, 24]. Whitecell deposition has been implicated in the pathogenesis of pulmonary injury during cardiopulmonary bypass [20, 23, 25]. Whitecell deposition in the heart and superoxide cytotoxicity could contribute to postoperative reperfusion injury. Oxygen free radical scavengers (superoxide dismutase and catalase) have been shown to improve myocardial recovery after cardioplegic arrest [26—28].

Although the results of coronary bypass surgery are excellent, perioperative myocardial protection remains incomplete. In recent studies, we have demonstrated anaerobic myocardial metabolism during aortic occlusion and during reperfusion [29, 30]. Perioperative ischemic injury had no longterm sequelae in patients undergoing elective cardiac surgery, but incomplete perioperative myocardial protection could account for the increased incidence of ventricular dysfunction, myocardial infarction and death in highrisk patients [31]. Reperfusion injury potentiates intraoperative cellular damage. Intraoperative ischemia injures myocardial membranes and permits further cellular dysfunction during reperfusion. The pathogenesis of reperfusion injury remains obscure but myocardial deposition of activated platelets and leukocytes could potentiate reperfusion injury [15, 26, 28].

Pharmacologic interventions by platelet-inhibiting agents may prevent platelet activation and its deleterious consequences. Dipyridamole is a pyridopyrimidine compound which limits platelet activation, aggregation and granular release. The mechanism of action may be related to inhibition of platelet phosphodiesterase activity, increase in platelet cyclic adenosine monophosphate concentrations and decrease in platelet calcium mobilization [32, 33]. Dipyridamole preserves platelet adhesion and therefore does not inhibit platelet hemostatic function [34]. Chesebro and associates demonstrated improved early postoperative coronary bypass graft patency employing preoperative dipyridamole and postoperative dipyridamole and aspirin [35]. The mechanism for the beneficial effect was not determined by their study, but may be related to prevention of platelet deposition in small diseased coronary arteries and ischemic myocardium.

We report our experience at the Toronto General Hospital with dipyridamole myocardial platelet and white cell deposition.

Prevention of myocardial platelet and leukocyte deposition and thromboxane release with dipyridamole

We recently performed a prospective, randomized trial in patients undergoing elective coronary bypass surgery to assess the effects of dipyridamole on myocardial platelet deposition and thromboxane release [36].

Forty patients scheduled for elective coronary artery surgery were randomly assigned to receive dipyridamole (n = 20) or to serve as controls (n = 20). In the dipyridamole group, and intravenous infusion dipyridamole was instituted 20 h before surgery at dose of 0.24 mg/kg/h. The infusion was continued intra-operatively and for 24 h postoperatively. The control group received dipyridamole. Cardiopulmonary bypass was instituted using and asanguinous prime and a membrane oxygenator. Multidose cold blood cardioplegia was employed for myocardial protection. An average of 3.7 ± 1.0 bypass grafts were constructed per patient.

Arterial platelet and leukocyte counts during cardiopulmonary bypass were greater in the dipyridamole group, suggesting that dipyridamole preserved platelets and leukocytes. Myocardial cellular deposition was assessed by autogenous, radio-labelled platelets (^{111}In), leukocytes (^{99m}Tc) and erythrocytes (^{51}Cr). Full thickness left ventricular muscle biopsies were obtained 10, 20 and 30 min after aortic cross-clamp removal. The radioactivity of the specimens, presenting cellular deoposition, was measured in a gamma counter.

Both platelets and leukocytes were deposited in the myocardium following aortic declamping and reperfusion (Fig. 1). Platelet deposition increased exponentially during the reperfusion period and leukocyte deposition peaked at 20 min and fell at 30 min of reperfusion. The magnitude of myocardial platelet deposition was significantly reduced by dipyridamole (Fig. 1). Myocardial leukocyte deposition also tended to be less with dipyridamole.

We also measured arterial and coronary sinus blood concentrations of thromboxane B_2 and 6-keto-PGF$_{1\alpha}$ (the stable metabolites of thromboxane A_2 and prostacyclin) by radioimmunoassay to determine the cardiac release of these prostanoids. 6-keto-PGF$_{1\alpha}$ was released during cardiopulmonary bypass, but no further cardiac production of 6-keto-PGF$_{1\alpha}$ was noted after discontinuation of bypass (Fig. 2). Dipyridamole had no significant effect on cardiac 6-keto-PGF$_{1\alpha}$ release. However, cardiac thromboxane release was observed after crossclamp release and persisted during the first 5 h of reperfusion. With dipyirdamole, the reduction in myocardial platelet deposition was associated with a decrease in cardiac thromboxane release during reperfusion (Fig. 2).

To assess platelet and leukocyte deposition in the severely ischemic myocardium, we employed a canine model of region ischemia, followed by reperfusion during cardioplegic arrest on cardiopulmonary bypass to simulate urgent coronary revascularization for acute myocardial ischemia [37]. Four dogs received dipyridamole (50 mg IV bolus preoperatively and 50 mg/h perioperatively) and four dogs served as controls. Severe regional myocardial ischemia was induced by snare occlusion of

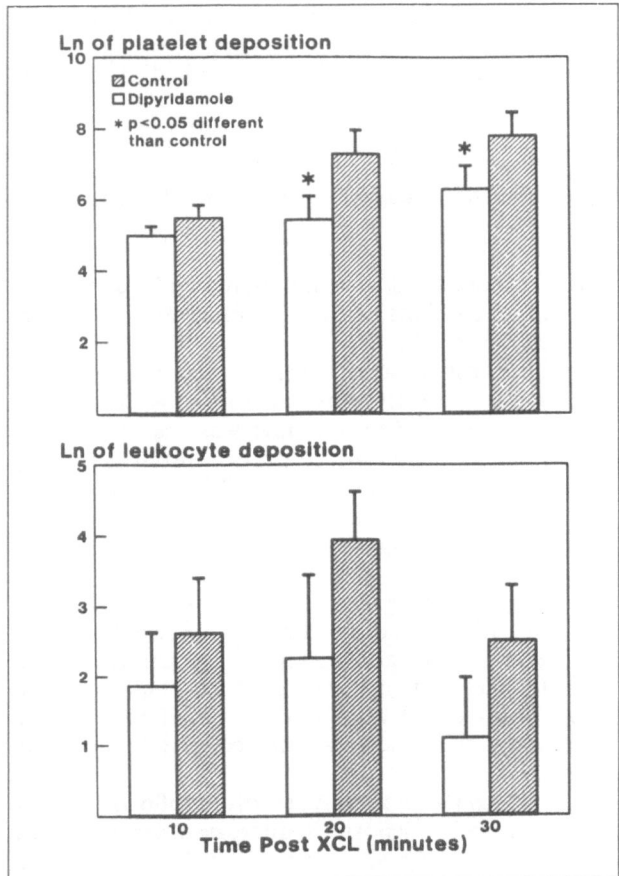

Fig. 1. The natural logarithm (Ln) of myocardial platelet and leukocyte deposition. Dipyridamole reduced myocardial platelet deposition.

the left anterior descending artery (LAD) for 45 min followed by cardiopulmonary bypass, cardioplegic arrest for 60 min and reperfusion. Platelet deposition (by radiolabelled platelets) was four times greater in the LAD region than in the non-ischemic circumflex region of the heart at 10, 20, 30 and 60 min of reperfusion (Fig. 3). Platelet deposition increased with time and was maximal at 30 min of reperfusion in the LAD region and 20 min of reperfusion in the circumflex region. Platelet deposition in the respiratory diaphragm was 30 times less than in the LAD region, suggesting that cardiopulmonary bypass was not the only factor inducing platelet deposition. Dipyridamole reduced platelet deposition significantly in both regions, but the magnitude of reduction was greater in the ischemic LAD region (Fig. 3).

Leukocyte deposition was also observed during reperfusion in the myocardium. The respiratory diaphragm had 500 times less leukocyte deposition than the LAD region of the heart. Dipyridamole reduced leukocyte deposition in the ischemic LAD, but not in the non-ischemic circumflex region. We found platelet and leukocyte deposition to be greatest in the subendocardium where vulnerability to ischemia was the greatest.

Postoperative bleeding and blood transfusion

Patients undergoing cardiac surgery with cardiopulmonary bypass are at risk of significant postoperative bleeding. Excessive bleeding remains a prominent complication after cardiac surgery, contributing to its mortality and morbidity. Re-exploration is required in 3—5% of patients [38]. In addition, most patients require blood-component therapy to correct postoperative anemia and coagulation defects. Administration of blood products exposes the patient to the risk of transfusion-related reactions and infections [39]. Since more than 200,000 cardiac operations are performed annually in North America [40], the magnitude of this problem is substantial. Interventions intended to reduce postoperative bleeding may reduce the mortality and morbidity of cardiac operations and decrease the demand for blood products.

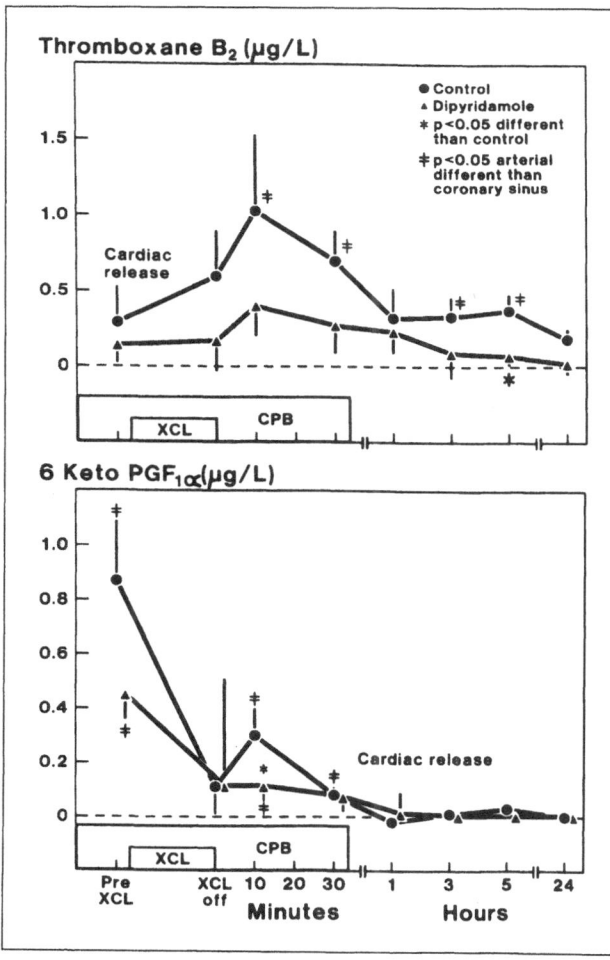

Fig. 2. Myocardial thromboxane B_2 and 6-keto-$PGF_{1\alpha}$ release. Significant thromboxane B_2 release was observed during reperfusion and in the early postoperative period in the control group, but not in the dipyridamole group. 6-keto-$PGF_{1\alpha}$ release was found during cardiopulmonary bypass in both groups.

199

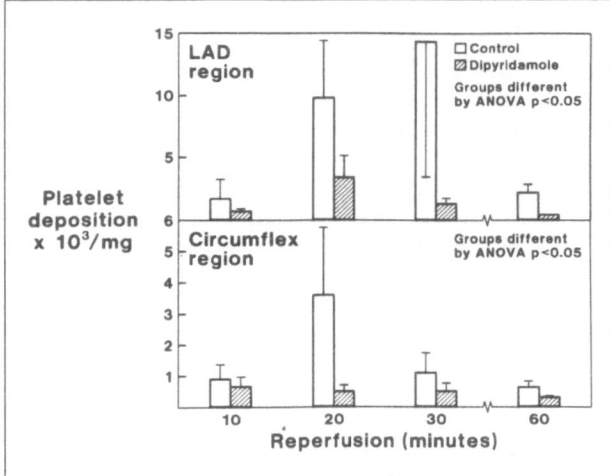

Fig. 3. Platelet deposition is depicted in the left anterior descending (LAD) and circumflex regions of the canine heart following crossclamp release (reperfusion). Platelet deposition in the LAD region was four times greater than in the circumflex region. Dipyridamole significantly reduced platelet deposition in both the LAD and circumflex regions.

Multiple complex changes in the hemostatic mechanism have been described after cardiopulmonary bypass. Some of these hemostatic defects may increase the hemorrhagic tendency [38]. Abnormal bleeding after cardiopulmonary bypass my be the result of excessive fibrinolysis and/or a transient impairment of platelet function.

Fibrinolysis during cardiac surgery has been postulated as a cause of postoperative bleeding [41—43]. Release of plasminogen activator may occur during manipulation of the heart [44] and secondarily, to activation of the coagulation and complement systems. The magnitude of fibrinolytic hemorrhage has been estimated to be responsible for 12—25% of the bleeding episodes [45, 46]. Antifibrinolytic agents such as aprotinin and transexamic acid have been employed to prevent or treat fibrinolytic hemorrhage following cardiac surgery with favorable results [47—50].

Transient impairment of platelet function mediated by platelet activation during passage through the oxygenator apparatus may promote postoperative bleeding. The etiology of this platelet dysfunction is unknown, but may be due to a transient depletion of a functional platelet component, generation of an unidentified labile platelet inhibitor [51], or a reversible membrane abnormality. Evidence for a membrane abnormality includes the results of in vitro studies which demonstrated that platelets exposed to the oxygenator apparatus in a recirculating system had reduced binding to fibrinogen [52, 53].

Fibrinogen receptors are part of glycoproteins IIb/IIIa complex, a major constituent of platelet membranes. In addition, patients undergoing cardiopulmonary bypass display a defect in ristocetin-induced platelet aggregation [54], suggesting the involvement of Von Willebrand factor in the hemostatic defect, since Von Willebrand factor is required for ristocetin-induced aggregation. Thrombocytopenia, largely the result of hemodilution, may exacerbate the bleeding tendency induced by platelet dysfunction.

The degree of impairment of platelet function is proportional to the duration of cardiopulmonary bypass and is likely related to the level of hypothermia [55]. In most patients, the platelet dysfunction is rapidly reversible after the completion of cardiopulmonary bypass, but there may be abnormal and excessive bleeding in patients in whom the functional platelet defect persists longer. Pharmacologic agents may modify this acquired platelet defect and reduce postoperative bleeding.

Desmopressin acetate (DDAVP) is a synthetic vasopressin analogue that lacks vasoconstrictor activity. DDAVP increases the plasma concentrations and activity of high molecular weight forms of factor VIII, Von Willebrand factor which is necessary for adhesion of platelets to subendothelial connective tissue [56]. Czer [57] and Salzmann [58] have reported shortening of bleeding time and reduction of postoperative bleeding in patients undergoing cardiac surgery.

Dipyridamole limits platelet activation, aggregation and granular release. Dipyridamole has been employed to improve postoperative coronary bypass graft patency [35] but its use as an agent to preserve platelets and reduce postoperative bleeding has not been previously demonstrated. We evaluated the effects of dipyridamole on postoperative platelet preservation and bleeding in a prospective, randomized clinical trial [59].

Platelet preservation and reduction of postoperative bleeding with dipyridamole

Fifty-eight patients undergoing elective coronary bypass surgery at the Toronto General Hospital were randomized to receive intravenous dipyridamole as described (n = 21), oral dipyridamole according to the Chesebro protocol [35] (n = 19) or no dipyridamole (n = 18). Since platelet counts may be affected by the type of oxygenator employed, patients were stratified to receive either a bubble (n = 25) or a membrane (n = 33) oxygenator to provide an equal number of each oxygenator in each treatment group.

Postoperative arterial platelet counts were lowest in the control group, intermediate in the oral dipyridamole group and highest in the intravenous dipyridamole group (Fig. 4). In the control group, only 25% (5/18 patients) had any postoperative platelet counts within the normal range ($150-350 \times 10^9$ platelets per liter at our institution) compared to 50% (9/19 patients) in the oral dipyridamole group and 71% (15/21 patients) in the intravenous dipyridamole group ($p < 0.05$). The intravenous dipyridamole group had significantly higher platelet counts on postoperative days 2 and 3 than either the oral dipyridamole or the control group, which had the lowest counts.

The superior platelet preservation by intravenous dipyridamole compared to oral dipyridamole may have resulted from the higher and more stable dipyridamole drug levels achieved wiht intravenous delivery (Fig. 5). Both oral and intravenous dipyridamole administration resulted in similar plasma drug levels (measured by high performance liquid chromatography) preoperatively. However, plasma levels fell during cardiopulmonary bypass and remained low in the early postoperative period in the oral dipyridamole group, whereas drug levels were maintained by intravenous administration. We also measured salicylate levels on the first postoperative day and found undetectable levels in 16 patients and very low levels in three patients (0.07 ± 0.2 mmol/L) despite aspirin administration into the nasogastric tube 11 hours postoperatively. This suggests that the platelet effects we observed were solely due to dipyridamole.

Postoperative blood loss and transfusion requirements were related to platelet preservation. Postoperative blood loss was greatest in the control group (1.6 ± 0.3 L) and was reduced 42% with oral and 46% with intravenous dipyridamole (p

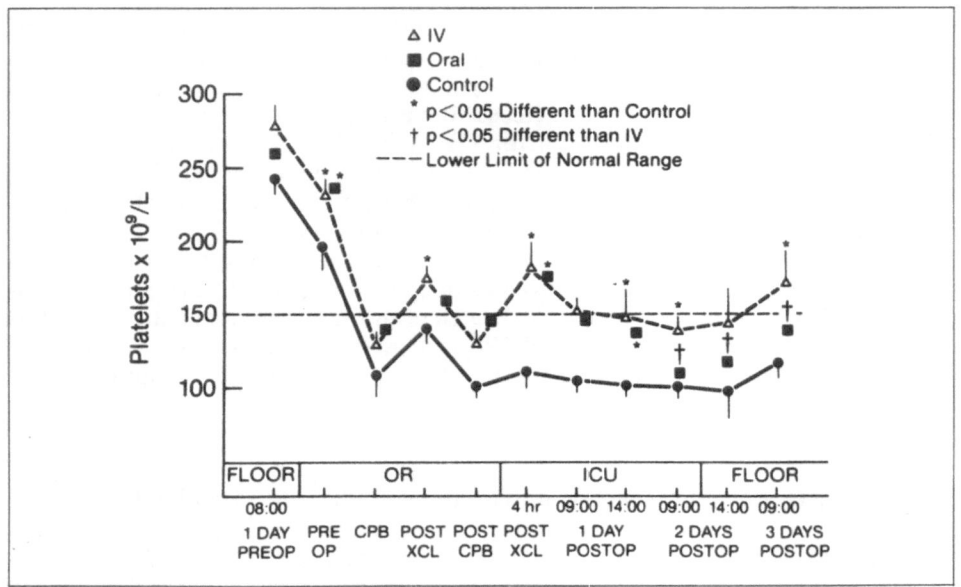

Fig. 4. Arterial platelet counts are illustrated. Dipyridamole preserved circulating platelets. Platelet counts were lowest in the control group, intermediate in the oral group, and highest in the intravenous dipyridamole group.

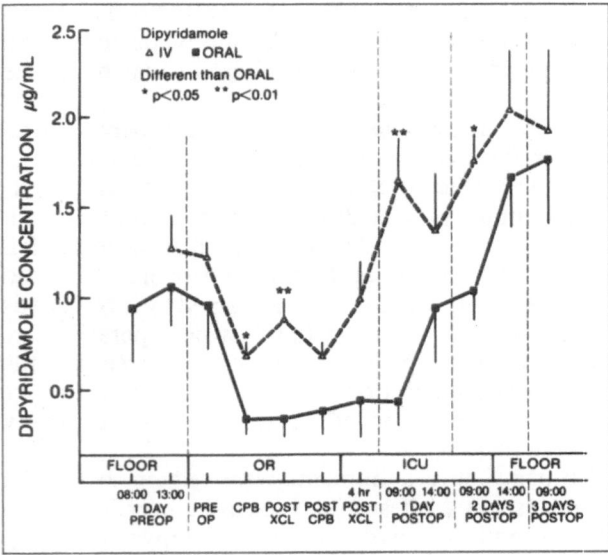

Fig. 5. Plasma dipyridamole concentrations are illustrated. Intravenous administration resulted in more stable drug levels perioperatively.

202

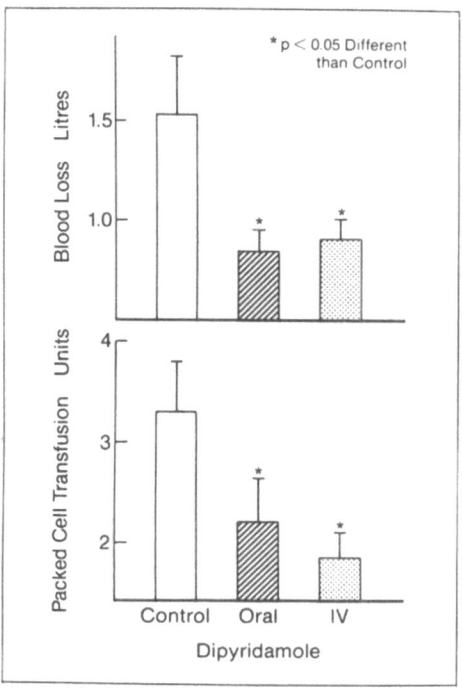

Fig. 6. Both oral and intravenous dipyridamole reduced total blood loss and packed red cell transfusions.

< 0.05, Fig. 6). Postoperative packed red cell transfusions were delivered to maintain the hemoglobin above 100 g/L. Packed red cell transfusions were significantly reduced by both oral and intravenous dipyridamole. Both postoperative bleeding and amount of red cells transfused correlated significantly with the postoperative platelet counts. A multivariate analysis indicated that two factors independently influenced postoperative platelet counts and bleeding. Platelet preservation and reduction in postoperative bleeding were affected by the use of a membrane oxygenator and dipyridamole [60]. We found reduction of postoperative bleeding least with a bubbler oxygenator and no dipyridamole, intermediate with either a membrane oxygenator or dipyridamole, intermediate with either a membrane oxygenator or dipyridamole and optimal when both a membrane oxygenator and dipyridamole were employed (Fig. 7).

Conclusions and recommendations

Platelet activation occurred during cardiac surgery and cardiopulmonary bypass. Myocardial platelet and leukocyte deposition with thromboxane release occurred despite apparently adequate myocardial protection. Myocardial platelet and leukocyte deposition had no serious sequelae in patients undergoing elective surgery, but may contribute to ischemia-reperfusion injury and increased mortality and morbidity in high risk patients. Dipyridamole reduced platelet activation, reduced myocardial cellular deposition and thromboxane release. This may be the mechanism

203

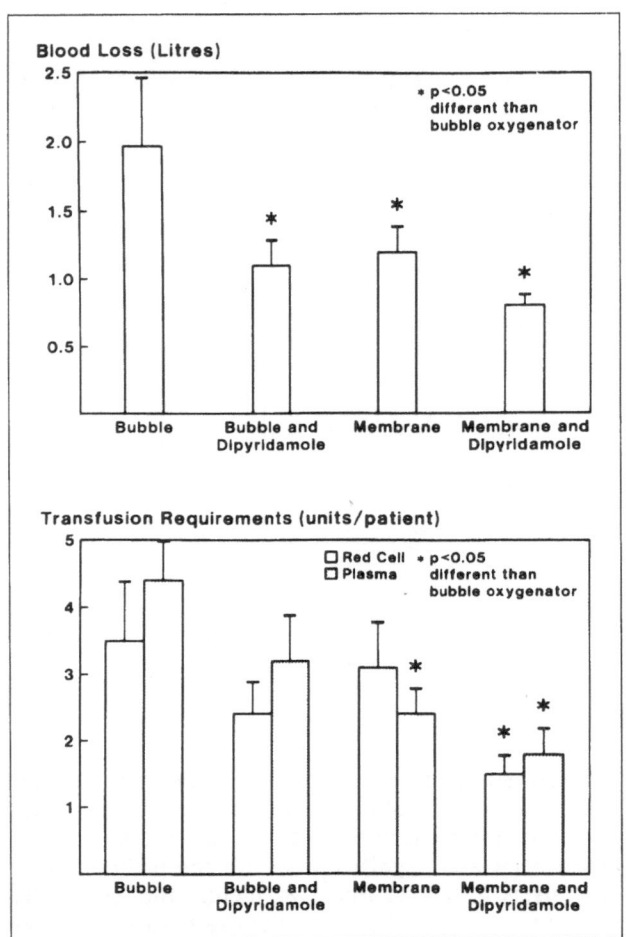

Fig. 7. Postoperative blood loss and transfusion requirements were reduced with the use of a membrane oxygenator or dipyridamole. Optimal reduction in blood loss was achieved with a membrane oxygenator and dipyridamole together.

for improved bypass graft patency. Dipyridamole may reduce ischemia-reperfusion injury following high risk coronary revascularization. Dipyridamole also preserved platelets and reduced postoperative bleeding and transfusion requirements. Intravenous dipyridamole provided more stable drug levels perioperatively and preserved platelets better than oral dipyridamole. Intravenous dipyridamole may be required to reduce postoperative bleeding in high-risk patients.

References

1. Harker LA, Malpass TW, Bronson HE, Hessel EA II, Slichter SJ (1980) Mechanism of abnormal bleeding in patients undergoing cardiopulmonary bypass: acquired transient platelet dysfunction associated with selective-granule release. Blood 56: 824--834
2. Addonizio VP Jr, Smith JB, Strauss JF III, Colman RW, Edmunds LH (1980) Thromboxane

systhetis and platelet secretion during cardiopulmonary bypass with a bubble oxygenator. J Thorac Cardiovasc Surg 79: 91—96

3. Edmunds LH, Ellison N, Colman RW, et al. (1982) Platelet function during cardiac operation: comparison of membrane and bubble oxygenators. J Thorac Cardiovasc Surg 83: 805—812

4. Davies GC, Sobel M, Salzman EW. (1980) Elevated plasma fibrinopeptide A and thromboxane A_2 levels during cardiopulmonary bypass. Circulation 61: 808—814

5. Dutton RC, Edmunds LH, Hutchinson JC, Roe BB. (1974) Platelet aggregate emboli produced in patients during cardiopulmonary bypass with membrane and bubble oxygenators and blood filters. J Thorac Cardiovasc Surg 67: 25

6. Allerdyce DB, Yoshida SH, Ashmore RG (1980) The importance of microembolism in the pathogenesis of organ dysfunction caused by prolonged use of the pump oxygenator. J Thorac Cardiovasc Surg 62: 936

7. DeBoer AC, Turpie AGG, But RW, Johnston RV, Genton E (1982) Platelet release and thromboxane systhesis in symptomatic coronary artery disease. Circulation 66: 327—333

8. Sobel M, Salzman EW, Davies GC et al. (1981) Circulating platelet products in unstable angina pectoris. 63: 300—306

9. Smitherman TC, MIlam M, Woo J, Willerson JT, Frenkel EP (1981) Elevated beta thromboglobulin in peripheral venous blood of patients with acute myocardial ischemia. Direct evidence for enhanced platelet reactivity in vivo. Am J Cardiol 48: 395—402

10. Baylet T, Clements J, Oshahr A (1967) Pulmonary and circulatory effects of fibrinopeptides. Circ Res 21: 469—474

11. Copley AL, Haning JP, Luchini BW (1967) On the capillary permeability enchancing activity of isolated fibrinonopeptides and their role in the physiology of the blood capillary wall. Bibl Anat 9: 475—477

12. Mehta J, Mehta P, Pepine CJ (1978) Platelet aggregation in aortic and coronary venous blood in patients with and without coronary artery disease. Role of tachycardia, stress and propanolol. Circulation 58: 881—886

13. Needleman P, Kulkarni PS, Raz A (1977) Coronary tone modulation: formation and actions of prostaglandins, endoperoxides, and thromboxanes (1977) Science 195: 409—415

14. Shimamoto T, Kobayashi M, Takahashi T, Numano F, Morooka S (1977) Myocardial infarction experimentally induced by thromboxane A_2. Abstract. Circulation 56 (suppl III): 3—23

15. Feinberg H, Rosenbaum DS, Levitsky S, Silverman NA, Kohler J, Le Brenton G (1982) Platelet deposition after surgically induced myocardial ischemia: An etiologic factor for reperfusion injury. J Thorac Cardiovasc Surg 84: 815—822

16. Rosenbaum D, Levitsky S, Silverman N et al. (1983) Cardioplegia does not prevent reperfusion injury induced by intracoronary platelet deposition. Circulation 58 (suppl II): 102—106

17. Teoh KH, Fremes SE, Weisel RD et al. (1987) Cardiac release of prostacyclin and thromboxane A_2 during coronary bypass surgery. J Thorac Cardiovasc Surg 93: 120—126

18. Chenoweth DE, Cooper SW, Hugh TE, Stewart RW, Blackstone EH, Kirklin JW (1981) Complement activation during CPB N Engl J Med 304: 497—503

19. Kirklin JK, Westaby S, Blackstone EH, Kirklin JW, Chenoweth DE, Pacifico AD (1983) Complement and the damaging effects of CPB. J Thorac Cardiovasc Surg 86: 845—857

20. Hammerschmidt DE, Stroncek DF, Bowers TK et al. (1981) Complement activation and neutropenia occurring during cardiopulmonary bypass. J Thorac Cardiovasc Surg 81: 370—377

21. Pfueller Sl, Lischer EF (1974) Studies of the mechanisms of human platelet release reaction induced by immunologic stimuli. I. Complement-dependent and complement-independent reactions. J Immunol 112: 1201—1210

22. Wautier JL, Ollier-Hartmann MP, Kadera H, Cohen F, Hartmann L, Caen JP (1981) First component of complement and thrombosis. Thromb Haemost 45: 247—251

23. Craddock PR, Hammerschmidt D, White JG, Dalmasso AP, Jacob HS (1977) Complement (C5a)-induced granulocyte aggregation in vitro. A possible mechanism of complement-mediated leukostasis and leukopenia. J Clin Invest 60: 260—264

24. Webster RO, Hong SR, Johnston RB Jr, Henson PM (1980) Biological effects of the human complement fragments C5a and C5a (des Arg) on neutrophil function. Immunopharm 2: 201—219

25. Fountain SW, Martin BA, Busclow CE, Cooper JD (1980) Pulmonary leukostasis and its relationship to pulmonary dysfunction in sheep and rabbits. Circ Res 46: 175—180

26. Gardner TJ, Stewart JR, Casale AS, Downey JM, Chambers DE (1983) Reduction of myocardial ischemic injury with oxygen-derived free radical scavengers. Surgery 94: 423—427
27. Shlafer M, Kane PF, Kirsh MM (1982) Superoxide dismutase plus catalase enhances the efficacy of hypothermic cardioplegia to protect the globally ischemic, reperfused heart. J Thorac Cardiovasc Surg 83: 830—839
28. Stewart JR, Blackwell WH, Crute SL, Loughlin V, Greenfield LJ, Hess ML (1983) Inhibition of surgically induced ischemia/reperfusion injury by oxygen free radical scavengers. J Thorac Cardiovasc Surg 86: 262—272
29. Fremes, SE, Chrsitakis GT, Weisel RD, Mickle DAG, Madonik MM, Ivanov J, Harding R, Seawright SJ, Houle S, McLaughlin PR, Baird RJ (1984) A clinical trial of blood and crystalloid cardioplegia. J Thorac Cardiovasc Surg 88: 726
30. Teoh KH, Mickle DAG, Weisel RD, Madonik MM, Ivanov J, Hardling RD, Romaschin AD, Wilson GJ, Mullen JC (1989) The effect of lactate infusion on myocardial metabolism and ventricular function following ischemia and cardioplegia. Can J Cardiol 5: 90—116
31. Teoh KH, Christakis GT, Weisel RD, Katz AM, Tong CP, Mickleborough LL, Scully HE, Baird RJ, Goldman BS (1987) Increased risk of urgent revascularization. J Thorac Cardiovasc Surg 93: 291
32. Best LC, McGuire MB, Jones PBB, et al (1979) Mode of action of dipyridamole on human platelets. Thromb Res 16: 367—377
33. Mills DCB, Smith JB (1971) The influence on platelet aggregation of drugs that affect the accumulation of adenosine 3:5-cyclic monophosphate in platelets. Biochem J 121: 185—196
34. Emmons PR, Harrison MJG, Honour AJ, Mitchell JRA (1965) Effect of dipyridamole on human platelet behaviour. Lancet 2: 603—606
35. Chesebro JH, Clements IP, Fuster V, et al (1982) A platelet-inhibitor-drug trial in coronary artery bypass operations: Benefit of perioperative dipyridamole and aspirin therapy on early postoperative vein graft patency. N Engl J Med 307: 73—78
36. Teoh KH, Christakis GT, Weisel RD, Mullen JC, Madonik MM, Invanov J, Henderson MJ, Warbick-Cerone A, Johnston LG, Mee AV, Wong PY, Reilly PA, Glynn MFX (1986) Prevention of myocardial platelet deposition and thromboxane release with dipyridamole. Circulation 74 (suppl III): 145—152
37. Teoh KH, Chrsitakis GT, Weisel RD, Madonik MM, Ivanov J, Warbick-Cerone A, Johnston LG, Cawthorn RH, Mullen JC, Glynn MFX, Wilson GJ, Salerno TA (1987) Dipyridamole reduced myocardial platelet and leukocyte deposition following ischemia and cardioplegia. J Surg Res 42: 642—652
38. Bachmann F, McKenna R, Cole ER, Najafi H (1975) The homostatic mechanism after openheart surgy. I. Studies on plasma coagulation factors and fibrinolysis in 512 patients after extracorporeal circulation. J Thorac Cardiovasc Surg 70: 76—85
39. Bove JR (1987) Transfusion-associated hepatitis and AIDS (1987) N Engl J Med 317: 242—246
40. Kennedy RH, McGoon DC, Smith HC, Kurland LT (1985) Trends in cardiac surgery in the United States.- N Engl J Med 312: 119—120
41. Bick RL (1985) Hemostasis defects associated with cardiac surgery prosthetic devices and other extracorporeal circuits. Semin Throm Hemostasis 11: 249—280
42. Kukuk O, Kwaan HC, Frederickson J, Wade L, Green D (1986) Increased fibrinolysis in patients undergoing cardiopulmonary bypass operations. AM J Hematol 23: 223—229
43. Umlas J (1967) Fibrinolysis and disseminated intravascular coagulation in open heart surgery. Transfusion 16: 460—463
44. Mayer M, Finci Z, Chaouat M (1986) Suppression of plasminogen activator activity by dexamethasone in cultured cardiac myocytes. J Mol Cell Cardiol 18: 1117—1124
45. Gilbert JW, Bronson WR, Brecher G (1964) Incidence of bleeding in cardiac surgery with extracorporeal circulation. Ann NY Aca Sci 115: 302—304
46. Tice DA, Reed GE, Clauss RH, Worth MH (1963) Hemorrhage due to fibrinolysis occurring with open heart surgery. J Thorac Cardiovasc Surg 46: 673—679
47. Van Oeveren W, Jansen NJG, Bistrup BP et al. (1987) Effects of aprotinin on hemostatic mechanisms during cardiopulmonary bypass. Ann Thor Surg 44: 640—645
48. Royston D, Bidstrup BP, Taylor KM, Sapsford RN (1987) Effect of aprotinin on need for blood transfusion after repeat open-heart surgery. Lancet II: 1289—1291

206

49. Bidstrup BP, Royston D, Taylor KM, Sapsford RN (1987) Effect of aprotinin on need for blood transfusion in patients with septic endocarditis having open-heart surgery. Lancet I: 366—367
50. Horrow JC, Hlavacek J, Strong MD, et al (1990) Prophylactic tranexamic acid decreases bleeding after cardiac operations. J Thorac Cardiovasc Surg 99: 70—74
51. Addonizo VP Jr, Strauss JF III, Colman RW, Edmunds LH Jr (1979) Effects of prostaglandin E_1 on platelet loss during in vivo and in vitro extracorporeal circulation with a bubble oxygenator. J Thorac Cardiovasc Surg 77: 119
52. Musial J, Niewiarowski S, Hershock D, Morinelli TA, Colman RW, Edmunds LH Jr. (1985) Loss of fibrinogen receptors from the platelet surface during simulated extracorporeal circulation. J Lab Clin Med 105: 514—522
53. Gluszko P, Rucinski B, Musial J, et al. (1987) Fibrinogen receptors in platelet adhesion to surfaces of extracorporeal circuit. Am J Physiol 252 (Heart Circ Physiol 21): H 615—621
54. Mammen EF, Koets MH, Washington BC, et al. (1985) Hemostasis changes during cardiopulmonary bypass surgery. Semin Thromb Hemost 11: 281—292
55. Harker LA (1986) Bleeding after cardiopulmonary bypass. N Engl J Med 314: 1446—1448
56. Ruggeri ZM, Mannucci PM, Lombardi R, Federici AB, Zimmerman TS (1982) Multimeric composition of factor VIII/von Willebrand factor following administration of DDAVP: implications for pathophysiology and therapy of von Willebrand's disease subtypes. Blood 59: 1272—1278
57. Czer L, Bateman T, Gray R, et al. Prospective trial of DDAVP in treatment of severe platelet dysfunction and hemorrhage after cardiopulmonary bypass. Circulation 72: 130
58. Salzman E, Weinstein M, Weintraub E, et al. (1986) Treatment with desmopressin acetate to reduce blood loss after cardiac surgery. N Engl J Med 314: 1402—1406
59. Teoh KH, Christakis GT, Weisel RD, Wong PY, Ivanov J, Madonik MM, Levitt DS, Reilly PA, Rosenfeld JM, Glynn MFX (1988) Dipyridamole preserved platelets and reduced blood loss after cardiopulmonary bypass. J Thorac Cardiovasc Surg 96: 332—341
60. Teoh KH, Christakis GT, Weisel RD, Madonik MM, Ivanov J, Wong PY, Mee AV, Levitt D, Benak A, Reilly PA, Glynn MFX. (1987) Blood conservation with membrane oxygenators and dipyridamole. Ann Thorac Surg 44: 40—47

Author's address:
Richard D. Weisel, M. D
Cardiovascular Surgery,
Toronto General Hospital,
200 Elizabeth Street
Eaton North 13—224
Toronto, Ontario
Canada

Clinical Effectiveness of Aprotinin in Heart Surgery

D. Royston

Consultant in Cardiothoracic Anaesthesia, Harefield Hospital, Harefield, Middlesex and Visiting Scientific Worker, Divisions of Anaesthesia and Vascular Biology, Clinical Research Centre, Harrow, Middlesex, U.K.

Introduction

The recent interest in blood-borne infections from donor blood has brought the subject of blood conservation to the attention of all surgeons, but particularly to cardiac surgeons.

In 1987, we described that a dramatic reduction in blood loss and blood usage could be achieved in patients having reoperation cardiac surgery by the use of aprotinin (Trasylol, Bayer A.G., FRG) in a large dose given over the period of surgery and bypass [1]. The reduction in postoperative bleeding was sufficient to ensure that over half of a group of patients having these complex reoperations received no donor blood; such patients otherwise would normally receive 2 to 8 units of donor blood. The purpose of this article is to review the background to this and subsequent papers in this symposium concerned with the use of aprotinin and to discuss the efficacy data collected thus far in cardiac surgical practice, concentrating on controlled double blind studies conducted in patients having non urgent primary surgery for aorto-coronary bypass grafting (CABG). These aspects are also discussed in other articles [2, 3] which have been recently published.

Background

Chemistry

Aprotinin is a basic (pK 10) polypeptide comprised of 58 amino acid residues and with a molecular weight of 6512 Daltons. The sequence biochemical structure and biophysical characteristics have been described and categorised [4]. Aprotinin is naturally occurring and was independently discovered and isolated from bovine lymph nodes by Kraut et al. in 1930 [5], who identified it as a kallikrein "inactivator", and by Kunitz and Northrop in 1936 [6], who defined its ability as a trypsin inhibitor in a preparation obtained from bovine pancreas. Aprotinin is a member of a family of serpins (serine protease inhibitors) which, as the name implies, are able to inhibit a range of proteases which have serine residues at their active site. Native aprotinin has this effect by forming reversible stoichiometric enzyme-inhibitor complexes between the active serine and the lysine residue found in position 15 of the aprotinin molecule. The concentration of aprotinin required to inhibit naturally occuring proteases such as trypsin, plasmin, tissue and plasma kallikrein has been documented in pure systems and varies between very low concentrations to inhibit trypsin to about 4 μMol to inhibit plasma kallikrein [4].

As a polypeptide, aprotinin is inactive when given orally and needs to be given by the intravenous route. The half-life in the plasma is biphasic with an initial elimination half-life of about 2 h. It follows that the compound has to be given by continuous infusion if the plasma concentration is to be maintained.

Its activity is expressed in "Kallikrein Inactivator Units" or KIU. The conversion factors are, therefore, that 1 milligram of protein is equivalent to 7143 KIU or 100 000 KIU is 14 mg protein. One µMol of aprotinin is 46.5 KIU/ml.

Aprotinin is available for human use as a preservative-free solution of 10 000 KIU/ml in 50 ml flasks under the trade name Trasylol (Bayer aG, Leverkusen, FRG).

Background to and results of pilot study

Our initial experience with aprotinin during open-heart surgery was not intended to investigate its use as an agent to prevent bleeding, but to prevent the damaging effects of extracorporeal circulation on certain tissues and organs, specifically the lung and pulmonary circulation. In particular, we wished to try to minimise kallikrein and complement activation and thereby to prevent cell activation. Our previous studies had shown that it was possible to demonstrate an increase in solute flux into and from the lungs of patients having open-heart surgery [7, 8]. In addition, there was evidence for increased oxygen-derived free radical activity, probably derived from neutrophils [9], and that there was a close relationship between the degree of pulmonary circulation free radical activity and protein leak into the lung [10]. A meeting on the use of Trasylol in cardiac and vascular surgery was held in Luxembourg in May of 1984, and at that meeting it was suggested that some of the damaging effects of cardiac surgery related to the cell activation outlined above and discussed [2, 3] could be reduced or abolished.

The rationale for this idea was that the contact of blood with the foreign surface of the oxygenator would stimulate a large number of "inflammatory cascades" which can act through humoral or cellular mechanisms, but which are ultimately controlled by amplification cascades of proteolytic enzymes, the vast majority of which are serine proteases.

During the period of extracorporeal circulation, the only inhibition of these potentially deleterious cascades is the routine administration of heparin given to inhibit the intrinsic pathway and prevent blood clotting by activating the naturally occuring serine protease inhibitor, antithrombin III. The hypothesis was that other limbs of these cascades particularly involved with complement activation and kinin release could also be blocked by giving reasonable amounts of an appropriate antiprotease. Aprotinin seemed a reasonable compound to try in this situation as it is the only serine antiprotease which is not only effective, but also has a sufficiently low toxicity to allow its use in humans in the high doses thought to be required to inhibit kallikrein. The concentration of aprotinin thought necessary to block the actions of kallikrein are about 4 µMol (200 KIU/ml of plasma). Based on studies of the use of continuous infusions of aprotinin in polytrauma patients [11], a dosage scheme was developed for use in cardiac surgery aimed at achieving this concentration of 200 KIU/ml throughout the period of extracorporeal circulation. The dose regime suggested was to give 2×10^6 KIU (280 mg) as a loading dose over a 20-min period after induction of anaesthesia and to follow this with a continuous infusion of 500 000 KIU (70 mg) an hour until the patient was returned to the intensive care unit. To overcome the dilution effect of the crystalloid prime in the oxygenator a further 1×10^6 KIU (140 mg) was added to this prime volume. The study was designed as a pilot investigation and, therefore, was not randomized — nor was it blinded to the observers. All the patients had CABG performed by one surgeon (B. P. Bidstrup) and one anaesthetist (the author DR). At the time of surgery it was obvious that whatever the biochemical and haematological changes resulting from the aprotinin infusion, the most striking effect was a reduction in bleeding which was, until then, a normal consequence of cardiopulmonary bypass. Certain results of this study have been published [12] and showed that there was a significant reduction in the blood loss into the postoperative drains in the day following surgery in those patients given the trial drug. The reduction was from a mean of 674 ml in the 11 patients designated as the control population and 357 ml in the 11 treated patients.

Analysis of plasma samples for aprotinin concentrations showed that the target kallikrein inhibiting concentration of about 200 KIU/ml was not achieved throughout the time of bypass and that the addition of the oxygenator prime volume produced a greater fall in concentration than predicted (shown in Fig. 1). It was subsequently decided that the addition to the prime volume be increased to a total of 2×10^6 KIU (280 mg) while maintaining the rest of the regime as outlined above. This has then been the dose regime used for all the subsequent studies to be discussed below.

Because of the foreign nature of aprotinin and earlier reports of anaphylactoid reactions to the drug the author has always given a "test dose" of 2 to 5 ml of solution (20 000 to 50 000 KIU) prior to administering the remainder of the loading dose. Thus far the author has observed no adverse effects on cardiovascular variables using this regime.

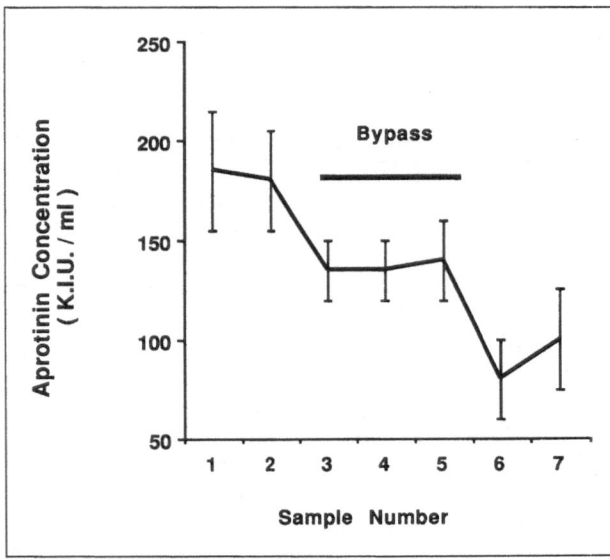

Fig. 1. Plasma concentrations of aprotinin obtained during pilot study (from [12]). Analysis of aprotinin concentrations was performed by Drs. M. Jochum and W. Muller-Esterl in Munich. Samples are from 1) after the infusion of the loading dose; 2) following sternotomy; 3) after 5 min of bypass; 4) following removal of the aortic cross clamp and reperfusion of the lungs; 5) at the end of the bypass; 6) 10 min after administration of protamine; 7) prior to transfer to the intensive care unit.

Studies of efficacy in open-heart surgery

Methods and measurements

All results from the London studies given below were performed using as standard a technique of anaesthesia and bypass as possible. The operations were performed by the same team of surgeons and anaesthetists.

Premedication was with papaveretum and scopolamine. Anaesthesia was standardized to include intermittent positive pressure ventilation with nitrous oxide and oxygen supplemented with a narcotic analgesic and, if necessary, a volatile agent, typically halothane. Bovine lung heparin (300 I.U./Kg) was injected prior to cannulation of the aorta and right atrium. Automatic clotting time (ACT) (Haemocron) was measured every 30 min and further heparin was administered if this ACT fell below 400 s. In all patients a Harvey 1700 (Bard Ltd, UK) bubble oxygenator was used and was primed with 1700—2000 ml of Hartmann's solution and 25 mM sodium bicarbonate. Bypass flows of 2.4 l/min/m2 were obtained with a minimally occlusive roller pump (Sarns Inc. Kalamazoo, Michigan, USA). Systemic hypothermia to 28—30 °C was maintained during the period of aortic occlusion. Myocardial preservation during aortic occlusion was maintained with St. Thomas's Hospital cardioplegic solution at 4 °C injected into the aortic root. Mean arterial pressure during bypass was maintained at 50—70 mmHg with nitroglycerin or nitroprusside infusion. Mean pressures were maintained at < 100 mmHg prior to and after surgery with the same agents. After rewarming to 37 °C the patients were weaned from bypass, decannulated and the residual heparinisation reversed with protamine sulphate (1 mg/100 I.U. total heparin administered).

Following transfer to the intensive care unit, intermittent positive pressure ventilation was continued until the patient was warm peripherally, was cardiovascularly stable and was not bleeding.

For all the studies except the double-blind study in primary coronary artery bypass patients a policy of normovolaemic haemodilution was used. In patients whose packed cell volume after induction of anaesthesia was more than 30% following sternotomy 1 unit (400—500 g) of blood was taken into acid citrate dextrose from a central vein and replaced with an equal amount of non haemic colloid (Hespan or Haemaccel). This blood was reinfused after surgery using the criteria set out below and was not counted in the transfused blood balance shown in the results section.

Postoperatively, all patients received an infusion of crystalloid at approximately 1 ml/kg/h and potassium supplements to maintain the plasma concentration between 4.5 and 6 mM.

The administration of blood in the postoperative period was according to predefined rules. All patients had right atrial or central venous filling pressures maintained at 5—15 mmHg depending on clinical considerations. Blood was only administered to maintain this pressure if the packed cell volume was < 30%. Otherwise, non haemic colloid as described above was administered.

Observations

In all patients the primary criteria for efficacy was the cumulative blood loss into the chest drains in the 24 h postoperatively. These losses were measured every hour until removal of the drains. In addition, the loss of haemoglobin into the drains was also determined, the haemoglobin being measured by the cyan methaemoglobin method. A record was made of all crystalloids, colloids, blood and blood products infused in the first 24 h. The urine output during the period of bypass and for each subsequent 6-h period of the first postoperative 24 h was also recorded.

In certain studies the template bleeding time (Simplate) was measured after induction of anaesthesia, and again 60—90 min after skin closure of the chest wound.

The studies of efficacy of aprotinin in reducing bleeding after cardiac surgery are presented in chronological order, starting with the studies in reoperation patients, and then discussing results in patients having primary surgery.

Results

Reoperations study

Patients having to have repeat open-heart surgery are well known to be at greater risk of bleeding after cardiac surgery and also are more likely to require donor blood transfusions than patients having primary surgery. Our original studies in this group of patients [1] showed that in the 11 patients comprising the non treated "control population the drains loss was 1509 (388) ml (mean S.D.)) and these patients all required blood transfusions; a total of 41 units of donor blood were given. In striking contrast, the 11 treated patients had a postoperative loss of 286 (48) ml; only four of the 11 patients received a total of five units of donor blood. This reduction in blood use was achieved without postoperative anaemia. The venous haemoglobin in the treated patients on the seventh day postoperatively were 11.9 (0.6) gr/dl (mean (SEM)) and 12.1 (0.5) gr/dl in the control population. Subsequent use of aprotinin in patients having complex repeat surgery has confirmed these results. In the UK, aprotinin has been available for clinical use on a so-called named patient basis. The criteria for using aprotinin is that the patient should be at greater risk of bleeding because they are having repeat surgery or have endocarditis (discussed below). About 40 % of the patients were having coronary artery bypass grafts, 25% aortic valve replacement, 20% mitral valve replacement, and the remainder more complex procedures such as double or triple valve replacements and heart-lung transplantation. Preliminary analysis of the data has shown that drains losses were comparable to those achieved in our studies above and that blood use was thereby subsequently reduced.

Double-blind studies in primary ACBG

Following the original pilot study five placebo controlled, randomised double-blind studies were established. The centres for these studies were the Onze Lieve Vrouvre Gasthuis, Amsterdam; University Hospital, Freiburg, FRG; University Hospital, Giessen, FRG; Humana Hospital (Wellington) London, and Deutsches Herzzentrum, Munich. Each of these centres have differences in the methods of cardiopulmonary bypass and surgery. Two of the centres used bubble-type oxygenators, two used hollow-fibre-type membrane systems, and one a flat-sheet type of membrane oxygenator.

Table 1. Data for drains loss in the first 24 h from each of the individual centres in the studies in primary CABG. Data are for mean ± s.d.: median ranges and numbers in each group.

	London	Giessen	Amsterdam	Munich	Freiburg
Placebo	575±164; 540 270–930; n = 37	347±103; 335 210–690; n = 38	716±248; 725 295–1215; n = 35	1185±601; 1130 500–3200; n = 20	984±516; 805 220–2430; n = 38
Trasylol	308±132; 293 130–830; n = 40	257±69; 290 90–380; n = 38	507±206; 495 220–1075; n = 35	548±290; 600 210–1400; n = 19	488±297; 390 140–1350; n = 38

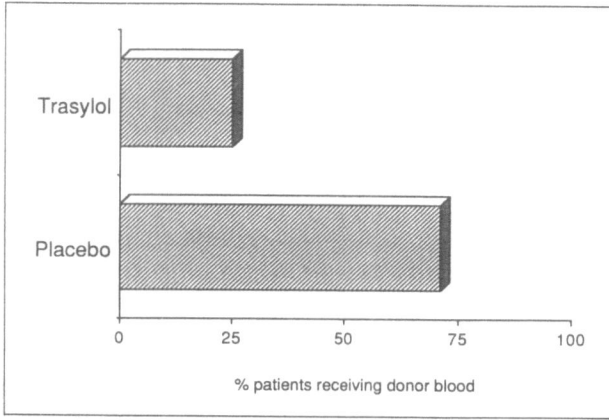

Fig. 2. Proportion of patients receiving donor blood in the five double-blind studies of aprotinin therapy in primary CABG.

The results from the study undertaken in London showed that the loss from the pericardial drains in the 18 to 24 h after surgery (after which the drains were removed) was 573 (166) ml (mean S.D.)) in the control patients and 309 (133) ml in the treated patients [13]. This reduction in drains loss was reflected in a major reduction in the need for donor blood transfusions. In the 37 control patients, 35 received a total of 75 units of donor blood. In contrast of the 40 patients in the treated group, only eight received donor blood; only 13 units being given in total.

Table 1 shows the data for drains loss in the first 24 h in the five centre studies. The remarkable reduction in bleeding and blood usage reported in our London studies was amplified by these results. The proportion of patients receiving donor blood and the blood used in those patients for the combined results from these five randomised controlled studies are shown in Figs. 2 and 3

It is obvious that the use of aprotinin was able to produce dramatic reductions in bleeding and blood transfusion requirements, despite different conditions and techniques of cardiopulmonary bypass and surgery. Certain of the data from these other centres has been published [14–16]. With continuing experience it is possible with the use of aprotinin to virtually guarantee that a patient having primary myocardial revascularisation will not require donor blood transfusions. What is also remarkable is that this can be achieved without the patient having to endure a period of anaemia postoperatively. The venous haemoglobin on the seventh day postoperatively in the patients in the London studies was 13.1 (1.4) g/dl (mean (S.D.)) compared to 12.5 (1.2) in the control patients [28].

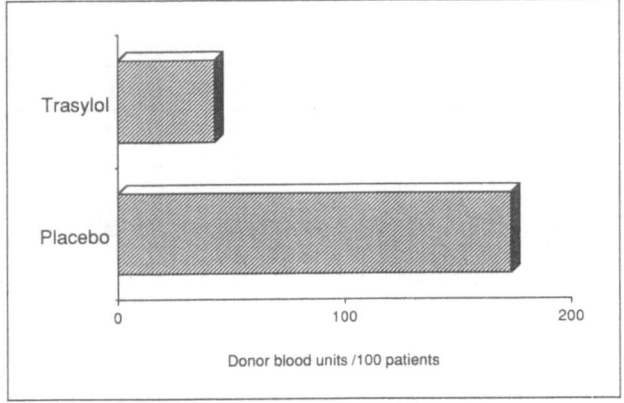

Fig. 3. Donor blood transfusions to patients in the five primary ACBG studies. Data has been normalised to give transfusions for each 100 patients in each group.

Septic patients

A small proportion of patients present for cardiac surgery with infections of native or prosthetic heart valves. These patients represent a considerable risk as they often have multiple organ dysfunction as part of the septicaemic process. In particular, they often have gross disturbances of clotting and haematological variables. Aprotinin has been used in a number of such cases with great benefit. Data from 15 treated patients showed that only six required perioperative blood transfusions. The blank-blood need of an average of less than 1 unit per patient contrasts with our previous experience of needing 8 or 9 units per patient [17]. The individual patient blood transfusions are shown in Fig. 4.

As can be seen, only four patients had postoperative blood transfusions. The remainder of the transfusions were given during surgery, usually to maintain an adequate haematocrit throughout bypass in those patients who had anaemia due to haemolysis prior to surgery. Data from these patients is described in detail elswere [11].

Comment

These data show that aprotinin given in a novel high-dose regime over the period of cardiac surgery is able to reduce the need for donor blood transfusions in this group of patients, who are more likely to need donor blood transfusions. In addition, this effect was achieved without the patients becoming anaemic in the postoperative period.

A number of issues arise from these observations. The first relates to minimising the normal bleeding which occurs after open-heart surgery. It is apparent from these results that there was a great variability in the blood losses in the control groups for each centre. These differences are difficult to relate to any specific feature. For example, the type of oxygenator used appeared not to be related to the degree of bleeding; the Munich and London studies were performed using Harvey 1700 bubble-type oxygenators and the control losses were quite different. In addition, the losses in the aprotinin-treated, primary operation patients exceeded our London

214

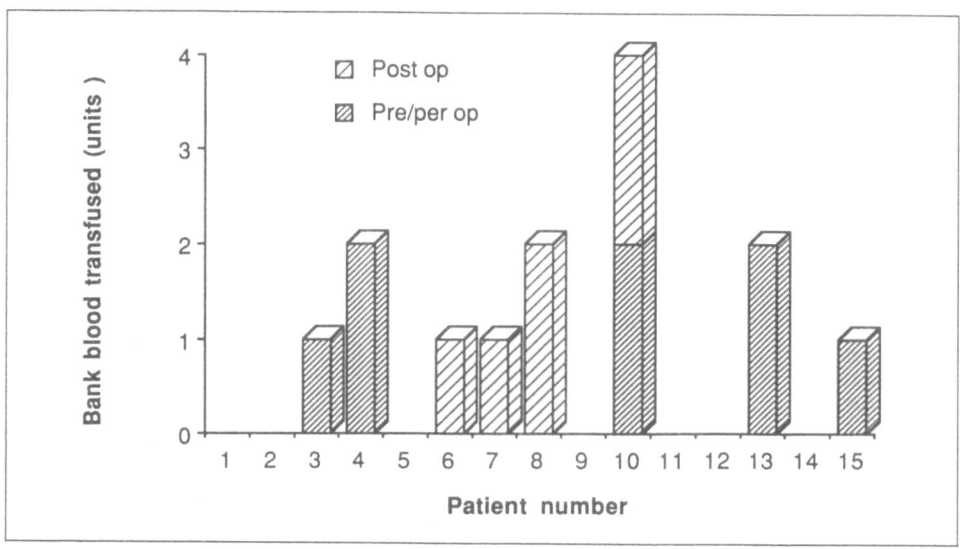

Fig. 4. Data for individual donor blood transfusions in the 15 patients operated on with endocarditis. The effect of aprotinin to prevent bleeding postoperatively is shown as only four of the patients required postoperative transfusions. The remainder of the donor blood use was to maintain the haematocrit in patients who had severe haemolysis or anaemia prior to surgery.

(and now UK data) for losses in complex reoperations patients. Additionally, there was no apparent correlation between the degree of bleeding and the times of bypass for the various centres. It is obvious that this particular aspect of the damaging effects of cardiopulmonary bypass still requires much further study.

The second question to address is related to the criteria for transfusion and the level of the safe haemoglobin. In the studies mentioned here there was a strict limit for the haematocrit before a blood transfusion was given. However, this strictly enforced policy highlighted two other difficulties. In our London study in primary CABG patients, of the eight patients in the aprotinin-treated group who received donor blood, four received all or part of only a single unit. This incidence of single-unit transfusions was mainly due to our strictly enforced transfusion policy, so that a patient who had just returned to the intensive care unit from theatre might have had a filling pressure of 3 mmHg and a haematocrit of 28 %. According to the protocol, a unit of blood would have been started to increase the filling pressure to our predefined level. The excretion of the crystalloid load from the oxygenator prime together with the minimal bleeding would mean that subsequent measurements of the haematocrit would be above the predetermined intent-to-transfuse value of 30% and the unit of blood would, therefore, not be completely administered.

One area of difficulty and debate is to define a suitable haematocrit for the intent-to-transfuse boundary. With a limit of 30% in the immediate postoperative period the patients were able to be discharged from hospital with an average venous haemoglobin concentration of about 12 grams per decilitre. If a discharge haemoglobin of 10 grams is accepted [18], then this means that the early postoperative haematocrit can be allowed to fall to about 25%. Acceptance of this level reduces considerably the need for donor blood in the control population, and we have shown that this policy completely removes the need for donor blood in those patients treated with Trasylol.

A number of other points need to be addressed related to the safety of this regime and also its mode of action. These aspects will be discussed more fully in the next two contributions in this volume, but at this time, the major issues appear to be related to assessing the degree of anticoagulation of patients during heparinisation. As aprotinin was given to reduce the contact activation of blood, then it is not surprising that coagulation times measured using this method (e.g. the Haemochron time of ACT) are prolonged in patients given aprotinin therapy. The relationship between aprotinin and heparin on coagulation is complex and requires much further study, but previous studies have shown that, despite prolonged Haemochron times, there is no need to give extra protamine to reverse this effect [19].

A second concern is about the effects of this regime on renal function (which are described later in this volume). Thirdly, as this is a non-human agent there is a possibility of an adverse reaction to the agent on first or subsequent usage. It is well known that all patients receiving drugs will develop some antibody of the IgG- and Ig M-class to that drug, and it is assumed that aprotinin will be no exception; indeed, none of the drug assays using radioimmune assay or enzyme-linked immunoab-sorbence assays are possible without such an antibody being formed. Whether any such IgG or IgM antibody is relevant to any subsequent adverse reactions remains to be investigated. As mentioned previously, it has been the authors' practice since the very first use of this drug to give a small "test dose" of aprotinin prior to the first loading bolus dose. Prior to this test dose the patient has intravenous access with a wide-bore cannula and intra-arterial pressure monitoring is established. A fourth area of concern is to the effects on graft patency. It is difficult to concept-ualise, and more difficult to comprehend, that aprotinin can apparently reduce clot-ting and thrombosis (as shown by the prolonged ACT) and yet improve haemostasis. Despite the now increasingly common usage of aprotinin therapy in Europe, there have been very few reports of early graft occlusions using this regime. However this is an important area of concern which is undergoing more formal study.

The final area to address is the need to give the dose described above. It is obvious that the dose regime I described in 1987, is highly effective, but it is still based on theoretical inhibitory concentrations for the enzyme kallikrein and is in essence an empirical regime. To define the need to give this high dose requires a brief review of previous studies using aprotinin in lower doses.

The use of aprotinin in patients having cardiac surgery has been described since the 1960s. At that time excessive bleeding after cardiac surgery was thought to be mainly due to increased fibrinolysis. Early studies showed that aprotinin could re-duce fibrinolytic activity during open-heart surgery. Tice published anecdotal re-ports of the beneficial effects of aprotinin given in a total dose of 200 000 KIU [20]. In 1968, Mammen [21] reported results from nonrandomised studies (using historic controls) in adults having valve replacements. These reports indicated that Trasylol was able to significantly reduce fibrinolytic activity, but with no effect on postop-erative bleeding. The dose regime was to give 100 000 KIU into the prime of the oxygenator together with an infusion of 100 000 KIU over 60 min and a further 100 000 KIU as a bolus at the end of the procedure (i.e. 300 000 KIU in total).

In a randomised, prospective, double-blind comparison of the effects of Trasylol (100 000 KIU/h through the surgery) and epsilon amino caproic acid (EACA) (100 mg/kg given prior to sternotomy) Ambrus et al. [22] reported a significant reduction in blood transfusions in the Trasylol-treated patients. The control population had 3502 (1846) (mean (SD)) ml blood transfused compared to the Trasylol group's need for 2749 (1500) (p < 0.05). The EACA patients transfusion need of 4055 (2310) was not significantly different from the control group.

In the late 1970s and early 1980s, a number of reports appeared to again suggest that aprotinin may be able to reduce bleeding after cardiac surgery. Particularly active in this respect were the group in Bonn. Hack et al. [23] reported the results from a retrospective non-randomised series of investigations in adults having aortic — or mitral — valve replacement. Three dose regimes where used, each for a 1-year period. In the first year the patients received a dose of 30 000 KIU/kg at the end of bypass; this regime had been shown by others to have no effect on coagulation variables nor on post-operative blood loss [24]. The following year patients received an additional 500 000 KIU into the oxygenator prime volume with a further 500 000 KIU after 1 h of bypass. The next year the regime had a further addition of 30 000 KIU/kg given 2 days preoperatively and the same dose just prior to surgery. The blood transfusion requirements for patients having mitral valve repair fell from about 2400 ml to 1400 ml over the time period of these studies. The results for aortic valve replacements followed the same trend, but the changes were of a lesser magnitude. Since the study was not randomised and other factors contributing to the adequacy of haemostasis could have changed over the time of the study then no definite conclusions can be drawn as to the efficacy of aprotinin.

In a retrospective study reported in 1984 [25], Huth and Hoffmeister compared two dose regime schedules for aprotinin in patients having primary myocardial re-vascularisation. The first group received a single dose of 5000 KIU/kg after induction of anaesthesia. The second group received an additional 10 000 KIU/kg into the oxygenator prime volume and a further 5000/kg at the end of the period of extracorporeal circulation. The results showed that the postoperative drainage losses were significantly lower in the higher dose-regime patients: 5.5 (1.9) ml/kg/24 h compared to 7.4 (4.1) ml/kg/24 h in the single-dose group. This was also reflected in the transfusion data with a reduction in blood transfused to 4.9 (1.9) units compared to 6.0 (3.6) units in the lower dose patients. As with the study of Hack et al., these data were from a non randomized open study and therefore definite conclusions regarding the efficacy of aprotinin are difficult to draw.

Aprotinin has also been reported to have a beneficial effect in paediatric heart surgery. Again, the anecdotal nature of the reports makes interpretation of certain aspects of the data highly complex. However, of some interest are the reports in neonates and small children (weighing 2—8 kg). Those given aprotinin in divided doses to a total of about 45 000 KIU/kg over the period of surgery had about a 60% reduction in blood loss and transfusion needs compared with those given nothing at the time of surgery. This former group also had a reduction in mortality with a group mortality of 14.7% compared to 23.6% in the group without intraoperative intervention.

Finally, two prospective, randomised, double-blind studies were reported prior to 1987. In the first of these [26], 47 patients having primary surgery for replacement of their aortic or mitral valve were randomised to receive placebo or aprotinin in a dose of 20 000 KIU/kg prior to surgery and 10 000 KIU/kg at the end of extracorporeal circulation. An additional 500 000 KIU was added into the oxygenator prime volume. The reduction in post-operative blood loss from a mean of 596 ml to 443 ml in the treated group did not achieve statistical significance. However, there was a statistically significant reduction in transfusion requirements from 2500 ml in the control group to 2000 ml in the treated group.

In the second prospective randomised study from Bonn [27, 28], patients were allocated to receive aprotinin placebo or C1 esterase inhibitor. The aprotinin dose regime was to give a loading dose of 1.5×10^6 KIU prior to surgery, 0.5×16^6 KIV added to the priming solution of the heart-lung machine, and a further 1×10^6 at the end of the surgery (following the administration of protamine). The reduction in post-operative drains volume from a median of 885 ml in the placebo group to 680 ml in the Trasylol group was statistically significant ($p < 0.01$). The loss of 900 ml in the C1 esterase treated patients suggested a lack of effect of that agent at the dose used (2500 units over the time of surgery). Nonetheless, the patients in both of the active therapy arms of the study had significantly lower blood transfusion requirements than the placebo patients (1800 ml cf 2500 ml). The data are more difficult to interpret due to the idiosyncratic nature of the protocol. Because of the authors' previous experiences with aprotinin the protocol allowed additional aprotinin to openly be given immediately after surgery in any patient deemed to be bleeding excessively (defined as > 1 ml/kg/h). This additional aprotinin was given without breaking the random code, 9/18 placebo, 4/18 C1 esterase inhibitor, and 4/17 aprotinin patients received the extra aprotinin in doses ranging from 0.5 to 8.5×10^6 KIU.

It is interesting to speculate as to the "best dose" of aprotinin to stabilise blood loss so that donor blood replacement will not be required. If data from a number of controlled studies of the use of aprotinin in patients having primary open-heart surgery are analysed, then some interesting relationships and speculations are apparent. Data from three such studies are shown in Fig. 5 where the postoperative drains' loss (shown on the vertical axis) is plotted against the total dose of aprotinin administered over the operative period (corrected for body weight).

These data point to there being a dose-response effect which has not as yet achieved a maximum. However, it is clear that the three studies from which these data were extracted are not likely to be directly comparable. It is probable that the most beneficial effects of aprotinin therapy will be greater at greater doses and in those centres and patients with the greatest postoperative losses due to non surgical

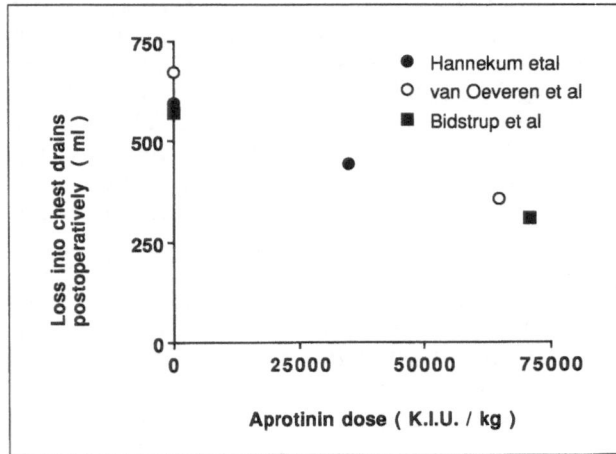

Fig. 5. Results for postoperative drains' losses compared to total dose of aprotinin recieved during the course of surgery from three prospective studies (from [12, 13, 26]). The losses in the control groups are very similar and there appears to be a suggestion that the reduction in postoperative bleeding is related to the dose of aprotinin given.

causes. The data from the studies outlined in this article show that there is a wide discrepancy in the normal volumes of drains losses between centres. It is also obvious that it will be necessary to perform a formal dose-response study in the future to compare, not only the losses, but also biochemical and haematological endpoints of safety and efficacy.

In conclusion, aprotinin has been shown to have major beneficial effects to prevent bleeding in patients having open-heart surgery. While it is also able to prevent bleeding following a number of other different types of surgery [2], it is probable that its major impact in blood conservation programs will be in this role. The future investigations with this drug must concentrate on aspects of safety related primarily to its role in open-heart surgery and also its mode of action in all different forms of surgery with the aim of determining the way forwards to the next generation of serine protease inhibitors that will thereby have improved efficacy and no adverse effects.

Acknowledgements

The author wishes to thank the Bayer company for support of the studies undertaken in London, and in particular, Mr. G. Hein and Dr. F. Schumann, without whom these studies would not have been performed. The earlier studies on lung injury were supported by The British Heart Foundation and The British Lung Foundation. I also wish to thank the principal authors from the studies conducted in Europe for allowing me to use some of their data.

References

1. Royston D, Bidstrup BP, Taylor KM, Sapsford RN (1987) Effect of aprotinin on need for blood transfusions after repeat open heart surgery. Lancet (ii): 1289—1291
2. Royston D (1990) The serine protease aprotinin (Trasylol): a novel approach to reducing postoperative bleeding. Blood coagulation and fibrinolysis 1: 55—69
3. Royston D (1990) Aprotinin in open-heart surgery: background and results in patients having aortocoronary bypass grafts. Perfusion 5 (suppl): 63—72
4. Fritz H, Wunderer G (1983) Biochemistry and applications of aprotinin, the kallikrein inhibitor from bovine organs. Arzneimittelforsch 33 (1): 479—494
5. Kraut E, Frey EK, Werle E (1930) Über die Inaktivierung des Kallikreins. Hoppe-Seyler's Zeitschrift für Physiologische Chemie 192: 1—21
6. Kunitz M, Northrop JH (1936) Isolation from beef pancreas of crystalline trypsinogen, trypsin, atrypsin inhibitor and an inhibitor trypsin compound. Journal of General Physiology 19: 991—1007
7. Royston D, Minty BD, Wallwork J, Higenbottam T, Jones JG (1985) The effects of surgery with cardiopulmonary bypass on alveolar-capillary barier function in man. Ann Thorac Surg 40: 133—142
8. Royston D, Braude S, Nolop Kb, Hughes JMB (1989) 113m Indium protein flux does not reflect degree or outcome in respiratory failure. Am Rev Respir Dis 139: A380
9. Royston D, Fleming JS, Desai JB, Westaby S, Taylor KM (1986) Increased peroxide product generation associated with open heart surgery; evidence for free radical generation. J Thorac Cardiovasc Surg 91: 759—766
10. Braude S, Nolop KB, Fleming JS, Krausz T, Taylor KM, Royston D (1986) Increased pulmonary transvascular protein flux after canine cardiopulmonary bypass; Association with lung neutrophil sequestration and tissue peroxidation. Am Rev Respir Dis 134: 867—872

11. Clasen C, Jochum M, Mueller-Esterl W (1987) Feasibility study of very high dose aprotinin in polytrauma patients. In: Schlag G, Redl H (eds.) First Vienna Shock Forum; Pathophysiological role of mediators inhibitors in shock. New York. Alan R, Liss Inc: 175—183
12. van Oeveren W, Jansen NJ, Bidstrup BP, Royston D, Westaby S, Neuhof H & Wildevuur Ch (1987) Effects of aprotinin on haemostatic mechanisms during cardiopulmonary bypass. Ann Thorac Surg 44: 640—645
13. Bidstrup BP, Royston D, Sapsford RN, Taylor KM (1989) Reduction in blood loss and blood use after cardiopulmonary bypass with high dose aprotinin (Trasylol) J Thorac Cardiovasc Surg 97: 364—372
14. Fraedrich G, Weber C, Bernard A, Hettwer A, Schlosser V (1989) Reduction of blood transfusion requirement in open heart surgery by administration of high dose aprotinin — preliminary results. Thorac and Cardiovasc Surg 37: 89—91
15. Dietrich W, Barankay A, Dilthey G, Henze R, Niekau E, Sebening F, Richter JA (1989) Reduction in homologous blood requirement in cardiac surgery by intraoperative aprotinin application-clinical experience in 152 cardiac surgical patients. Thorac and Cardiovasc Surg 37: 92—98
16. van Oeveren W, Harder MP, Roozendaal KJ, Eijsman L, Wildervuur CRH. Aprotinin protects platelets against the initial effect of cardiopulmonary bypass. J Thorac Cardiovasc Surg (In Press)
17. Bidstrup BP, Royston D, Taylor KM; Sapsford RN (1988) Effect of aprotinin on need for blood transfusion in patients with septic endocarditis having open heart surgery. Lancet (i): 366—367
18. Perioperative Red Cell Transfusion (1988) National Institutes of Health Consensus Development Conference Statement 7, Number 4
19. Royston D, Bidstrup BP, Taylor KM, Sapsford RN (1989) Reduced blood loss following open heart surgery with aprotinin is associated with an increase in intraoperative ACT. J Cardiothorac Anesth 3 (suppl 1): 80
20. Tice DA, Worth MH, Clauss RH, Reed GH (1964) The inhibition by Trasylol of fibrinolytic activity associated with cardiovascular operations. Sur Gynae Obst 119: 71—74
21. Mammen EF (1968) Natural protease inhibitors in extracorporeal circulation. Ann NY Acad Sci 146: 754—762
22. Ambrus JL, Schimert G, Lajos TZ et al (1971) Effect of antifibrinolytic agents and estrogens on blood loss and blood coagulation factors during open heart surgery. J Med 2: 65—81
23. Hack G, Kirchhoff PG, Popov-Cenic S, Kulzer R, Schlemminger B, Piepho A (1983) Aprotinin bei Operationen am offenen Herzen. Med Welt 34: 726—731
24. Koestering H, Kirchhoff PG, Voelker P, Warmann E, Koncz J (1973) Untersuchungen der Blutgerinnungsveränderungen während und nach Operationen mit Hilfe der Herz-Lungen-Maschine. Thoraxchirurge 21: 534—543
25. Huth C, Hoffmeister HE (1985) Einsatz von Proteinaseninhibitoren während der extrakorporalen Zirkulation-Wirkungsverbesserung durch Optimierung der Dosis in einer klinischen Studie. In: Dudziak et al (eds) Proteolyse und Proteinasen-inhibition in der Herz- und Gefäßchirurgie. Stuttgart and New York. Schattauer 1985; 243—253
26. Hannekum A, Reuter HD, Dalichau H, Horpacsy C, Selbherr J (1985) Anlage und zusammenfassendes Ergebnis einer Klinischen Doppelblindstudie bei Operationen am offenen Herzen. Einfluß von Aprotinin auf Thrombozytenzahl und -funktion. In: Dudziak et al (eds) Proteolyse und Proteinasen-inhibition in der Herz- und Gefäßchirurgie. Stuttgart and New York. Schattauer, 222—233
27. Popov-Cenic S, Murday H, Kirchhoff PG, Hack G, Fenyes J (1985) Anlage und zusammenfassendes Ergebnis einer klinischen Doppelblindstudie bei aorto-koronaren Bypass-Operationen. In: Dudziak et al (eds) Proteolyse und Proteinasen-inhibition in der Herz- und Gefäßchirurgie. Stuttgart and New York. Schattauer, 171—186
28. Murday H, Orellano L, Fenyes J, Popov-Cenic S, Kirchoff PG (1984) Sind postoperative Blutungen in der Herzchirurgie durch Behandlung mit Aprotinin bzw. C1 inhibitor vermeidbar? Thorac Cardiovasc Surg 44: 88

Author's address:
Dr. D. Royston, M.B.Ch.B., FFARCS
Harefield Hospital
Hill End Road
Harefield, Middlesex UB9 6JH, U.K.

Safety and Risk/Benefit Assessment of Aprotinin in Primary CABG

G. Fraedrich, K. Neukamm, T. Schneider, [2]M. Haag-Weber, [3]D. Schmidt, C. Weber and V. Schlosser

Abteilungen für Herz- und Gefäßchirurgie und [2]Nephrologie der Albert-Ludwigs-Universität Freiburg und [3]Institut für Klinische Chemie, München-Bogenhausen, FRG

Introduction

High-dose aprotinin administration in open-heart surgery has been proved to offer a major reduction in the need for donor blood [1, 2, 10]. We have performed several studies that all revealed a decrease of homologous blood requirement by 75% [4, 5].

However, potential risks associated with high-dose aprotinin administration are suspected. Therefore, an increased risk of bypass-graft occlusion is cited, in addition to an impairment in renal function, and the risk of sensitization. Occasionally, cost considerations of this treatment arise.

It is the aim of this presentation to discuss, based on the present knowledge, the safety and risk/benefit assessment of aprotinin treatment in patients undergoing primary coronary surgery.

Bypass-graft patency

To demonstrate the protective effect of aprotinin during and after cardiopulmonary bypass, we refer to findings from two randomized studies on 80 and 48 male coronary patients receiving either aprotinin (Trasylol, Bayer AG, Leverkusen, FRG), according to the London protocol [1] or placebo medication, respectively [5].

The surface contact by cardiopulmonary bypass leads to an activation of proteinases of the kallikrein-kinin cascade, as well as the coagulation and complement systems [3]. Aprotinin is well known as an inhibitor of serine proteinases [7].

An inhibition of the intrinsic coagulation system by aprotinin seems to be provable by the significantly prolonged partial thromboplastin time, whereas the further influence on the system may be masked by the marked heparin effect during bypass, a possible reason for the lacking difference between the two groups regarding further clotting and fibrinolysis parameters. However, there is a significant prolongation of the activated clotting time during cardiopulmonary bypass (Fig. 1).

An inhibition of the kallikrein-kinin system by high aprotinin plasma levels may be substantiated by the significantly lowered release of elastase complexed to α-proteinase-inhibitor (Fig. 2).

221

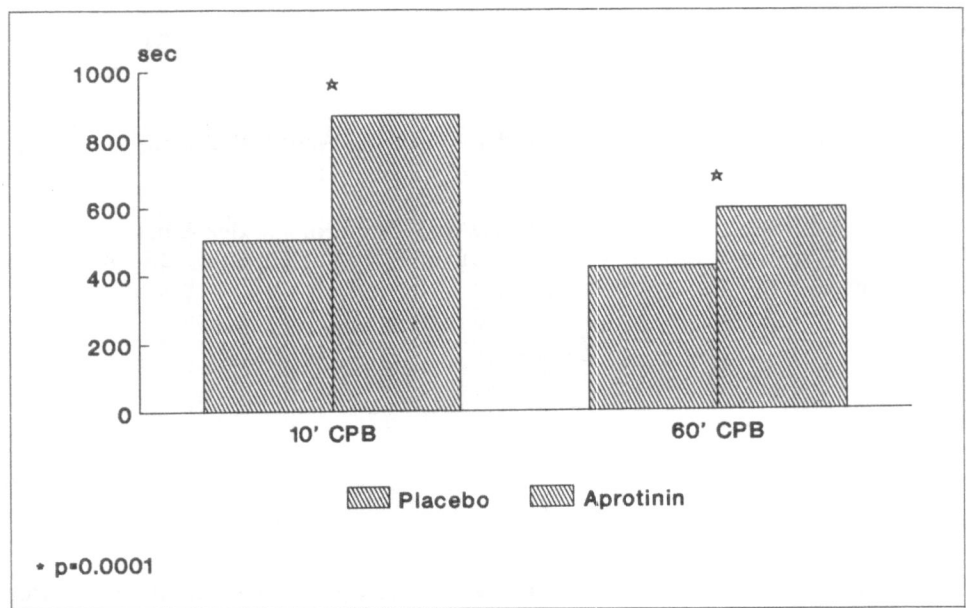

Fig. 1. Activated clotting time.

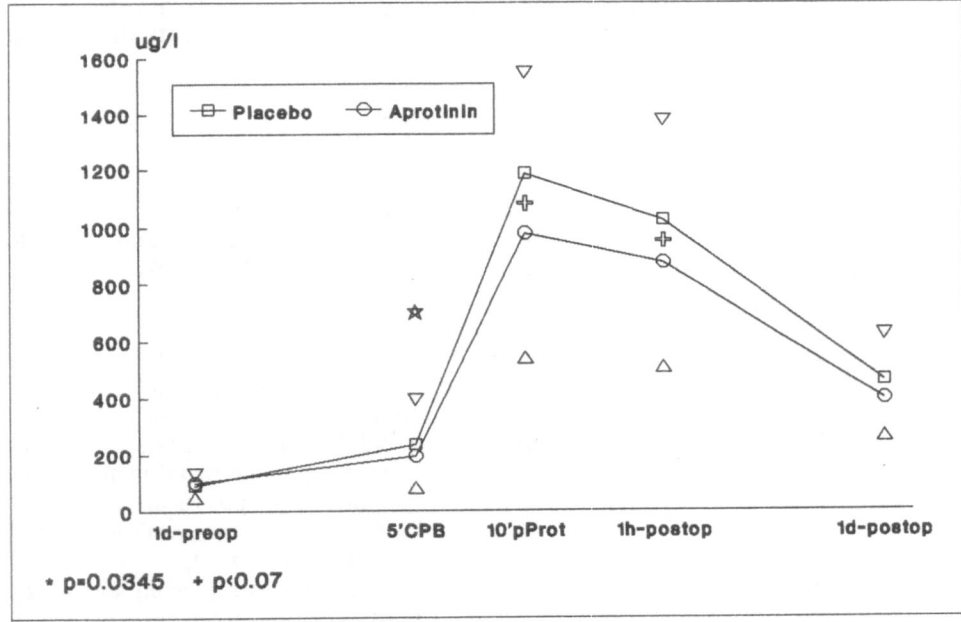

Fig. 2. Elastase-alpha-1-Pl (corrected for hemodilution).

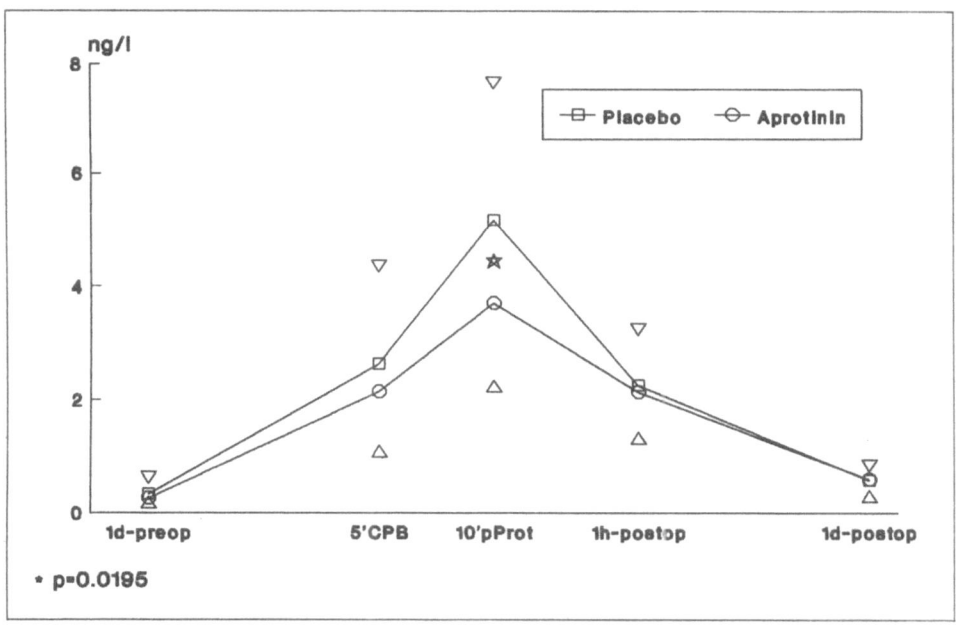

Fig. 3. Complement C3a des Arg (corrected for hemodilution).

A marked inhibition of the anaphylatoxin formation seems to be provable by the significant lowered release of complement C3a (Fig. 3).

Whether a direct platelet protection by aprotinin may play an additional role, as suggested by the findings that release of α-granule compounds and thromboxane B2 (Fig. 4) is significantly lowered, cannot be answered at this time. However, we suppose that the deleterious effect of proteinases on platelets seems to be mitigated by aprotinin, thus leading to a less disturbed hemostasis and not, as mentioned by several groups, to an increased coagulability of patients' blood after cardiopulmonary bypass [5].

These laboratory data seem to be supported by a follow-up investigation performed on patients treated with aprotinin or placebo who had been operated on for coronary-artery bypass at least 6 months previously. We could not perceive a significant difference between both groups regarding the occurrence of complaints or angina, as well as the need for nitrate medication. Even so, the routinely performed postoperative intraarterial substraction angiography of mammary artery grafts did not reveal different results between the two groups (Table 1). Moreover, we did not encounter an increased graft occlusion or myocardial infarction rate in more than 350 patients treated with aprotinin at our institution up to now.

Given that these data represent only indirect parameters, we would conclude that there is no evidence for an increased bypass occlusion rate in aprotinin-treated patients.

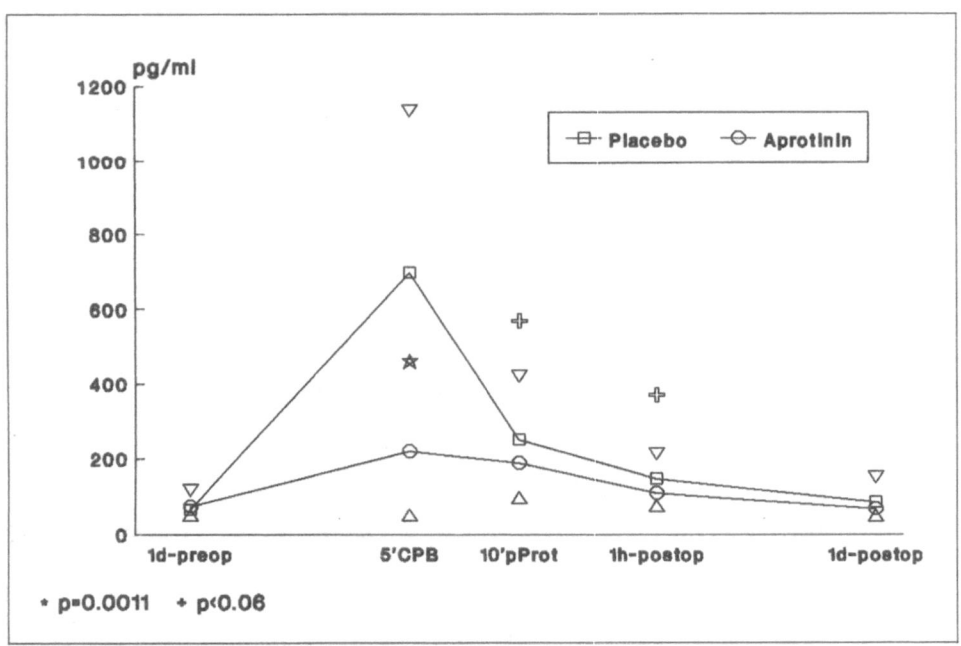

Fig. 4. Thromboxane B2 (corrected for hemodilution).

Table 1. Follow-up Data CABG > 6 months.

	Aprotinin	Placebo
Patients (n)	73	51
Late mortality	2 (2.7%)	1 (1.9%)
Without complaints	62 (84.9%)	45 (88.2%)
Nitrate medication	7 (9.6%)	4 (7.8%)
Angina < 75 W	9 (12.3%)	5 (9.8%)
i.a.DSA IMA-graft	22 (30.1%)	13 (25.5%)
IMA-graft patent	20 (90.1%)	12 (92.3%)

Renal function

Since aprotinin is virtually completely reabsorbed from the proximal tubular fluid [7], the question of whether renal disturbances may be induced by high concentrations of aprotinin seemed to be of interest. Therefore, of 60 male patients who underwent primary coronary surgery, 30 were randomized to receive a high dosage of aprotinin [1]. Urine samples and serum probes were collected preoperatively, 6 h postoperatively, and on the first, third, and fifth postoperative days.

Although protein loss was widely in a normal range, a differentiated analysis of proteinuria was performed, focussing on markers out of the prerenal, glomerular and tubular systems [8].

224

The original graphs in Fig. 5 illustrate the curves of glomerular and tubular markers obtained from two patients.

When compared to the placebo-group, aprotinin-treated patients showed a significantly increased diuresis of α-1-microglobulin (Fig. 6), of N-acetyl-glucosaminidase (Fig. 7), both representing lysosomal enzymes — and of aminopeptidase (Fig. 8), standing for the brush-border turnover. These changes were most pronounced on the first post-operative day and returned widely to normal ranges up to the sixth postoperative day.

We interpret these findings as signs of a tubular overload leading to a likely reversible tubular damage by aprotinin, that seems to be substantiated by the transient significant reduction of sodium resorption (Fig. 9).

Nevertheless, the mean values for serum-creatinine (Fig. 10) and the creatinine-clearance were in a normal range in both groups at all times.

However, a decrease of creatinine-clearance below 50 ml/min and a simultaneous rise of serum-creatinine levels occurred four times in the treated and three times in the untreated group; it improved in two placebo patients and in one aprotinin patient (Table 2). Aprotinin patients with reduced clearance on the sixth postoperative day revealed a preoperative serum-creatinine above 1.5 mg/dl.

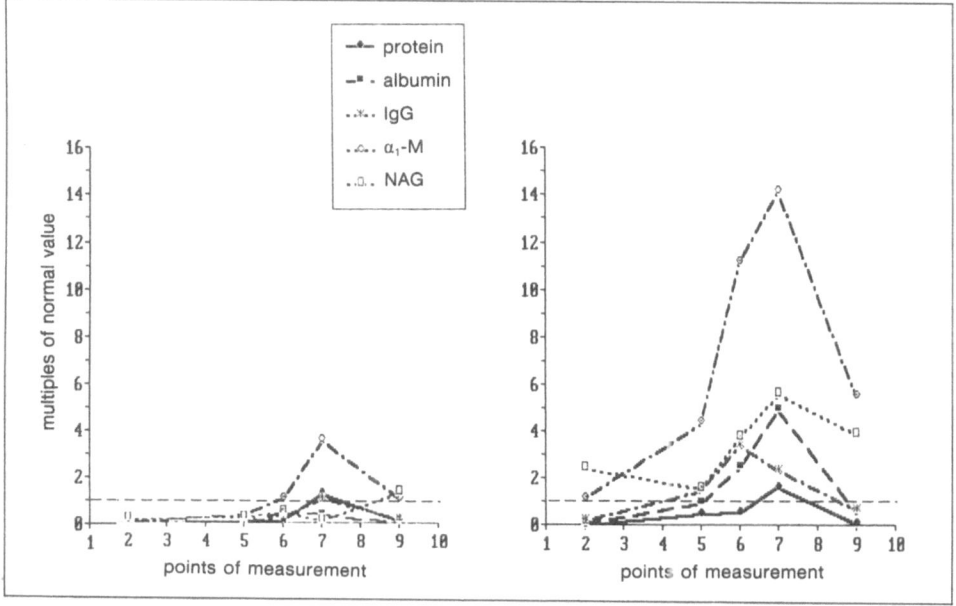

Fig. 5. Original graphs of differentiated proteinuria diagnostics; left side: placebo patient; right side: aprotinin patient.

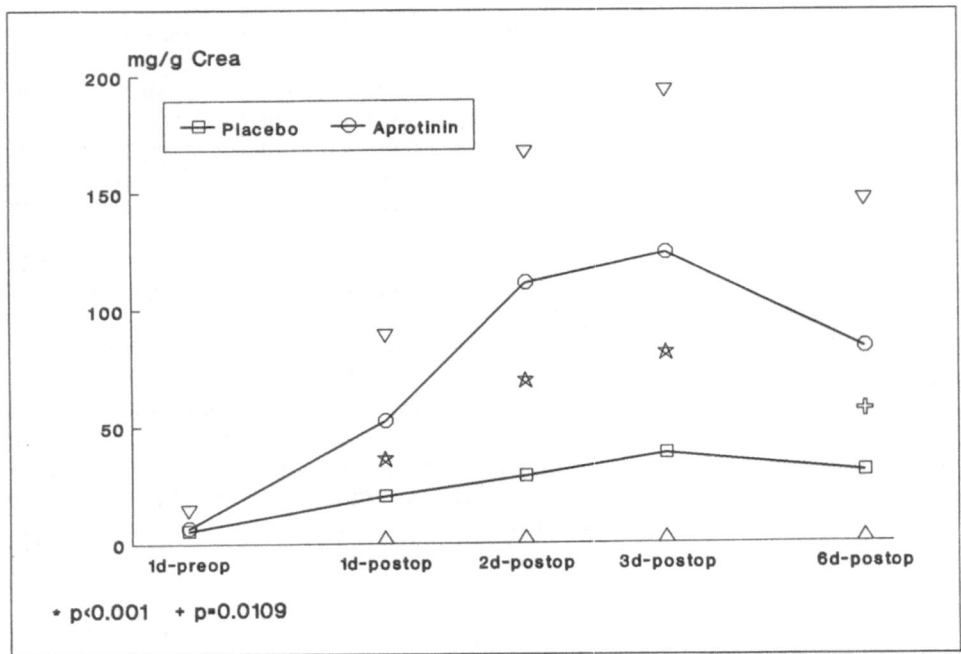

Fig. 6. alpha-1-microglobulin/urine.

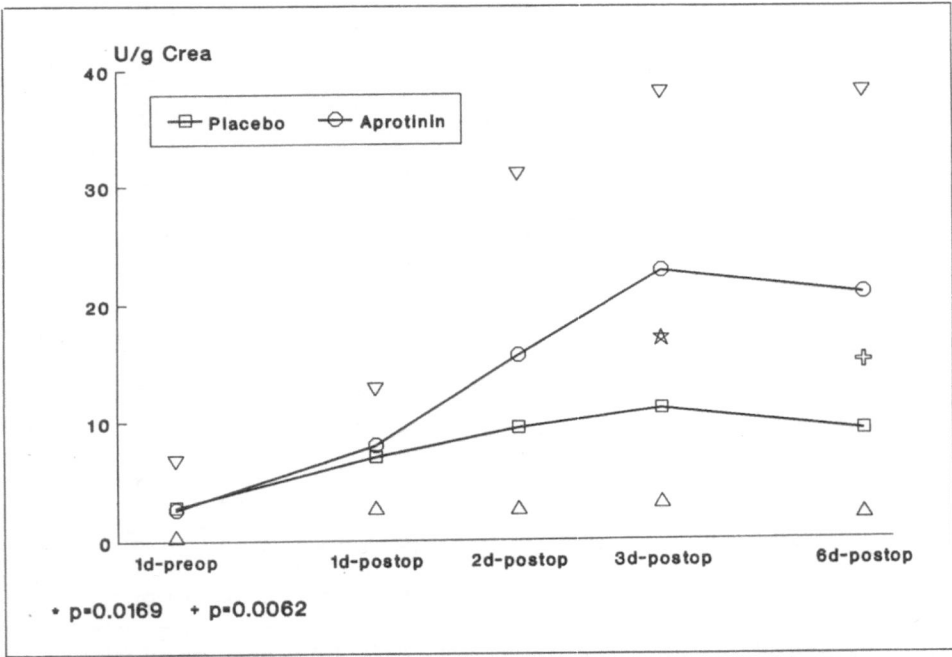

Fig. 7. N-acetyl-beta-D-glucosamidase.

226

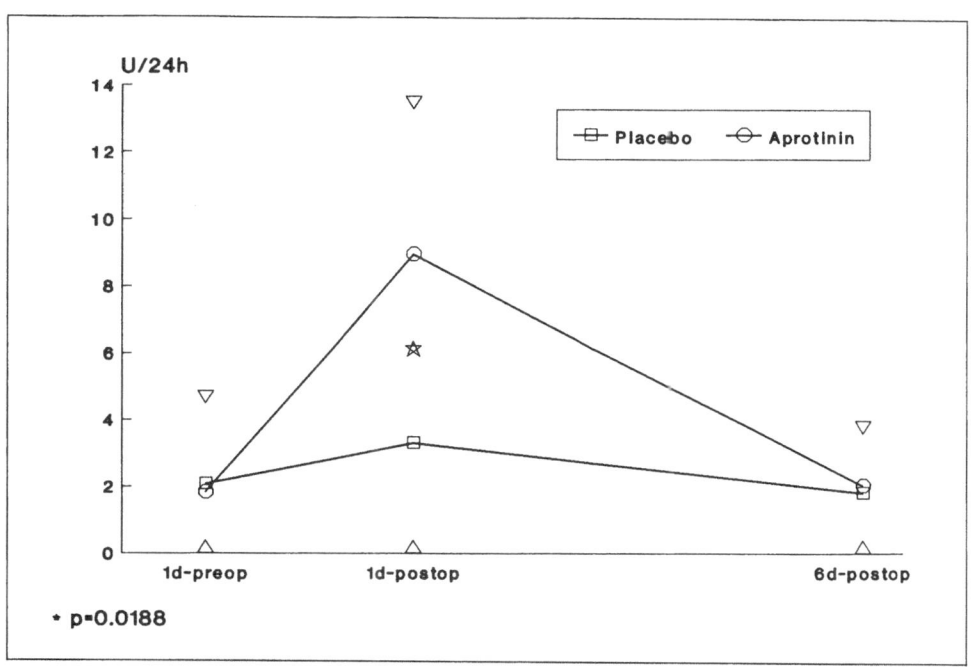

Fig. 8. Leucine-aminopeptidase/urine.

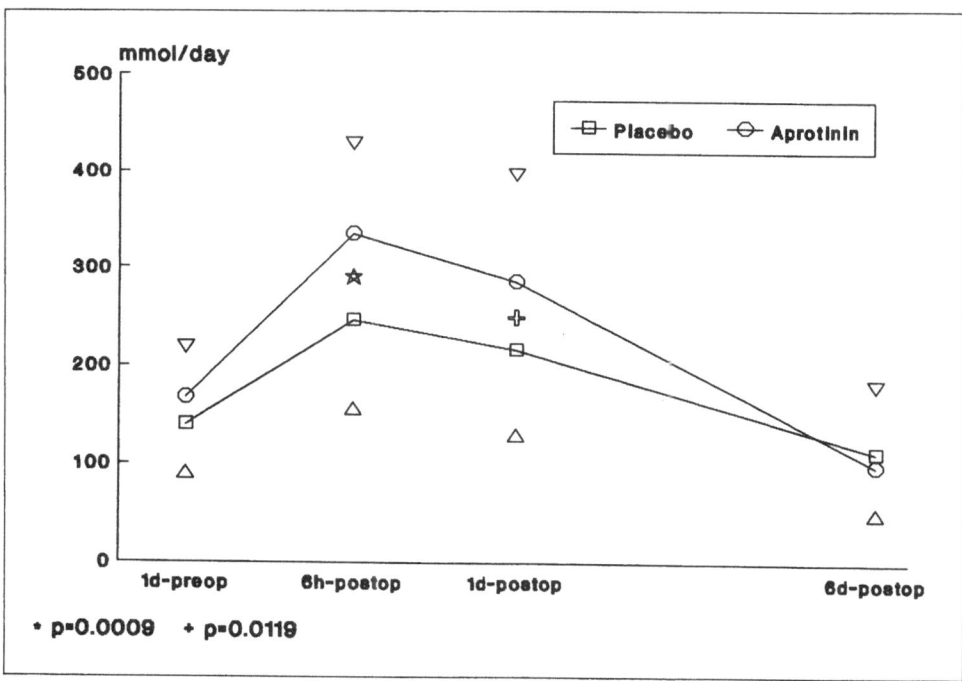

Fig. 9. Sodium excretion/urine.

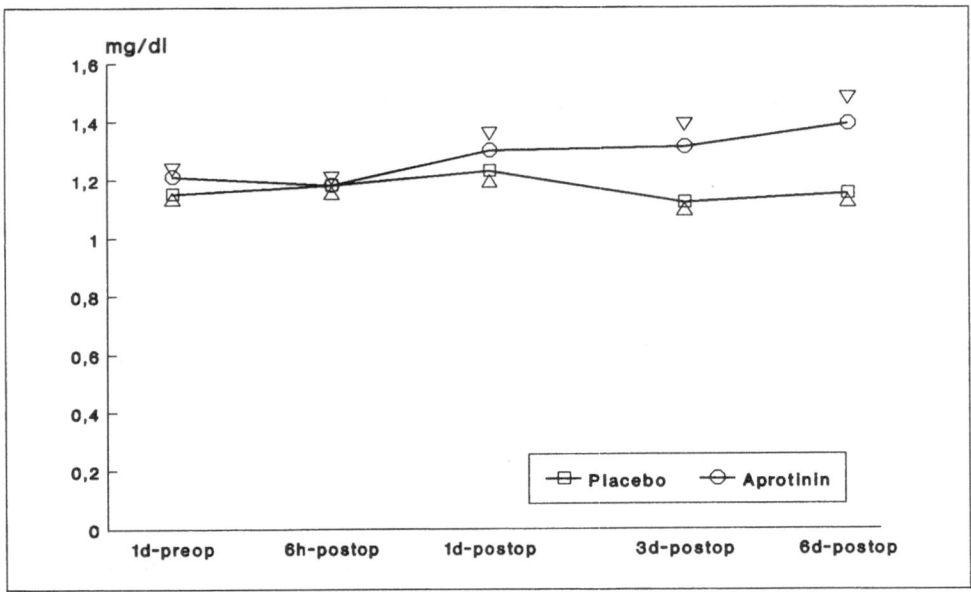

Fig. 10. Serum creatinine.

Table 2. Postoperative renal function.

	Aprotinin (n = 28)	Placebo (n = 28)
Crea-Clea < 50 ml/min	4	3
Improvemt <6 d postop	1	2
SCrea preop > 1,5 mg%	3	1

We therefore conclude that high-dose aprotinin can be administered with little risk in patients with preoperative unimpaired renal function, but patients with preoperative disturbed renal function probably have an increased risk for developing renal complications after high dose aprotinin. In regards to this recommendation, an increased renal-risk standing that offsetts the marked blood-saving effect of aprotinin seems to be widely excludable.

Sensitization

Since aprotinin is a basic proteinase from bovine organs [7] it seems capable of producing specific antibodies in humans. A Japanese group could detect specific immunglobulin E antibodies in 24 out of 62 aprotinin-treated patients [12]. A preliminary evaluation of the immunological response to aprotinin by our group revealed a distinct formation of specific immunglobulin G antibodies by 30%, and an occurrence of specific immunglobulin M antibodies by 40%, in patients operated at least 6 months previously (Fig. 11).

However, such antibody formation in about 40% is known for numerous drugs [11] and the clinical relevance cannot yet be determined. Moreover, the hypersensitivity incidence is reported with less than 1% and allergic reactions appear to be rare, although aprotinin has been administered in large groups of patients suffering from pancreatitis and other indications [6].

We have seen two cases of aphylactic reactions in our 350 cases, both had prior aprotinin administration.

Therefore, some precaution is indicated in patients that have been pretreated with aprotinin, in particular if there is a need for cardiac reoperation. A skin test or, if available, a specific antibody-test should be performed in patients at risk.

Cost/benefit assessment

Regarding the cost/benefit assessment, hard data are difficult to obtain in view of the problem in calculating costs for all potential infections induced by homologous transfusions. We proceeded to calculate for our department, in collaboration with Health-Econ (Basel, Switzerland), the cost amount for a changing number of donor blood units, and the potential incidence and outcome of nonA/nonB hepatitis, the most common infection associated with homologous blood transfusions.

Assuming a nonA/nonB hepatitis risk of 1%, the need for 3 units of blood in non-treated patients, and a donor blood economization by aprotinin of 50%, any blood-saving procedure will lower the costs by 159 DM. This difference has to be reduced by the particular cost of aprotinin in each institution. This cost-benefit increases up to 264 DM, when 5 units of donor blood have to be transfused. When a blood-saving effect of 75% is presumed, these differences will rise to 238 and 396 DM, respectively (Table 3).

Adding to this cost assessment the non-quantifiable costs for other transfusion-induced infections, we conclude from this pattern that a potential cost-benefit by

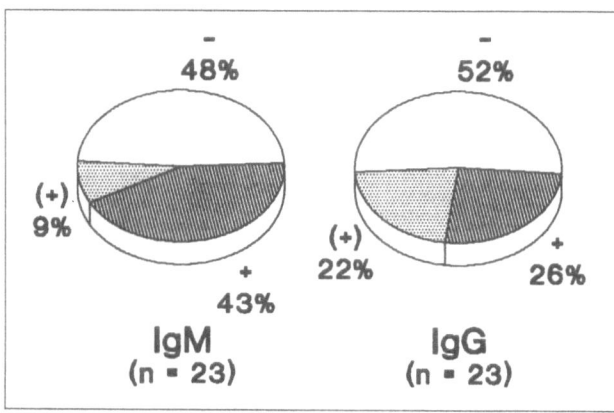

Fig. 11. Immunological response to Aprotinin. Operation > 6 months.

aprotinin depends on the number of homologous blood units transfused on the average in the respective institution.

Conclusions

In an attempt to comment on the potential risks listed at the beginning of this presentation, it can be stated that there seems to be no evident risk of bypass-graft occlusion. Patients with preoperative disturbed renal function probably have an increased risk for developing renal complications after high dose aprotinin. The risk for sensitization seems to be of some importance but not quantifiable at this time; nevertheless, one has to consider it in case of reoperation. The cost-benefit assessment seems to speak in favor of aprotinin treatment.

As mentioned in the introduction, we performed randomized studies focusing on the need of homologous blood requirement. Even conceding the fact that, as a result of the more frequent application of all blood-saving procedures and increased attention at our institution, the need for donor blood could even be reduced by nearly 35% in the placebo group within 1 year; the homologous blood saving rate amounted to 75% in both studies (Fig. 12).

Table 3. Cost/Benefit — Assessement, HealthEcon Basel (CH).

	Transfusion of 3 units	Transfusion of 5 units
Transfusion < 50%	159 DM	264 DM
Transfusion < 75%	238 DM	396 DM
Risk of nonA/nonB hepatitis 1 %		

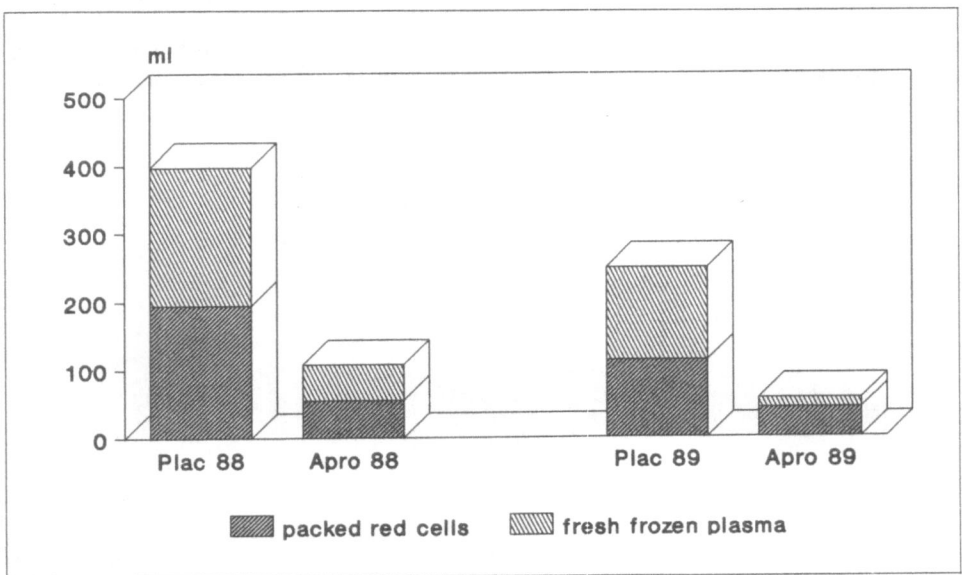

Fig. 12. Donor Blood Requirement units/100 patients.

Therefore, the benefits associated with aprotinin treatment are the highly significant decrease in donor blood requirement and, therefore, a reduced risk for transfusion-induced infections. Moreover, a recently published study [9] suggests that aprotinin may be effective in preserving cardiac viability and function after prolonged cardioplegia.

In conclusion, the highly significant blood-saving effect of a high-dose aprotinin regimen in open-heart surgery does not seem to reveal evident risks, and may be safe when some recommendations are observed regarding renal function and potential sensitization. The indications at our institution for aprotinin administration in order to reduce postoperative donor blood requirements are, at present, re-do procedures, a preoperative impaired coagulation system, and patients who refuse blood transfusions.

References

1. Bidstrup BP, Royston D, Sapsford RN, Taylor KM (1989) Reduction in blood loss and blood use after cardiopulmonary bypass with high dose aprotinin (Trasylol). J Thorac Cardiovasc Surg 97: 364—372
2. Dietrich W, Barankay A, Dilthey G, Henze R, Niekau E, Sebening F, Richter JA (1989) Reduction of homologous blood requirement in cardiac surgery by intraoperative aprotinin application — Clinical experience in 152 cardiac surgical patients. Thorac Cardiovasc Surgeon 37: 92—98
3. Edmunds LH, Addonizio VP (1987) Extracorporeal circulation. In: Colman RW, Hirsh J, Marder VJ, Salzman EW (eds) Hemostasis and thrombosis — Basic principles and clinical practice. JB Lippincott Co, Philadelphia, pp 901—912
4. Fraedrich G, Weber C, Bernard C, Hettwer A, Schlosser V (1989) Reduction of blood transfusion requirement in open heart surgery by administration of high doses of aprotinin — Preliminary results. Thorac Cardiovasc Surgeon 37: 89—91
5. Fraedrich G, Engler H, Weber C, Schlosser V (1990) Effect and potential mechanism of high dose aprotinin regimen in open heart surgery — a prospective randomised double blind trial. In: Birnbaum D, Hoffmeister HE (eds) Blood saving in open heart surgery. Schattauer, Stuttgart—New York, in press
6. Freeman JG, Turner GA, Venables CW, Latner AL (1983) Serial use of aprotinin and incidence of allergic reactions. Curr Med Res Opin 8: 559—561
7. Frith H, Wunderer G, Jochum M (1983) Biochemie und Anwendung des Kallikreininhibitors Aprotinin aus Rinderorganen. Arzneim Forsch Drug Res 33: 479—494
8. Hofmann W, Guder WG (1989) A diagnostic programme for quantitative analysis of proteinuria. J Clin Chem Clin Biochem 27: in press
9. Sunamori M, Innami R, Amano J, Suzuki A, Harrison CE (1988) Role of protease inhibition in myocardial preservation in prolonged hypothermic cardioplegia followed by reperfusion. J Thorac Cardiovasc Surg 96: 414—320
10. van Oeveren W, Jansen NJ, Bidstrup BP, Royston D, Westaby S, Neuhof H (1987) Effects of aprotinin on hemostatic mechanisms during cardiopulmonary bypass. Ann Thorac Surg 44: 640—645
11. Weiss ME, Adkinson NF, Hirshman CA (1989) Evaluation of allergic drug reactions in the perioperative period. Anesthesiology 71: 483—486
12. Yanagihara Y, Shida T (1985) Immunological studies on patients who received aprotinin therapy. Jpn J Allergol 34: 899—904

Author's address:
Dr. med. G. Fraedrich
Abt. Herz- und Gefäßchirurgie
Universitätsklinikum
Hugstetter Str. 55
D-7800 Freiburg

Investigation on the Mechanisms of Action of Aprotinin in Cardiac Surgery

W. Dietrich[1], M. Spannagl[2], M. Jochum[3], P. Wendt[4], A. Barankay[1],
J. A. Richter[5]

[1] Staff Anesthesiologist, Institute for Anesthesiology, German Heart Center, Munich, [2] Research Fellow, Internal Medicine, University Clinic Munich, [3] Research Fellow, Department of Surgery, Division of Clinical Chemistry, University Clinic Munich, [4] Research Fellow, Department of Experimental Surgery, Technical University Munich, [5] Chairman, Institute for Anesthesiology, German Heart Center Munich

Introduction

Blood loss and bleeding tendency with the consequence of homologous blood transfusion still present a major problem in cardiac surgery. Many efforts have been made to influence the bleeding tendency in open-heart surgery by pharmacological means. Aprotinin is a naturally occurring enzyme inhibitor derived from bovine lungs. It acts on trypsin, plasmin, tissue-kallikrein and, to lesser degree, on plasma-kallikrein [1, 2]. Moreover, it is reported to have direct platelet-preserving properties in very high dosages [3]. Aprotinin has been used in Europe for a long time in varying indications, but only since the results published by Royston et al. [4] who applied very high dosages of aprotinin, has this drug been regarded with increased interest. Recently, these results were corroborated by several studies [5—9].

Based upon previous investigations [7], we postulated that the clinical effect of aprotinin is mainly due to the inhibition of the contact phase of coagulation. During CPB this system is activated by contact of blood with artificial surfaces of the extracorporeal circuit [10]. However, the postoperative bleeding tendency after cardiac surgery seems to be primarily due to impaired platelet function [11]. But the mechanism underlying the benefit from aprotinin has not yet been elucidated completely.

The aim of our present prospective, double-blind, placebo controlled study was to obtain further information about the mode of action of aprotinin.

Methods

Forty patients scheduled for elective primary myocardial revascularization gave informed consent to participate in this study, which had been approved by the local ethics committee. The study group comprised only male patients with preoperative normal left ventricular function (EF > 40%, LVEDP < 20 mmHg), with a preoperative hemoglobin concentration > 13.5 g/dl, and who were not receiving preoperative anticoagulant treatment or antiplatelet medication.

Patients were randomly assigned to one of two groups: the aprotinin group (group A) and the control (group C). The following dosage regime of aprotinin was applied:

after induction of anesthesia and prior to surgery, patients received a loading dose of 2×10^6 KIU aprotinin over a 15-min period, followed by a continuous infusion of 5×10^5 KIU per hour administered by an infusion pump during the whole time of surgery. An additional bolus of 2×10^6 KIU was added to the pump prime of the heart-lung machine. Patients of group C received an equal volume of saline.

The indication for intra- and postoperative transfusion of homologous blood or blood products was defined in the study protocol as a hematocrit of less than 30 %.

Anesthetic, operative, and bypass management were standardized. Patients were heparinized with 125 units/kg mucosa heparin. Further heparin (125 units/kg) was administered if the activated clotting time (ACT) decreased below 400 s. The extracorporeal circuit consisted of a bubble oxygenator, which was primed with 1400 ml crystalloid solution. After completion of CPB, residual heparin was neutralized with protamine chloride in a ratio of 1.5 mg per 125 units of the initial heparin dosage.

Blood transfusions needed until discharge from the hospital were recorded. Intraoperative blood loss was assessed by weighing the gauzes and sponges and measuring the content of the suction reservoir. Postoperative blood loss was measured as cumulative chest tube output 6, 12, and 24 h postoperatively, as well as at the removal of the chest tubes.

Blood samples were taken at the following times: 1) after induction of anesthesia and prior to aprotinin infusion; 2) prior to heparin administration; 3) 5 min and 4) 30 min after start of CPB; 5) at the end of CPB; 6) after chest closure. After discarding the first 10 ml, blood was drawn into EDTA tubes or into ACC solution (4 : 1).

Tissue plasminogen activator (tPA) concentration, the split products of crosslinked fibrin (D-dimers), total degradation products of fibrinogen and fibrin (FSP), and the complex of thrombin with antithrombin III (TAT) [12] were determined by sandwich ELISA's using polyclonal as well as monoclonal antibodies. Results are given in ng/ml. Aprotinin plasma concentrations were quantified by means of a competitive ELISA, according to Müller-Esterl et al. [13]. Spontaneous fibrinolytic activation in the native samples, as well as in their euglobulin fraction, was estimated on plasminogen containing human fibrin plates [14].

To determine the ACT, the Hemochron 800 (International Technidine Corp., New Jersey, USA) was used. ACT measurements were performed every 30 min and at all intraoperative measurement times.

Summary data of all variables are expressed as means $\pm$ standard deviation (SD). Analysis of variance (ANOVA) was used if appropriate. Chi-square test was applied for categorical data. A p value less than 0.05 was considered statistically significant.

Results

Patients' demographic data were comparable in terms of age, weight, operation, and CPB time. Thirteen patients in group C and 11 patients in group A had an additional internal mammary artery implantation.

The assessed intraoperative blood loss was 636 ± 322 ml in group C and 363 ± 159 ml in group A ($p < 0.05$). The mean cumulated loss 6, 12 and 24 h postoperatively was 721 ± 471 ml, 894 ± 491 ml, and 1169 ± 605 ml in group C, and 303 ± 209 ml, 399 ± 251 ml, and 584 ± 295 ml in group A. The total postoperative blood loss until removal of the chest tubes was 1431 ± 760 ml in group

C, and 738 ± 411 ml in group A (p < 0.05) (Fig. 1). The mean amount of intra- and postoperatively transfused homologous blood was 838 ± 963 ml/patient in group C and 163 ± 308 ml in group A, respectively (p < 0.05). 2.3 ± 2.2 units of homologous blood or blood products were given in group C and 0.63 ± 0.96 units/patient in group A (p < 0.05). Twenty-five % of the patients in group C and 63% in group A were discharged from the hospital without receiving any banked blood or homologous blood products. The intraoperative blood loss correlated significantly with CPB time in group C, whereas it did not in group A.

The ACT, which was in a comparable range preoperatively in the two groups, was significantly increased 5 min prior to administration of heparin in group A (141 ± 13 vs 122 ± 25 s) and remained significantly higher until antagonizing the effect of heparin after CPB. The aPTT was also significantly increased before heparin in group A (34 ± 2.8 vs 74 ± 7.3 s) (p < 0.05) and remained significantly prolonged until 2 h post surgery (66 ± 23 vs 45 ± 25 s).

The concentration of the TAT complex 30 min after the start of CPB and at the end of CPB showed significant differences (p < 0.05) with 48 ± 21 and 82 ± 42 ng/ml (group C) compared to 24 ± 11 and 42 ± 14 ng/ml in group A.

The concentration of the split products of the cross-linked fibrin (D-dimers) increased in both groups during surgery. However, the increase was less in the aprotinin group and was 532 ± 1425 and 497 ± 1398 ng/ml, 30 m in after onset of CPB and at the end of CPB, respectively, significantly less than the values of group C (2155 ± 2300 and 3131 ± 2755 ng/ml). The FSP concentrations showed a similar course (Fig. 2). At the end of CPB the concentration was 10 824 ± 7261 ng/ml in group C and 2510 ± 3932 ng/ml in the aprotinin group (p < 0.05).

The fibrin plates revealed increased fibrinolytic activity during the entire course of CPB in the control group. In the native samples fibrinolytic activity was evident

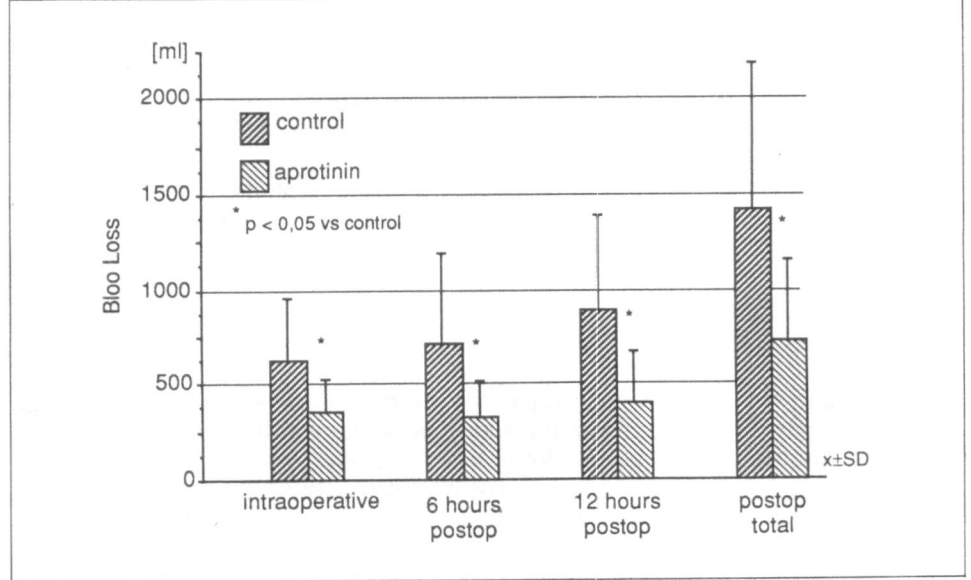

Fig. 1. Intra- and postoperative blood loss. The postoperative data are cumulative values.

234

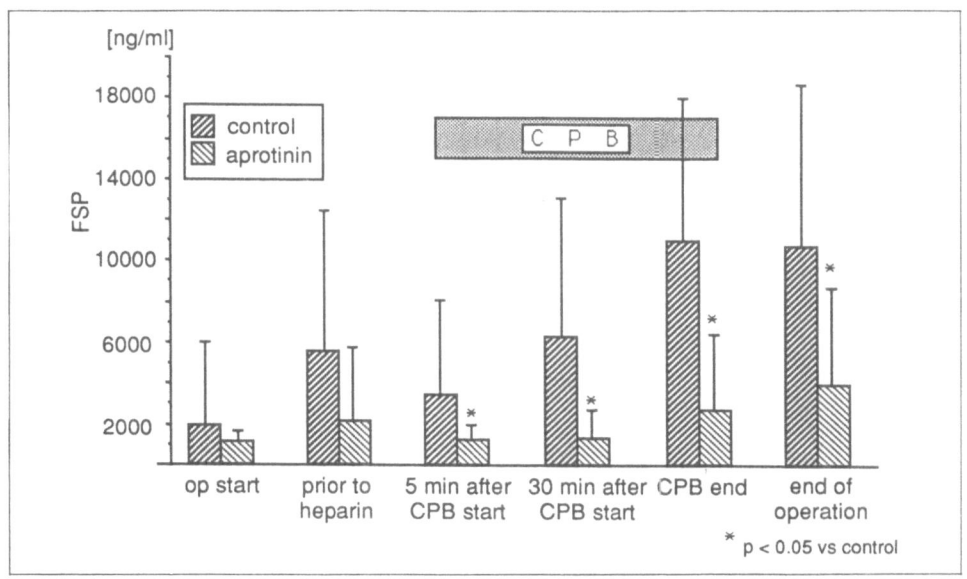

Fig. 2. Total degradation products of fibrinogen and fibrin. Values shown in the graph are mean ± SD. There was a significant increase during the whole period of CPB in the control group compared to the aprotinin group.

in 12 patients/5 min and in 13 patients/30 min after onset of CPB in the control group, whereas this could not be demonstrated 5 min after start of CPB, and in 8 patients/30 min after start of CPB in the aprotinin group ($p < 0.05$). The tPA concentration was not significantly different during the course of surgery.

The aprotinin plasma concentration (Fig. 3) demonstrated an increase from 152 ± 61 KIU/ml prior to heparin to 335 ± 106 KIU/ml 5 min after onset of CPB. Thereafter, a continuous decrease was found until the end of CPB (191 ± 62 KIU/ml).

The postoperative course of all patients was uneventful. There were no clinically relevant side effects that could be attributed to aprotinin treatment.

Discussion

The present study demonstrates the influence of high-dose aprotinin treatment on intra- and postoperative blood loss. Comparing homogeneous patient groups, a significant reduction of intra- and postoperative blood loss was found in the aprotinin-treated group. This reduction led to a concomitant saving of homologous blood. The postoperative blood loss was reduced by 48%, whereas the banked blood requirement was diminished by nearly 80%.

The differences between the two groups with regard to bleeding and banked blood requirement agree with the results of other authors applying the same or a similar aprotinin dosage regime. The blood-saving effect in these studies varied between 43% [7] and 88% [4] (Table 1). All studies using aprotinin during coronary artery bypass grafting showed nearly identical reductions in blood loss.

235

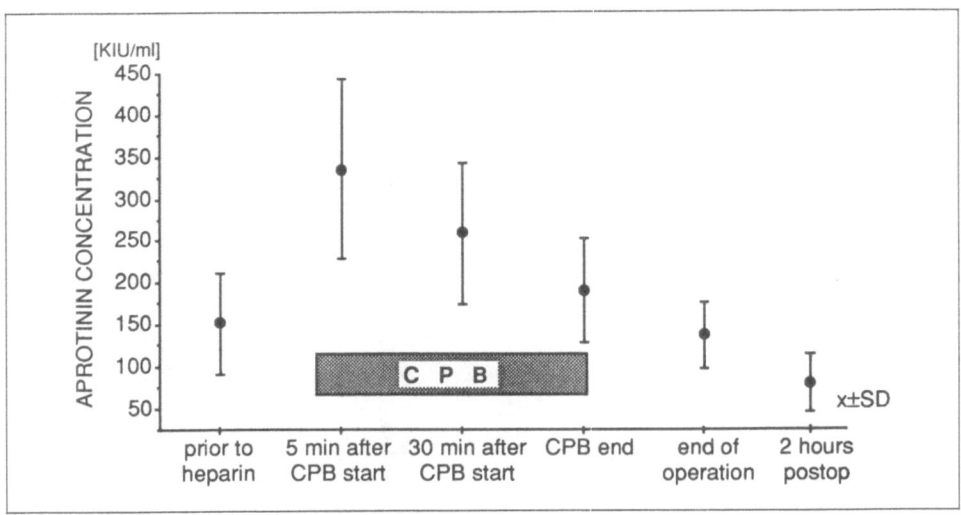

Fig. 3. Aprotinin plasma level. The peak value 5 min after the onset of CPB represents the bolus of 2×10^6 KIU aprotinin given to the pump prime. Despite the continuous infusion of 5×10^5 KIU aprotinin/h the concentration decreased towards the end of CPB and towards the end of operation.

Table 1. Studies on aprotinin in open-heart surgery.

Autor	Year	Type of operation	No. of patients	Blood loss	Blood saving
Royston et al. [4]	1987	Redos	22	− 80%	88%
v. Oeveren et al. [15]	1987	CABG	22	− 47%	− 50%
Bidstrup et al. [6]	1989	CABG	80	− 46%	− 83%
Dietrich et al. [7]	1989	Miscellaneous	152	− 29%	− 43%
Fraedrich et al. [8]	1989	CABG	80	− 46%	− 43%
Henze et al. [16]	1989	Miscellaneous	380	− 35%	− 40%
Dietrich et al. [17]	1989	CABG	40	− 48%	− 80%
Dietrich et al. [18]	1990	Miscellaneous	1784	− 34%	− 53%

Nevertheless, the mode of action of aprotinin is not yet completely clear. Capillary bleeding and oozing in cardiac surgery are supposed to be due to impaired platelet function [11, 19]. The most important consequence of CPB is the loss of platelet aggregability [10]. The influence of aprotinin on platelet adhesive receptors could be demonstrated in one study [9]. Consequently, a direct platelet-preserving property of aprotinin has been postulated [9, 15].

The surface-mediated activation of the contact system of coagulation involves the interaction of Factor XII (Hageman factor) and kallikrein (besides high molecular weight kininogen and Factor XI) [20]. Aprotinin may inhibit kallikrein. Without the amplifying effect of kallikrein on the conversion of Factor XII to XIIa the contact phase activation is inhibited or takes place only slowly. Major consequences of the surface-mediated activation are the stimulation of both the intrinsic pathway of coagulation [21] with the effect of thrombin formation and the propagation of the fibrinolytic pathway leading to plasminogen activation. Thrombin is a powerful platelet activator. Therefore, it is conceivable that the effect of aprotinin on platelets is secondary to the inhibition of the contact system of coagulation (Fig. 4)

Aprotinin is a strong plasmin inhibitor [22]. While we observed differences in the results of the fibrin plates between the groups, we could no detect any significant difference in the course of tPA concentration. The current findings indicate, that endothelial activation of fibrinolysis is not inhibited by aprotinin, whereas the activation via plasma kallikrein is attenuated. The course of the ACT, which is an indicator of contact activation [23], as well as the aPTT elevation with aprotinin treatment refer to the inhibition of the contact phase of coagulation. These hemostasiological results strongly suggest, that the inhibition of the contact phase of coagulation is the primary effect of aprotinin and is thus responsible for its blood-saving effect. This finding is in contrast to the interpretation given by van Oeveren et al. [9, 15], who focused on the direct platelet protective effect of aprotinin on the specific platelet receptors.

The rationale for choosing the given aprotinin dose regime was to get a constant aprotinin plasma level of more than 200 KIU/ml, which is supposed to be the threshold of plasma kallikrein inhibition [24]. The course of plasma aprotinin level revealed that aprotinin dosage was not able to maintain a stable concentration throughout CPB. However, the concentration exceeded 200 KIU/ml after onset of CPB. The course of the fibrin-fibrinogen split products and the results of the fibrin plates demonstrated that aprotinin was not able to suppress the ongoing hemostatic activation totally. All parameters showed an increase towards the end of CPB. Further investigation is needed to ascertain whether this tendency can be prevented with an even higher dose regime of aprotinin during CPB.

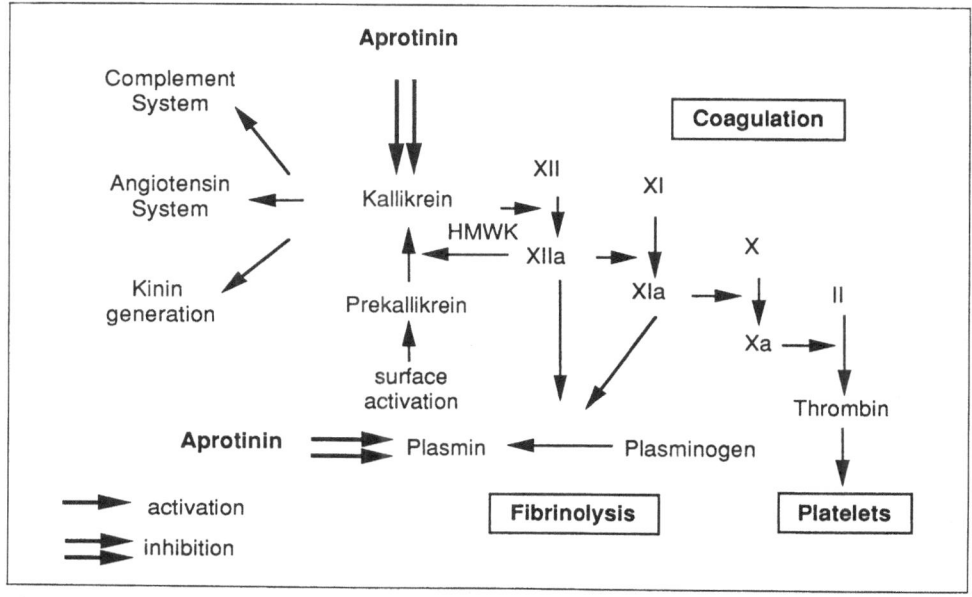

Fig. 4. Aprotinin action on the hemostatic system.

The results of this study suggest that the most likely mechanism of action of aprotinin is the inhibition of the contact phase of coagulation. This is due to the ability of aprotinin to inhibit kallikrein. It acts supplementary to heparin on coagulation. The combination of both drugs provides an enhanced anticoagulatory effect. However, because aprotinin only acts on the contact phase of coagulation, it is not recommended to reduce the heparin dosage under aprotinin. The better preserved platelet function and the inhibition of fibrinolysis is secondary to the better preserved coagulation system.

In conclusion, high-dose aprotinin treatment has a highly beneficial effect on the hemostatic mechanism during and after CPB, leading to a substantial reduction of intra- and postoperative bleeding tendency. The most likely mechanism of aprotinin action is the inhibition of kallikrein and not a direct platelet-preserving property.

References

1. Emerson FE (1989) Pharmacology of aprotinin and efficacy during cardiopulmonary bypass. Cardiovasc Drug Rev 7: 127—140
2. Fritz H (1985) The target enzymes of aprotinin in vitro and in vivo. Proteolyse und Proteinaseinhibition in der Herz- und Gefäßchirurgie, 143—154
3. Aoki N, Naito K, Yoshida N (1978) Inhibition of platelet aggregation by protease inhibitors. Possible involvement of proteases in platelet aggregation. Blood 52: 1—12
4. Royston D, Taylor KM, Bidstrup BP, Sapsford RN (1987) Effect of aprotinin on need for blood transfusion after repeat open-heart surgery. Lancet, ii: 1289—1291
5. Alajmo F, Calamai G, Perna AM et al (1989) High-Dose Aprotinin: Hemostatic effects in open-heart operations. Ann Thorac Surg 48: 536—539
6. Bidstrup BP, Royston D, Sapsfort RN, Taylor KM (1989) Reduction in blood loss and blood use after cardiopulmonary bypass with high dose aprotinin (Trasylol). J Thorac Cardiovasc Surg 97: 364—372
7. Dietrich W, Barankay A, Dilthey G, et al (1989) Reduction of homologous blood requirement in cardiac surgery by intraoperative aprotinin application — clinical experience in 152 cardiac surgical patients. Thorac Cardiovasc Surgeon 37: 92—98
8. Fraedrich G, Weber C, Bernard C, Hettwer A, Schlosser V (1989) Reduction of blood transfusion requirement in open-heart surgery by administration of high doses of aprotinin — preliminary results. Thorac Cardiovasc Surgeon 37: 89—91
9. van Oeveren W, Harder MP, Roozendaal KJ, Eijsman L, Wildevuur CRH (1990) Aprotinin protects platelets against the initial effect of cardiopulmonary bypass. J Thorac Cardiovasc Surg 99: 788—797
10. Edmunds LH, Ellison N, Colman WR, et al (1982) Platelet function during cardiac operation — comparison of membran and bubble oxygenators. J Thorac Cardiovasc Surg 83: 805—812
11. Harker LA (1986) Bleeding after cardiopulmonary bypass. N Engl J Med 314: 446—448
12. Bauer KA, Rosenberger RD (1984) Thrombin generation in acute promyelocytic leukemia. Blood 64: 64
13. Müller-Esterl W, Oettl A, Trucheit E, Fritz H (1984) Monitoring of aprotinin plasma levels by an enzyme-linked immunosorbent assay (ELISA). Fresenius Z Anal Chem 317: 718
14. Wendt P, Fritsch A, Schulz F, Wunderlich G, Blümel G (1984) Proteinases and inhibitors in plasma and peritoneal exudate in acute pankreatitis. Hepato-gastroenterol 31: 277—281
15. van Oeveren W, Jansen NJG, Bidstrup BP, et al (1987) Effects of aprotinin on hemostatic mechanisms during cardiopulmonary bypass. Ann Thorac Surg 44: 640—645
16. Henze R, Dietrich W, Hähnel C, Sebening F, Richter JA (1989) Verminderter Blutverbrauch in der Herzchirurgie durch intraoperative Aprotininapplikation. Anästhesist 38: 510
17. Dietrich W, Spannagl M, Jochum M, Wendt P, Sebening F, Richter JA (1989) Reduction of homologous blood requirement in cardiac surgery using high-dose aprotinin. Anesthesiology (Suppl)

238

18. Dietrich W, Hähnel C, Richter JA (1990) Routine application of high-dose aprotinin in open-heart surgery — a study on 1784 patients. Anesthesiology (Suppl), in press
19. Edmunds LH (1989) Letter to the editor: Blood platelets and bypass. J Thorac Cardiovasc Surg 97: 470—477
20. Colman RW (1984) Surface-mediated defense reactions. The plasma contact activation system. J Clin Invest 73: 1249—1253
21. Carvalho AC, De Marinis S, Scott CF, Silver LD, Schmaier AH, Colman RW (1988) Activation of the contact system of plasma proteolysis in the adult respiratory distress syndrome. J Lab Clin Med 112: 270—277
22. Verstraete M (1985) Clinical application of inhibitors of fibrinolysis. Drugs 29: 236—261
23. Hattersley PG (1966) Activated coagulation time of whole blood. JAMA 196: 436—440
24. Fritz H, Wunderer G, (1983) Biochemistry and applications of aprotinin, the kallikrein inhibitor from bovine organs. Arzneim Forsch/Drug Res 33: 479—494

Authors' address:
W. Dietrich, M.D.
Institute for Anesthesiology
German Heart Center Munich
Lothstraße 11
8000 Munich 2, FRG

High-dose Aprotinin Reduces Bleeding in Patients Taking Aspirin at the Time of Aorto-Coronary Bypass Surgery

B. P. Bidstrup

Humana Hospital Wellington, London, England

Introduction

Antiplatelet medication is widely used in the treatment of cardiovascular disease today. The cheapest and least toxic of these is aspirin. It has been shown to reduce myocardial infarction and death in unstable angina [9, 11], vascular mortality after acute myocardial infarction [8] and, to a lesser extent, late after myocardial infarction. Improved results after coronary angioplasty [1] as well as better aorto-coronary vein graft patency [3, 7] have been demonstrated. With increasing frequency, patients admitted for coronary artery surgery have continued to take aspirin. It is now well established that aspirin is associated with an increased risk of bleeding and the need for blood-component therapy after extracorporeal circulation [6, 7, 10]. High-dose aprotinin (Trasylol, Bayer) is effective in reducing blood-transfusion needs in patients undergoing primary aorto-coronary bypass surgery, re-operations, and with infective endocarditis [2]. This paper reports our initial experience in a preliminary open study of the effect of aprotinin on bleeding in patients taking aspirin at the time of aorto-coronary bypass surgery.

Patients and methods

Forty-four adult patients (mean age 58 ± 7.9 years) underwent elective aorto-coronary bypass surgery over a 6-month period. All patients had been taking aspirin for a period of greater than 2 weeks prior to their surgery. Twenty-six patients were randomly allocated to receive high-dose aprotinin. Informed consent was obtained from patients receiving the drug (Trasylol) which was supplied by Bayer (Newbury, Berkshire). They received an intravenous loading dose of 280 mg (= equivalent to 2 000 000 kallikrein inactivator units) after induction of anaesthesia and a constant infusion of 70 mg/h during the operation. A further 280 mg was added to the pump prime. The remaining 18 patients did not receive the drug and constituted the control group.

Anaesthetic, operative and perfusion techniques were standardised within the limitations of clinical practice. Heparin (300 IU/kg body weight) was administered before cannulation and further doses were given if the activated clotting time fell below 400 s. A Harvey H1700 S bubble oxygenator primed with 2000 ml Hartmann's solution was used in all patients. Patients were cooled to a core temperature of 28 °C and rewarmed to 37 °C, commencing with removal of the aortic clamp. Myocardial protection during aortic cross-clamping was achieved with St. Thomas's crystalloid cardioplegia. All blood shed intraoperatively during systemic heparinisation was returned to the heart/lung machine. Postoperatively, mean arterial pressure was controlled with nitroglycerine and nitroprusside to maintain levels between 70 and 90 mm Hg. Volume replacement to maintain satisfactory haemodynamic status was carried out with non-haemic plasma expanders (Haemaccel). Regular estimations of the haemoglobin levels were made and blood was administered only if the haemoglobin fell below 10 g/dl. Careful measurements were made of the total drainage from the mediastinal drains which were usually removed 18—24 h postoperatively. The use of blood and blood products was checked with the transfusion laboratory for accuracy. The haemoglobin content of the drains was determined as previously described [2]. Template bleeding times were carried out using the Simplate device preoperatively and 60—90 min after patients' return to the intensive care unit. Data are presented as mean ± standard deviation where appropriate and were analysed using non-parametric methods.

Results

Both groups were similar in regard to age, weight, sex distribution, bypass time, the number of grafts and the use of the internal mammary artery (Table 1). Four patients

Table 1. Demographic data.

	Control n = 18	Aprotinin n = 26
Age (years)	58 (8)	59 (8)
Weight (kg)	77 (10)	78 (9)
Sex (F/M)	3/15	5/21
Bypass Time (min	73 (23)	66 (19)
Number of Grafts	3.7 (0.5)	3.3 (0.7)
Number of IMA	12	17

Data are expressed as mean (standard deviation). IMA = internal mammary artery

Table 2. Use of blood and blood components.

	Control n = 18	Aprotinin n = 26
Red Cells (units/patient)	2.7(2.1)	0.8(0.8) p<0.001
range	0—8	0—3
Fresh frozen plasma (units/patent)	0.8(1.4)	
range	0—4	0
Platelets	1 pt	0
Patients not requiring transfusion	2	11
Patients with 1-unit transfusion	2	11

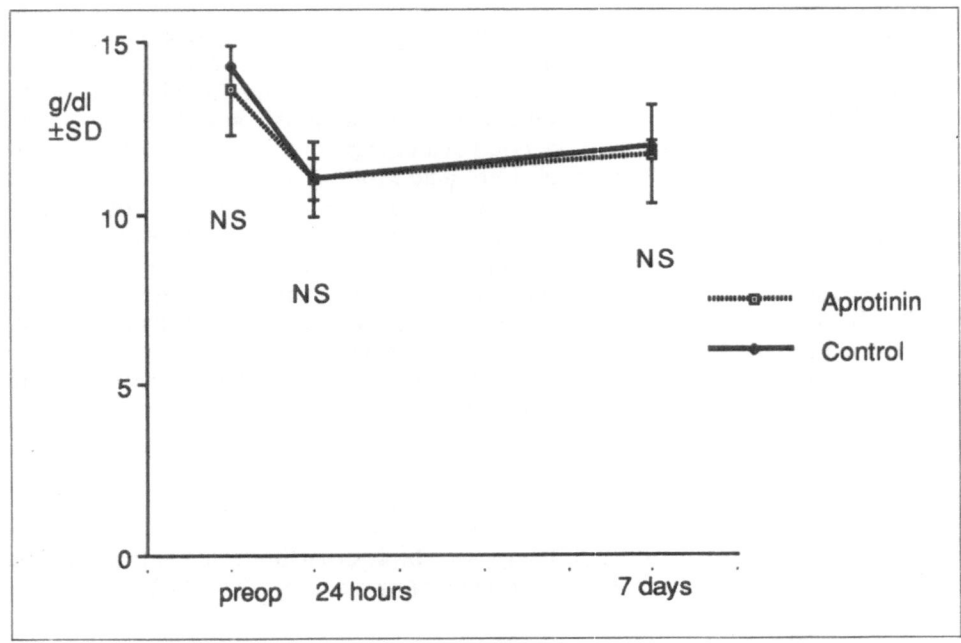

Fig. 1. Venous haemoglobin levels preoperatively, 24 h post operatively and prior to discharge from hospital.

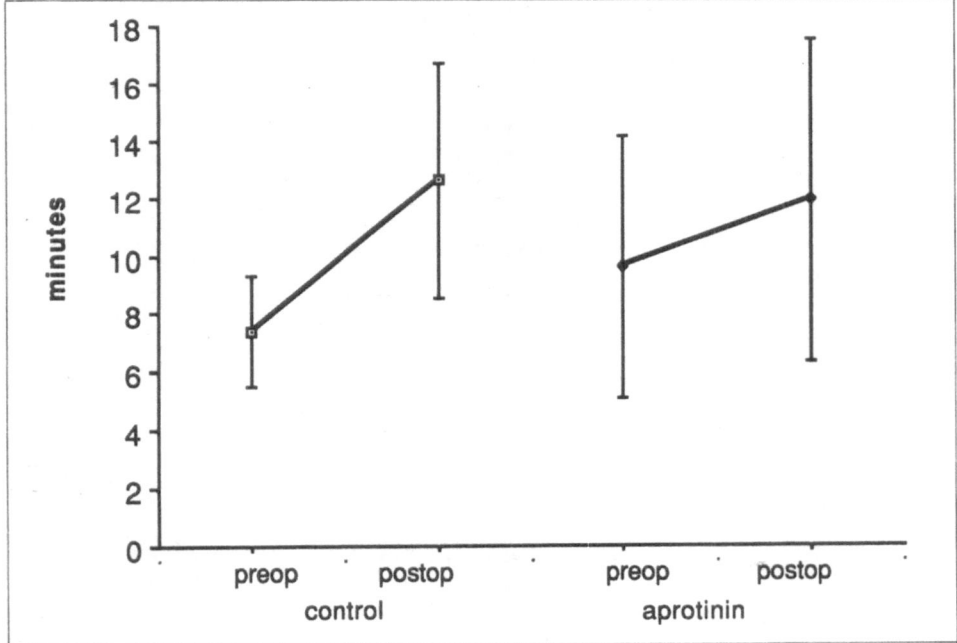

Fig. 2. Template bleeding times. There was no significant difference between the preoperative measurements. The increase in the control group was significant, whereas that in the treated group was not.

in the control group and one patient in the aprotinin group were re-explored for bleeding. Two of the four control patients and the one aprotinin patient had surgical causes for the bleeding. Total blood loss was significantly reduced by the administration of aprotinin from 1393 ± 979 ml to 352 ± 138 ml, $p < 0.001$ (Mann-Whitney U-test). When the blood loss data was analysed excluding the reopened patients the difference between these two groups remains highly significant, $p < 0.001$ (Mann-Whitney U-test). Haemoglobin loss into the chest drains was reduced to 9.3 ± 9.9 g in the aprotinin group from 44 ± 20.8 g, $p < 0.001$. The use of red cells, fresh frozen plasma and platelet concentrates is shown in Table 2. There was a marked reduction in the use of all blood products in the aprotinin-treated patients. In spite of the reduction in use of red cells, haemoglobin levels did not differ significantly preoperatively, 24 h postoperatively and on discharge from hospital (Fig. 1). There was a significantly smaller increase in template bleeding time in the aprotinin-treated patients, although the initial bleeding time was higher (Fig. 2). No adverse effects due to the use of aprotinin were seen in these patients.

Discussion

Many centres follow the policy of deferring operations on patients taking aspirin for about 10 days, the time it takes for most of the affected platelets to be replaced. This policy is not always possible because of logistic problems, emergency referrals and the belief that benefit of aspirin outweighs potential risks. Comparison of the control group in this study and that in a previous study carried out by the same team under the same conditions shows a greater use of blood and blood products [2]. This has been confirmed in other reported studies [6, 7, 10]. The use of aprotinin offers a reliable method to combat this risk.

The action of aspirin is to irreversibly acetylate platelet cyclo-oxygenase, the enzyme responsible for production of thromboxane A2. Aggregation induced by ADP and collagen is partially inhibited but response to thrombin and the initial adherence to exposed subendothelium is unaffected. Further aggregation is inhibited, explaining the increase in skin-bleeding time and tendency for disturbed haemostasis. Several pathways for platelet aggregation exist and they are not all dependent on thromboxane synthesis. It is possible that in the presence of aprotinin during bypass, receptors to, say, thrombin are now able to respond, allowing more normal platelet responses.

Not all patients seem to have the same risk of bleeding after aspirin. There appears to be a bimodal distribution of bleeding in the control group although the numbers in this study are small. This suggests that there is a subset of patients who are particularly sensitive to aspirin. They may have the syndrome of intermediate platelet dysfunction described by Czapek [5]. Further work is needed in this area to identify those at greater risk.

Of the treated patients, 11 received no blood and 11 received single-unit transfusions. This is a possible deficiency in our algorithm for giving red cell transfusions. Many centres accept haemoglobin levels of 7 g/dl postoperatively and do not transfuse unless the patient is symptomatic [4]. How many patients get re-admitted to a local hospital after discharge from the cardiac centre and transfused because of their "anaemia" is unknown. A safe level is still subject to some debate [12], but around 8.5 g/dl is suitable for most adults. This would result in nearly all the treated patients and about 40% of the untreated patients avoiding transfusion. There is probably no justification in the majority of patients for transfusing to haemoglobin levels of > 11 g/dl immediately postoperatively. Aprotinin allows higher haemoglobin levels to be maintained without transfusion.

Those involved in cardiac surgery need to address the problems of reducing bleeding rather than attempting to deal with it after it is well established. The use of fresh frozen plasma given in most instances is not justified empirically. Further work needs to be done on the identification of individual patients at risk of bleeding. The use of aprotinin will complement the armamentarium of the cardiac surgical team in improving the results of open-heart surgery.

References

1. Barnathan E, Schwartz J, Taylor L (1987) Aspirin and dipyridamole in the prevention of acute coronary thrombosis complicating coronary angioplasty. Circulation 76: 125—134
2. Bidstrup BP, Royston D, Sapsford RN, Taylor KM (1989) Reduction on blood loss and blood use after cardiopulmonary bypass using high dose aprotinin (Trasylol). J Thorac Cardiovasc Surg 97: 364—372
3. Chesebro J, Clements I, Fuster V, Elveback L, Smith H, Bardsley W, Frye R, Holmes D Jr, Vlietstra R, Plutz J, Wallace R, Puga F. Orszulak T, Piehler J, Schaff H, Danielson G (1982) A platelet inhibitor drug trial in coronary artery bypass operations: benefit of perioperative dipyridamole and aspirin therapy on early postoperative graft patency. N Engl J Med 307: 73—78
4. Cosgrove DM, Loop FD, Lytle BW, Gill CC, Golding LR, Taylor PC, Forsythe SB (1985) Determinants of blood utilization during myocardial revascularization. Ann Thorac Surg 40: 380—384
5. Czapek EE, Deykin D, Salzman E, Lian EC, Hellerstein LJ, Rosoff CB (1978) Intermediate syndrome of platelet dysfunction. Blood 52: 103—112
6. Ferraris VA, Ferraris SP, Lough FC, Berry WR (1988) Preoperative aspirin ingestion increases operative blood loss after coronary artery bypass grafting. Ann Thorac Surg 45: 71—74
7. Goldman S, Copeland J, Moritz T, Henderson W, Zadina K, Ovitt T, Doherty J, Read R, Chesler E, Sako Y, Lancaster L, Emery R, Sharma G, Josa M, Pacold I, Montoya A, Parikh D, Sethi G, Holt J, Kirklin J, et al. (1988) Improvement in early saphenous vein graft patency after coronary artery bypass surgery with antiplatelet therapy: results of a Veterans Administration Cooperative Study. Circulation 77: 1324—1332
8. ISIS-2 (Second International Study of Infarct Survival) Collaborative Group (1988) Randomized trial of intravenous streptokinase, oral aspirin, both or neither among 17,187 cases of suspected acute myocardial infarction: ISIS-2. Lancet 2: 349—360
9. Lewis H, Davis J, Archibald D, et al. (1983) Protective effects of aspirin against acute myocardial infarction and death in men with unstable angina: results of a Veterans Administration Cooperative Study. N Engl J Med 309: 396—403
10. Michelson E, Morganroth J, Torosian M, Mac Vaugh H III (1978) Relation of preoperative use of aspirin to increased mediastinal blood loss after coronary artery bypass surgery. J Thorac Cardiovasc Surg 76: 694—697
11. Theroux P, Ouimet H, McCans J (1988) Aspirin, heparin, or both to treat acute unstable angina. N Engl J Med 319: 1105—1111
12. Weisel R, Charlesworth D, Mickleborough L, Fremes S, Ivanov J, Mickle D, Teasdale S, Glynn M, Scully H, Goldman B, Baird R (1984) Limitations of blood conservation. J Thorac Cardiovasc Surg 88: 26—38

Author's address:
B. P. Bidstrup
66 Harley Street
London W1N 1AE

Preserved Hemostasis During the Combined Use of Aprotinin and Aspirin in CABG Operations

N. Tabuchi[1], W. van Oeveren[1], L. Eijsman[2], K. J. Roozendaal[2], Y. J. Gu[1], Ch. R. H. Wildevuur[1]

[1] Department of Cardiopulmonary Surgery, Research Division, University Hospital, Groningen
[2] Department of Cardiopulmonary Surgery and of Hematology, Onze Lieve Vrouwe Gasthuis, Amsterdam, The Netherlands

Introduction

After the remarkable improvement of hemostasis in cardiopulmonary bypass (CPB) obtained with the proteinase inhibitor aprotinin [17], its use spread rapidly in cardiac clinics throughout Europe [2, 3]. Although the mode of action has not been completely revealed, we concurrently showed the relation of improved hemostasis with preserved platelet adhesive receptors [18, 19]. Increasing numbers of patients with coronary artery diseases are now treated with aspirin [14] and are submitted with this treatment for coronary artery bypass grafting operation (CABG).

To accept these patients for immediate operation is of great concern, because of the complication of severe bleeding [6]. Since we have demonstrated that aprotinin improves hemostasis in CPB by preserved platelet adhesive (hemostatic) receptors and that aspirin inhibits platelet aggregation (thrombosis) [5, 10], the combined use would be advantageous in preserving hemostasis and improvement of graft patency would be achieved.

This study was performed to evaluate the effect of preoperative aspirin on platelet function and hemostasis with or without use of perioperative aprotinin.

Methods

Patients

After obtaining informed consent, 80 otherwise healthy patients undergoing elective coronary revascularization surgery entered this study. Forty patients took aspirin before operation and 40 patients did not take aspirin.

Twenty patients of the aspirin group and 20 patients of the non-aspirin group were selected in random manner and aprotinin was added to the pump prime solution (2 million KIU).

N. Tabuchi is a visiting fellow from the Department of Cardiothoracic Surgery, Tokyo Medical and Dental University, Tokyo, Japan. Y. J. Gu is a visiting fellow from the Department of Cardiothoracic Surgery, Shanghai Second Medical University, Shanghai, China.

Thus, the patients are divided into four groups: control, aspirin, aprotinin, aspirin and aprotinin.

Aprotinin (Trasylol) was supplied by Bayer AG (Leverkusen, FRG) in bottles containing 50 ml of saline solution without any additives or preservatives; each milliliter contained 10 000 kallikrein inactivator units (KIU). The anesthetic technique, heparinization, extracorporeal circuit, and use of cardioplegia were standardized, as previously published [19].

Blood loss and requirement: Blood loss after operation was determined by the drainage volume from the pleural cavities in the ICU for 24 h after operation. Blood transfusion of packed red cells in the ICU was documented.

Hematology and biochemical assays: In a subpopulation of 10 patients, chosen randomly from each group, blood samples were taken from the radial artery or arterial line of the extracorporeal circuit after induction of anesthesia, 5 min before CPB, at 5 or 30 min of CPB, at the end of CPB, and 30 min after protamin sulphate administration.

Thromboxane B_2: The generation was measured in citrate blood by an enzyme immunoassay (Cayman Co. Ann Arbor, Michigan, USA).

von Willebrand Factor/Factor VIII complex (vWF/FVIII) was determined in citrated plasma by a sandwich-type fluoroimmunoassay (FIA) with specific anti-FVIII related antigen (Behring Diagnostica) and anti-vWF antiserum (DAKO-PATTS).

Platelet glycoprotein Ib (GPIb) receptors: Platelet-rich plasma was equilibrated with Ca^{++} free Tyrode's buffer and the receptors were determined by FIA with specific antibodies and compared with measurements in platelet-poor plasma. Platelet-rich plasma was prepared by centrifuging citrate blood (3.2%) at $90 \times g$ for 10 min.

Platelet aggregation: Platelet-rich plasma aggregometry was performed with a platelet count higher than $150 \times 10^9/L$, by addition of collagen (Ethicon, Inc., Somerville, New Jersey, USA; final concentration 0.1 mg/ml).

Statistical analysis was performed with Student's *t*-test for independent samples. Results are expressed as the mean $\pm$ SEM. A p value of less than 0.05 was considered significant.

Results

Blood loss: Aprotinin significantly ($p < 0.05$) decreased blood loss from 980 ± 67 ml to 571 ± 28 ml in non-aspirin treated patients, and from 1096 ± 121 ml to 672 ± 65 ml in aspirin-treated patients, respectively.

Blood requirement: Postoperative red-blood-cell transfusion was decreased by aprotinin from 0.61 ± 0.21 U to 0.18 ± 0.10 U in non-aspirin patients, and from 0.71 ± 0.23 U to 0.38 ± 0.15 U in aspirin patients, respectively.

Thromboxane B_2 (Fig. 1): In control patients, thromboxane production was increased during CPB with a peak at the end of CPB. In the two aspirin groups, it was suppressed during and after CPB ($p < 0.05$). With aprotinin treatment alone, thromboxane was suppressed, but not as profoundly as with aspirin.

vWF/FVIII (Fig. 2): Aspirin treatment had no effect on the vWF/FVIII serum concentration during surgery. In the non-aprotinin groups, vWF/F VIII was generated and released in the early phase of CPB ($p < 0.05$), but it was decreased in the

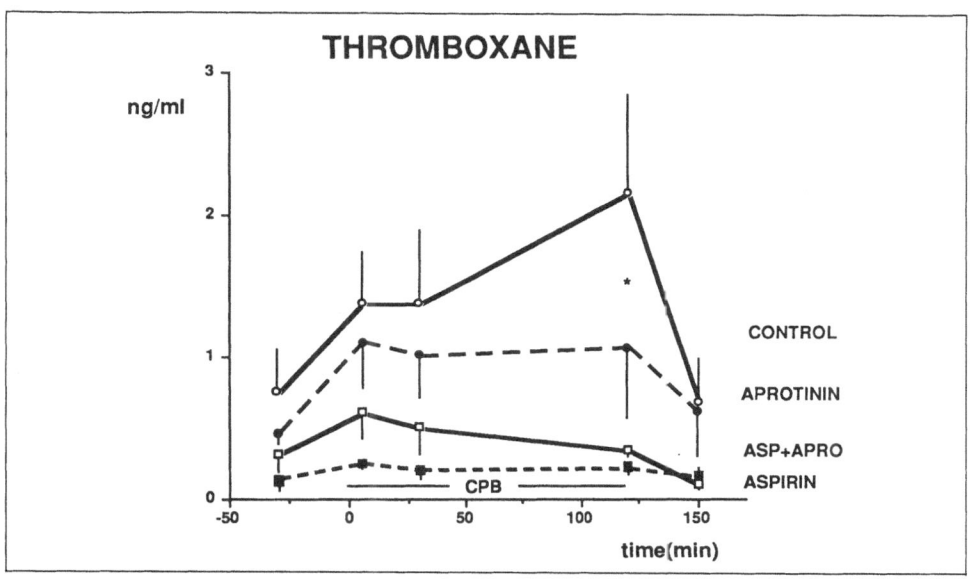

Fig. 1. Thromboxane B_2 production, corrected for hemodilution, was higher during CPB in the control group and it was significant at the end of CPB compared with aspirin or the combined use group (*p < 0.05). With aprotinin it was moderately decreased. In two aspirin groups it was completely suppressed before, during, and after CPB.

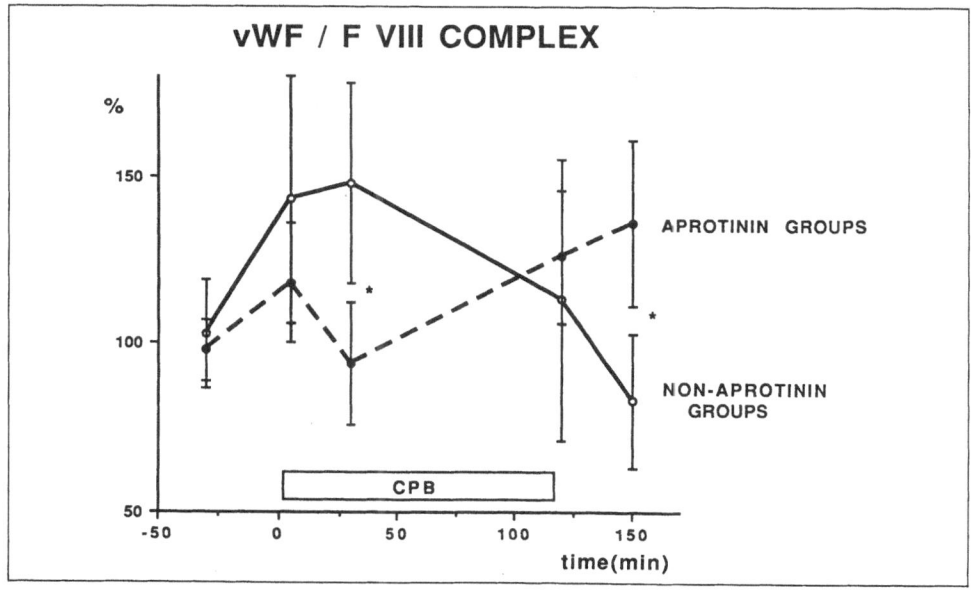

Fig. 2. Plasma level of von Willebrand Factor / Factor VIII complex (vWF/FVIII), corrected for hemodilution, was higher at start of CPB and decreased toward the end of surgery in non-aprotinin groups. With aprotinin treatment it was significantly suppressed at the initial phase and increased after CPB (*p < 0.05). Results are presented as percentage of standard human serum.

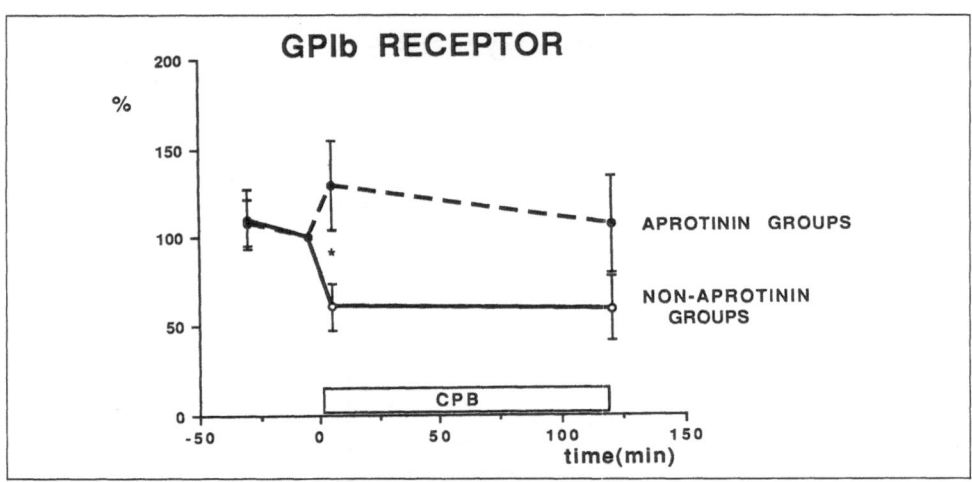

Fig. 3. Antigen determination of the platelet glycoprotein Ib (GPIb) receptor showed the reduction of the receptor at the initial phase of CPB in non-aprotinin groups. GPIb antigen was kept significantly higher with aprotinin treatment, (*p < 0.05).

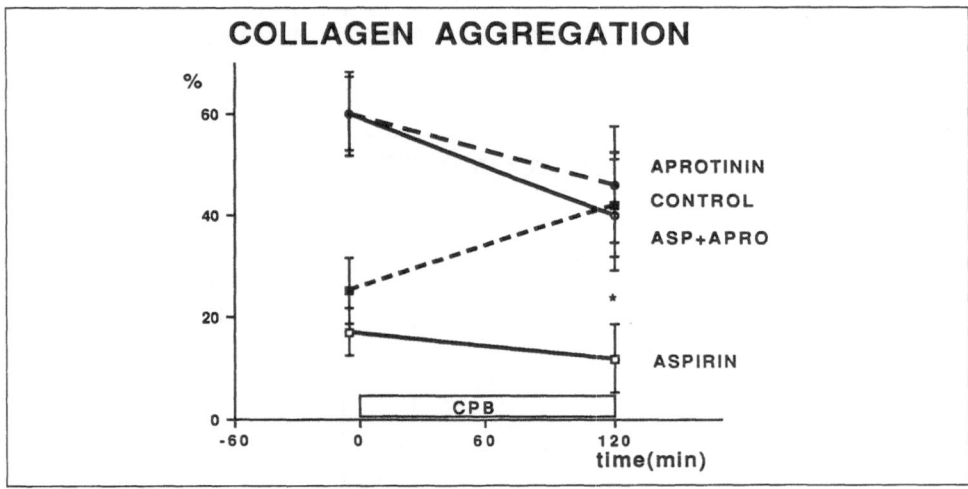

Fig. 4. Collagen aggregation was decreased with aspirin treatment and it was recovered to become significantly higher with addition of aprotinin, compared to the aspirin group (*p < 0.05).

late phase of CPB, and it was significantly lower after CPB (p < 0.05), compared with the aprotinin groups.

GPIb receptor (Fig. 3): Aspirin treatment had no effect on the receptor numbers. In the non-aprotinin groups, the number of the receptor was decreased after the start of CPB, and was decreased further toward the end of CPB. Contrasting with the aprotinin groups, GPIb receptor was maintained at a high level during CPB (p < 0.05).

248

Collagen aggregation (Fig. 4): Aspirin-treated platelets had a low aggregatory response (less then 40%) to collagen before CPB, but with the concomitant use of aprotinin, the response to collagen recovered significantly after CPB (p < 0.05). In the aprotinin and non-treated patients the response was decreased slightly during CPB from 60% to 46% and to 40%, respectively.

Discussion

The remarkable beneficial effect of aprotinin on hemostasis after cardiac surgery has now been substantiated in various institutes [2, 3, 17]. In this study the same effectiveness was experienced in patients treated with aspirin. Several reports proved that aspirin is the most effective anti-platelet drug and that it increases graft patency after coronary revascularization operations [5, 10]. However, to have the most beneficial effect for early graft patency, aspirin therapy should preferably be started before surgery to cover the most vulnerable period for thrombosis of the grafts, that is, immediately after revascularization [10]. In particular, the endothelial cells of vein grafts are damaged during surgery [1], generating a high thrombogenicity for 8 h after injury [11]. It is assumed, however, that in this early postoperative period there is an existing platelet dysfunction induced by the damage of CPB [9, 15]. This might be true if bubble oxygenators are used, but we found in this study that collagen aggregation was not significantly decreased during CPB with the use of membrane oxygenators, which indicates that the risk of thrombus formation on the deendothelialized vein grafts might exist [9]. These data are strongly supported by the results of autopsy which revealed the formation of fibrin microthrombi on the intima of vein grafts within hours after operation [4]. The pre- or perioperative use of an anti-platelet drug to reduce platelet deposition in these thrombogenic vein grafts is therefore meaningful [8, 12].

However, a serious adverse effect of aspirin is the increased bleeding tendency when aspirin is given before operation [6]. To solve this problem, it was proposed to administer aspirin 7 h after the operation with concomitant use of perioperative dipyridamole [10], but the effectiveness of dipyridamole in this regard is still controversial.

In the current study, we demonstrated that the inhibition of cyclo-oxygenase by aspirin and the consequent suppression of thromboxane production, still existed when aprotinin was used. Although aprotinin also inhibited thromboxane production [17], aspirin was far more effective and suppressed thromboxane production also after CPB, which might be important in regard to protecting graft patency.

The collagen aggregation inhibited by aspirin preoperatively was improved by aprotinin after CPB, which might reflect the positive effect of aprotinin on the platelet adhesive receptor, since aspirin does not inhibit platelet adhesion to collagen in physiological conditions [7, 13].

The most important finding of the present study was that hemostasis was improved by aprotinin independently of aspirin. In this regard the observation that after CPB the vWF/F VIII concentration was significantly higher and the GPIb platelet receptors were preserved in the aprotinin treated patients sufficiently explains the improved hemostasis after CPB with this treatment. This is in accordance with the study of Salzman et al. [16] who regarded low vWF concentrations as a cause of impaired hemostasis and found desmopressin acetate (DDAVP) to be effective in reducing postoperative blood loss.

The multiple properties of aprotinin, being plasmin inhibition, preservation of the platelet GPIb receptor and its ligand vWF can explain the hemostasis benefits of aprotinin treatment.

Conclusion

To determine the efficacy of aprotinin to preserve hemostasis in patients using aspirin prior to coronary artery bypass grafting, we compared control, aspirin users, aprotinin alone (2×10^6 KIU in the pump prime), and aspirin users plus aprotinin. Analysis of postoperative blood loss and requirements in 80 patients (20 in each group) revealed that aprotinin improved hemostasis independent of the use of aspirin.

The biochemical effects of aspirin and/or aprotinin were studied in a subpopulation of 10 patients in each group. In the two aspirin groups, thromboxane production was completely suppressed during and after cardiopulmonary bypass (CPB) ($p < 0.05$), but only partly in the aprotinin group as compared to the non-treated control group. Before CPB, serum concentrations of von Willebrand factor/Factor VIII complex (vWF/FVIII) and the number of platelet membrane glycoprotein Ib (GpIb) receptors on platelets were not affected by aspirin treatment. With aprotinin treatment, vWF/FVIII concentration remained constant during and after CPB, but without aprotinin treatment it was substantially released in the early phase of CPB ($p < 0.05$) and was decreased after CPB ($p < 0.05$).

The number of GPIb receptors decreased after the start of CPB, but with aprotinin treatment the numbers remained high ($p < 0.05$).

Since in the combined treatment, aspirin remained effective to suppress the thromboxane production during and after CPB, and aprotinin preserved the platelet GPIb receptors and prevented vWF/F VIII consumption during CPB, the combined use of perioperative aspirin with aprotinin seems to be the ideal treatment for optimal hemostasis and graft patency in patients undergoing CPB.

References

1. Adcock GD, Adcock OT Jr, Wheeler JR, Gregory RT, Snyder SO Jr, Gayle RG, Trivedi AN (1987) Arterialization of reversed autogenous vein grafts. J Vasc Surg 6: 283—295
2. Alajmo F, Calamai G, Perna AM, Melissano G, Pretelli P, Palmarini MF, Carbonetto F, Noferi D, Boddi V, Palminiello A, Vaccari M (1989) High-dose aprotinin: Hemostatic effects in open-heart operations. Ann Thorac Surg 48: 536—539
3. Bidstrup BP, Royston D, Sapsford RN, Taylor KM (1989) Reduction in blood loss and blood use after cardiopulmonary bypass with high dose aprotinin. (Trasylol) J Thorac Cardiovasc Surg 97: 364—372
4. Bulkley BH, Hutchins GM (1977) Accelated atherosclerosis. A morphologic study of 97 saphenous vein coronary artery bypass grafts. Circulation 55: 163—169
5. Chesebro JH, Clements IP, Fuster V, Elveback LR, Smith HC, Bardsley WT, Frye RL, Holmes DR Jr, Vliestra RE, Pluth JR, Wallace RB, Puga FJ, Orszulak TA, Piehler JM, Schaff HV, Danielson GK (1982) A platelet-inhibitor drug trial in coronary artery bypass operations. N Engl J Med 307: 73—77

6. Ferraris VA, Ferraris SP, Lough FC, Berry WR (1988) Preoperative aspirin ingestion increases operative blood loss after coronary artery bypass grafting. Ann Thorac Surg 45: 71—74
7. Feuerstein IA (1987) Aspirin does not inhibit platelet adherence to and detachment from collagen-coated glass. Thromb Res 46: 751—754
8. Fuster V, Dewanjee MK, Kaye MP, Josa M, Metke MP, Chesebro JH (1979) Noninvasive radioisotope technique for detection of platelet deposition in coronary artery bypass grafts in dogs and its reduction with platelet inhibitors. Circulation 60: 1508—1512
9. Fuster V, Chesebro JJ (1985) Aortocoronary artery vein-graft disease: experimental and clinical approach for the understanding of the role of platelets and platelet inhibitors. Circulation 72: V 65—70
10. Goldman S, and the Veterans administration group (1988) Improvement in early saphenous vein graft patency after coronary artery bypass surgery with antiplatelet therapy. Circulation 77: 1324—1332
11. Groves HM, Kinlough-Rathbone RL, Mustard JF (1986) Development of non-thrombogenicity of injured rabbits aorta despite inhibition of platelet adherence. Arterioslcerosis 6: 189—195
12. Josa M, Lie JT, Bianco RL, Kaye MP (1981) Reduction of thrombosis in canine coronary bypass vein grafts with dipyridamole and aspirin. Am J Cardiol 47: 1248—1254
13. Kinlough-Rathbone RL, Cazenave JP, Packham MA, Mustard JF (1980) Effect of inhibitors of arachidonate pathway on the release of granule contents from rabbit platelets adherent to collagen. Lab Invest 42: 28—34
14. Lewis HD Jr, and the Veterans administration cooperative study group (1985) Unstable angina: status of aspirin and other forms of therapy. Circulation 72: V — 155—163
15. Mohr R, Golan M, Martinowitz U, Rosner E, Goor DA, Ramot B (1986) Effect of cardiac operation on platelets. J Thorac Cardiovasc Surg 92: 434—441
16. Salzman EW, Weinstein MJ, Weintraub RM, Ware JA, Thurer RL, Roberston L, Donovan A, Gaffney T, Bertele V, Troll J, Smith M, Chute LE (1986) Treatment with desmopressin acetate to reduce blood loss after cardiac surgery. N Engl J Med 314: 1402—1406
17. Van Oeveren W, Jansen NJG, Bidstrup BP, Royston D, Westaby S, Neuhof H, Wildevuur CRH (1987) Effects of aprotinin on hemostatic mechanisms during cardiopulmonary bypass. Ann Thorac Surg 44: 640—645
18. Van Oeveren M, Eijsman L, Roozendal KJ, Wildevuur CRH (1988) Platelet preservation by aprotinin during cardiopulmonary bypass. Lancet 1: 644
19. Wildevuur CRH, Eijsman L, Roozendaal KJ, Harder MP, Chang M, Van Oeveren W (1989) Platelet preservation during cardiopulmonary bypass with aprotinin. Eur J Cardio-thoracic Surg 3: 533—538

Author's address:
W. Van Oeveren
Cardiopulmonary Surgery Research Division
University Hospital
Oostersingel 59
9713 EZ Groningen
The Netherlands

ACT and Aprotinin

D. U. Preiss, I. Witt*, H. Kiefer, P. Betz

Benedikt Kreutz Rehabilitation Center, Bad Krozingen, FRG
*University Children's Hospital, Freiburg, FRG

Introduction

Monitoring of the adequacy of anticoagulation is essential to the safe conduct of cardiopulmonary bypass (CPB). While there is no universally accepted heparin level or test of adequate anticoagulation during cardio-pulmonary bypass, the automated activated clotting time (Hemochron ACT) became the routine method of monitoring heparinization in most cardiac centers, because of its simplicity, rapidity, and an observed linear relationship to the heparin dose [2, 3, 10]. However, hemodilution, coagulation-factor depletion, and hypothermia have all been shown to influence ACT and, thus, may lead to a non-heparin-induced prolongation of ACT. Furthermore, there is also no universally accepted safe minimum ACT for CPB [6, 12].

Aprotinin has been demonstrated, both in vivo and in vitro, to prolong ACT, especially in the presence of heparin. In this study we have examined the effect of aprotinin upon the relationship of heparin concentration and ACT prolongation, the heparin sensitivity of ACT, and the heparin dosage related to the duration of extracorporeal circulation (ECC).

Methods

The patient populations of groups I–IV are described in Table 1. Patient characteristics were similar in all groups. Surgical procedures were the same in groups I and II. Nineteen patients had valves replaced in group IV, as compared to 16 in group III. Three patients in group III and one patient in group IV received aorto-coronary bypass grafts in addition. The mean time of ECC was 20 min longer in group II compared to group I (Table 2). Groups II and IV patients were treated with high doses of aprotinin (Trasylol) according to the protocol described by Bidstrup et al. [1]; patients of groups I and III served as controls. We followed an improved Bull protocol [3, 9] for heparinization and its reversal with protamine in patients of groups I and II. Patients of groups III and IV received a heparin loading-dose of 360 I.E. heparin/kg b.w. before CPB. Additional heparin was given, when needed, to reach a target ACT of 480 s. Heparin neutralization in groups III and IV was achieved with a protamine/heparin ratio of 0.68 ± 0.12 and controlled with test tubes of the Protamine Dose Assay (International Technidyne). Anesthesia management, CPB management, and the use of cardioplegia during aortic cross-clamp time were similar in all groups. Heparin concentrations were determined according to Witt et al. [11]. ACT was measured with a Hemochron 800 instrument (International Technidyne).

Table 1. Patient characteristics.

Group	I (Control)	II (Aprotinin)	p <	III (Control)	IV (Aprotinin)	p <
Sex (male/female)	8/1	6/3		40/10	38/11	
Mean Age (years)	57.2 ± 6.2	57.8 ± 6.3	n.s.	59.6 ± 8.6	60.8 ± 8.1	n.s.
Mean Height (cm)	171.5 ± 8.8	169.8 ± 10.4	n.s.	167.9 ± 8.4	167.8 ± 8.2	n.s.
Mean Weight (kg)	72.0 ± 9.1	73.5 ± 11.1	n.s.	68.5 ± 9.8	70.2 ± 8.7	n.s.

Table 2. Surgical procedures.

Group	I (Control)	II (Aprotinin)	p <	III (Control)	IV (Aprotinin)	p <
CABG	n = 7	7		33	31	
CABG + valve replacement	n = 0	0		3	1	
Valve replcement or repair	n = 2	2		13	18	
Operating time (min)	205 ± 38.9	263.3 ± 81.2	n.s.	199 ± 45	194 ± 52	n.s.
ECC (min)	86.1 ± 14.3	106.6 ± 20.6	0.05	95 ± 28	90 ± 29	n.s.

Results

Although ACT values of group II patients receiving aprotinin were significantly prolonged, as compared to group I patients (Fig. 1a), heparin concentrations did not differ (Fig. 1b) or were slightly, but not significantly, smaller in patients receiving aprotinin.

Since ACT during CPB is influenced by factors other than heparin concentration, i.e., hemodilution, hypothermia, and depletion of coagulation factors, a good linear relationship between plasma heparin concentration and ACT can only be found before CPB is initiated [4, 5, 7]. Accordingly, before ECC a linear relationship between plasma heparin concentration and increase in ACT was found in patients of group I (Fig. 2a). In patients treated with aprotinin, heparin concentration and increase in ACT (Δ ACT) were not correlated (Fig. 2b).

The finding that longer ACTs in patients treated with aprotinin are obviously not due to higher plasma heparin concentrations led us to investigate the heparin sensitivity of the ACT in larger groups of patients with and without aprotinin. In addition, in groups III and IV ACT during CPB and heparin dosages in relation to the duration of ECC were studied. Slopes of the ACT dose-response curves weres determined as a measure for the individual heparin sensitivity [6, 8]. A linear ACT dose-response curve that forms an angle of 45 ° with the x-axis has a slope of 1. Numbers < 1 signify slopes > 45 ° and, therefore, indicate a smaller effectiveness of heparin as compared to numbers > 1. Patients of group III had a mean slope of 0.82 ± 0.31; group IV patients, receiving aprotinin averaged 1.48 ± 0.65 (Fig. 3). This difference was highly significant ($p < 0.0001$).

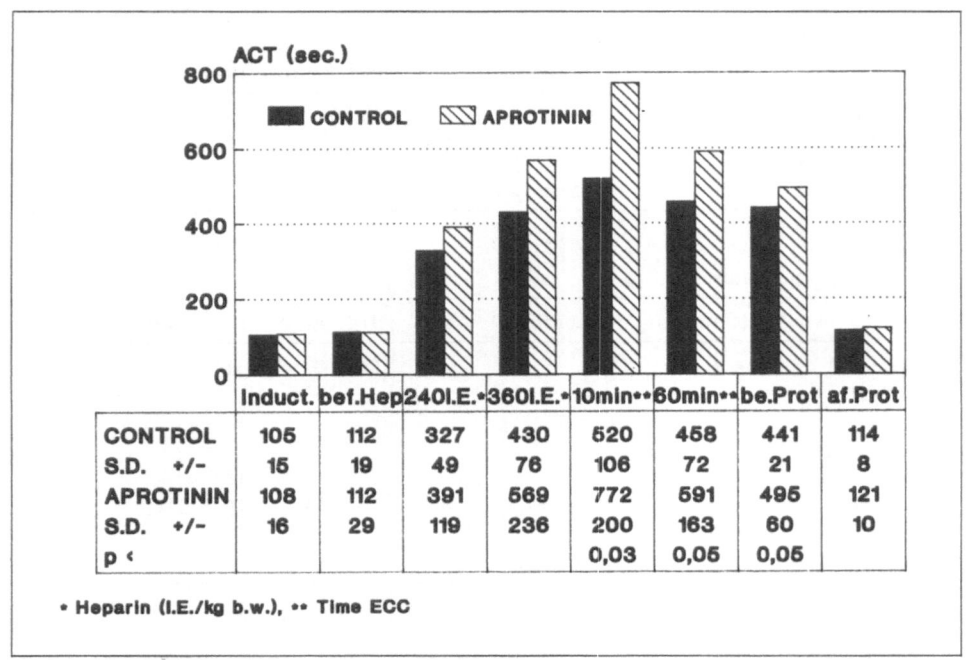

Fig. 1a. ACT-values throughout cardiac surgical procedures in patients with and without high doses of aprotinin.

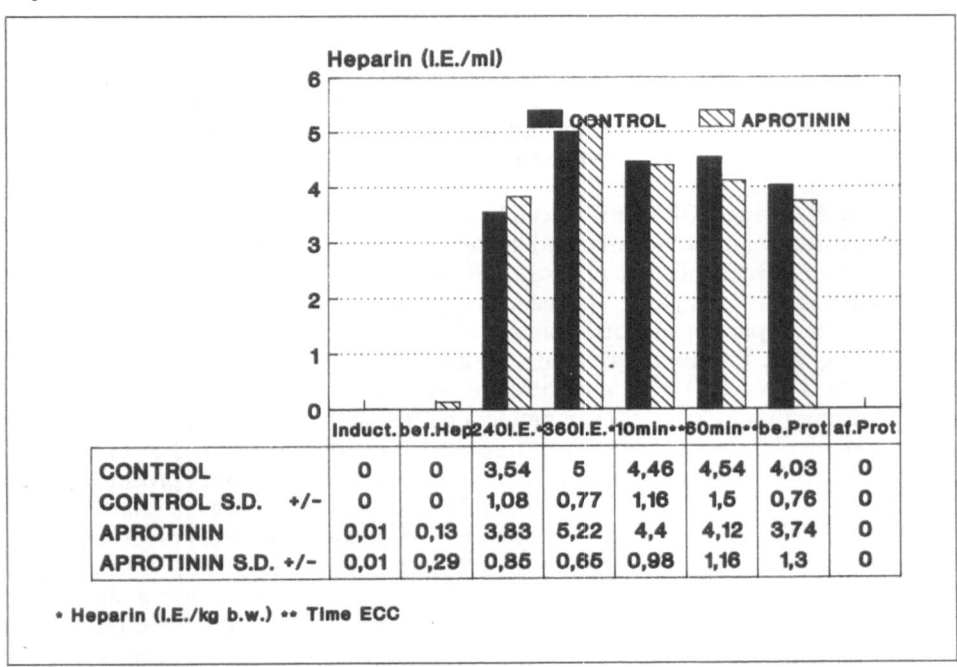

Fig. 1b. Plasma heparin-concentrations throughout cardiac surgical procedures in patients with and without high doses of aprotinin.

254

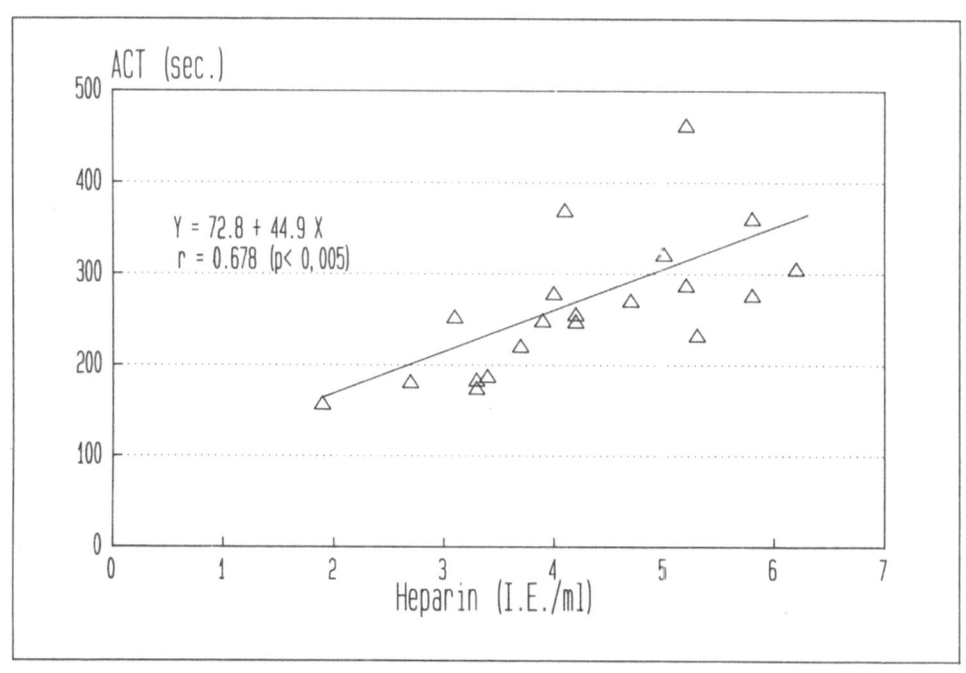

Fig. 2a. Relationship between plasma heparin-concentration and increase of ACT in patients without aprotinin.

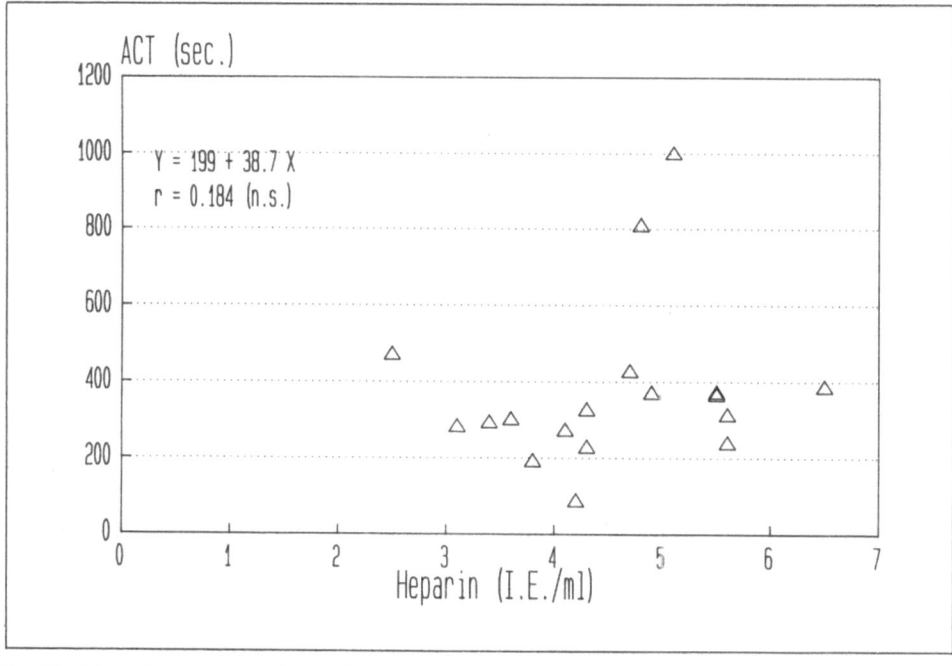

Fig. 2b. Disparity between plasma heparin-concentration and increase of ACT in patients treated with high doses of aprotinin.

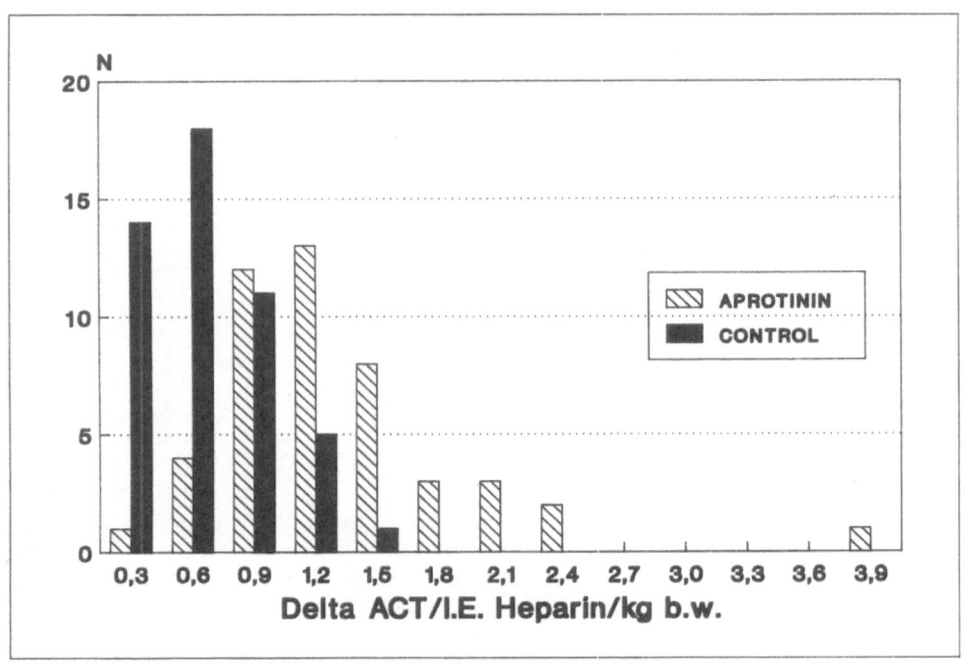

Fig. 3. Distribution of the slopes ($\triangle$ ACT/I.E./kg b.w.) of the heparin-ACT dose-response curves of patients with and without high doses of aprotinin.

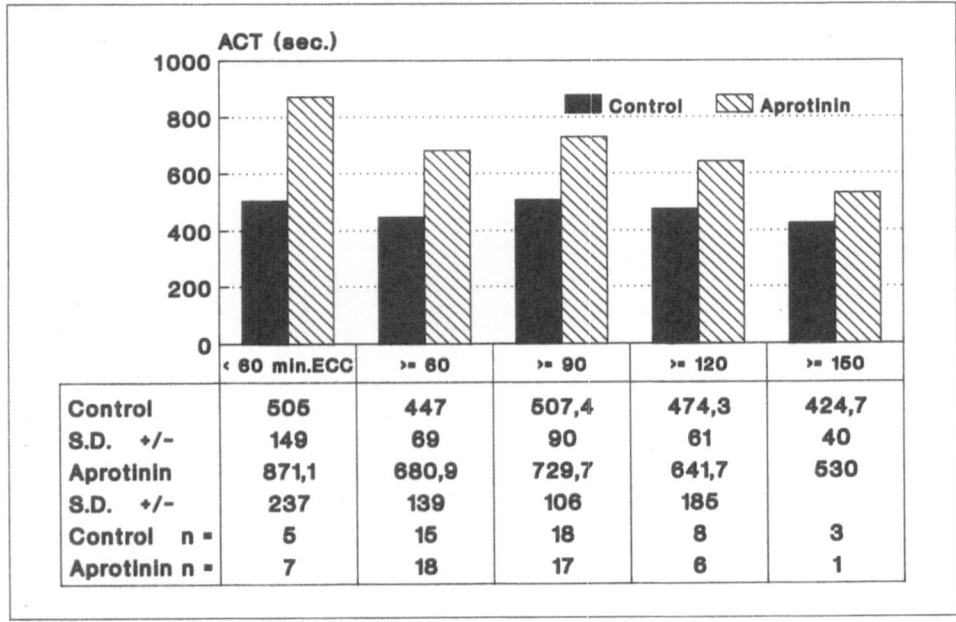

	< 60 min.ECC	>= 60	>= 90	>= 120	>= 150
Control	505	447	507,4	474,3	424,7
S.D. +/-	149	69	90	61	40
Aprotinin	871,1	680,9	729,7	641,7	530
S.D. +/-	237	139	106	185	
Control n =	5	15	18	8	3
Aprotinin n =	7	18	17	6	1

Fig. 4. Mean values of the ACT ($\overline{m}$ ACT) during the time of heparinization in relation to the duration of extracorporeal circulation (ECC) of patients with and without high doses of aprotinin.

In group IV patients mean ACT values during the period of heparinization were longer, as compared to group III patients, irrespective of the duration of ECC (Fig. 4). This difference was highly significant (p < 0.0001). Mean ACT values within group IV were longer in patients with shorter cardiopulmonary bypass times (p < 0.01). But in group III patients duration of ECC had no influence on mean ACT values. This finding could be explained by taking into consideration the method of maintenance and control of anticoagulation during ECC. Additional doses of heparin are given when ACT values, determined every 30 min, tend to fall below 480 s. In consequence, if aprotinin prolongs ACT considerably, fewer or smaller additional heparin doses are given, and towards the end of prolonged bypass times ACT values of aprotinin-treated patients might tend to approach ACT values of controls. If this were true the heparin dosage in group IV would have to be smaller in comparison with group III.

This is precisely what we found in the larger groups of patients. Group III patients required minimally, but significantly, more heparin per kg of body weight and min of ECC than group IV patients: 7.94 ± 2.64 vs 6.79 ±2.52 I.E./kg b.w./min (p < 0.03). The length of cardiopulmonary-bypass time influenced the dosage in both groups, but had no influence on the difference between heparin dosages among patients of group III and IV (Fig. 5).

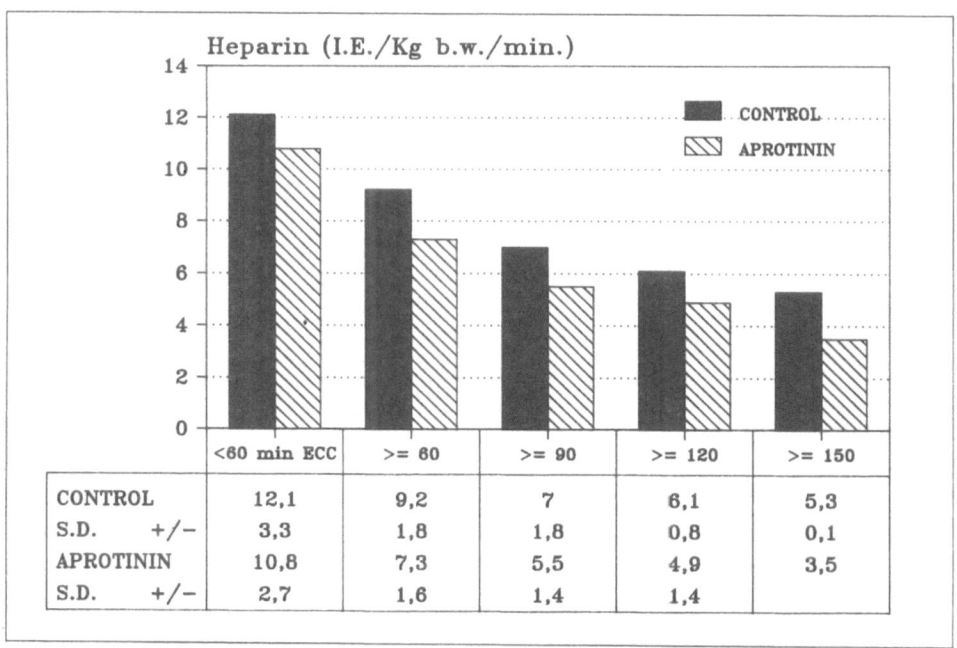

Fig. 5. Heparin doses (I.E./kg b.w./min) in relation to the duration of extracorporeal circulation (ECC) of patients with and without high doses of aprotinin.

257

Discussion and conclusion

Our study demonstrates that high doses of aprotinin result in a greatly increased heparin sensitivity of the ACT and a loss of correlation between heparin concentration and ACT. Subsequently, patients treated with aprotinin received smaller doses of heparin compared to controls, because heparin doses were adjusted by ACT. These findings raise — but cannot answer — the question: Does the ACT in patients treated with aprotinin still adequately reflect anticoagulation in cardiac surgical patients? Further studies are needed to answer that question. At present the following recommendations are made for the practical use of ACT measurements in cardiac surgical patients treated with high doses of aprotinin:

Recommendations

1) Borderline ACT values should not lead to the omission of a repeated heparin dose, especially with extended bypass procedures. Aprotinin should not be used to save heparin.
2) Increased ACT values (e.g., > 800 s) at the end of ECC should not lead to a higher dosage of protamine [9]. Basically, the amount of heparin given to the patient still determines the protamine dose required for neutralization.
3) There is no "over-dose" of heparin when ACT values appear to be high during ECC.
4) If ACT values after protamine administration still appear to be high, i.e., tending to suggest a surplus of heparin, residual heparin, if present, can easily, quickly, and reliably be detected by using the orange-stoppered test tubes of the protamine dose assay kit (manufactured by International Technidyne, distributed by Fresenius AG, Bad Homburg, FRG) and neutralized by giving additional doses of protamine.

References

1. Bidstrup BP, Royston D, Sapsford RN, Taylor KM (1989) Reduction in blood loss and blood use after cardiopulmonary bypass with high dose aprotinin (Trasylol). J Thorac Cardiovasc Surg 97: 364—372
2. Blohn von G, Hellstern P, Köhler M, Scheffler P, Wenzel E (1986) Klinische Gesichtspunke des erworbenen Antithrombin III-Mangels. Behring Inst Mitt 79: 200—215
3. Bull BS, Korpman RA, Huse WM, Briggs BD (1975) Heparin therapy during extracorporeal circulation. I. Problems inherent in existing heparin protocols. J Thorac Cardiovasc Surg 69: 674—684
4. Cohen EJ, Camerlengo LJ, Dearing JP (1980) Activated clotting times and cardiopulmonary bypass I: The effect of hemodilution and hypothermia upon activated clotting time. J Extra-Corp Tech 12: 139—141
5. Culliford AT, Gitel SN, Starr N, Thomas ST, Baumann FG, Wessler S, Spencer FC (1981) Lack of correlation between activated clotting time and plasma heparin during cardiopulmonary bypass. Ann Surg 193: 105—111
6. Esposito RA, Culliford AT, Colvin SB, Thomas SJ, Lackner H, Spencer FC (1983) The role of the activated clotting time in heparin administration and neutralization for cardiopulmonary bypass. J Thorac Cardiovasc Surg 85: 174—185

7. Hughes DR, Faust RJ, Didisheim P, Tinker JH (1982) Heparin monitoring during cardiopulmonary bypass in man: Use of fluorogenic heparin assay to validate activated clotting time.
   Anesthesia and Analgesia 61: 189—190
8. Preiss DU, Schmidt-Bleibtreu H, Berguson P, Metz G (1985) Blood transfusion requirements
   in coronary artery surgery with and without the activated clotting time (ACT) technique. Klin
   Wochenschr 63: 252—256
9. Preiss DU, Zobeley R (1983) Individuelle Heparin- und Protamindosierung in der Herzchirurgie. Klin Wochenschr 61: 1141—1146
10. Schriever HG, Epstein SE, Mintz MD (1973) Statistical correlation and heparin sensitivity of
    activated partial thromboplastin time, whole blood coagulation time and an automated coagu-
    lation time. Am J of Clin Path 60: 323—329
11. Witt I, Herz R, Lill H (1984) Heparin. In: Methods of enzymatic analysis. HU Bergmeyer (Ed)
    Verlag Chemie, Weinheim, Bergstr. p 477—486
12. Young JA, Kisker CT, Doty DB (1978) Adequate anticoagulation during cardiopulmonary by-
    pass determined by activated clotting time and the apparance of fibrin monomer. Ann Thorac
    Surg 26: 231—240

Author's address:
Dr. D. U. Preiss
Benedikt Kreutz Rehabilitation Center
Südring 15
D-7812 Bad Krozingen

Aprotinin : Effect on "Re-Do" Surgery

D. N. Ross and J. C. Simpson

National Heart Hospital, London, England

Introduction

The present early surgical treatment of congenital cardiac disease by palliative surgery in infancy entails the need for re-operation in later years. This is especially true of surgical treatment of congenital aortic stenosis and pulmonary atresia. The former condition can be palliated by aortic valvotomy — using inflow occlusion techniques — and the latter by modified Blalock shunt. In each case the infant is palliated to allow growth and thus a definitive repair of the diseased outflow tract.

This brief communication deals with blood loss and its prevention when these patients come for surgery to re-replace their outflow tract conduits.

The problem

During the last 25 years, Ross and coworkers developed a homograft service whereby both human aortic and pulmonary valves are available for surgical use. An extension of his work has enabled these valves to be used (often in combination with a pericardial or woven Dacron tube) successfully in the replacement of left or right ventricular outflow tract [2]. The use of these types of conduits obviates the necessity for longterm anticoagulation — the latter is undesirable and indeed dangerous in children and young people who should be encouraged, after surgery, to lead a normal and active life. The major problem encountered using human tissues and artificial conduits is one of tissue calcification, especially in the homograft valves, and the development of layers of fibrin desposit within the Dacron tubes - thus re-imposing the symptoms of outflow tract obstruction, and the need for further surgery. Because of the nature of the tissues and mediastinal adhesions from previous surgery, re-operation may cause major haemorrhage, and it is a well defined fact that the massive blood transfusion needed in this situation is a cause of morbidity and mortality - especially if accompanied by low cardiac output. Surgical haemorrhage may be contained by careful surgery, but there remains the problem of "medical bleeding" which may or may not be responsive to drug therapy, clotting factors and blood transfusion. Fresh donor blood is no longer available in the U.K.; however, aprotinin has been demonstrated to be of use in similar situations [1].

Study

A retrospective analysis was performed of such patients operated in the period 1987—1989. Forty patients were included, matched for age and weight, all of whom had undergone a clinical operation, using standard hypothermic cardiopulmonary bypass for surgical replacement of left or right ventricular outflow tract. Twenty patients (Group A) had not received aprotinin, whilst the remaining 20 patients (Group B) received aprotinin according to the manufacturer's protocol. Neither auto-transfusion nor the cell-saver was used in any of the patients.

Results

Operative mortality is defined, for the purpose of this paper, as death either in the operating room or the intensive care ward. Table 1 demonstrates four deaths in Group A and one death in Group B.

The four deaths in Group A were clinically related to uncontrollable bleeding, consequent low cardiac output, renal failure, tissue hypoxia, electrolyte imbalance, and in one case ARDS despite aggressive treatment. The single death in Group B was due to left ventricular infarction because of anatomical difficulty in coronary artery anastomosis during a third re-do aortic root replacement.

Table 2 aligns the quantity of whole blood, fresh frozen plasma and units of platelet concentrate used in the first 24 h post-operatively in the two groups.

The objectives of this part of transfusion therapy were to maintain adequate aterial filling pressures, achieving a haemoglobin level of 12 grams % and an adequate clotting time as judged by "bed-side" measurement of the activated clotting time using Haemochron Mark II. The results demonstrate that aprotinin reduced the volume, and thus the inherent dangers of transfusion of blood and blood-derived clotting factors.

The continuous clinical management of these patients necessitates frequent haemodynamic and laboratory investigation to assess progress. We have identified three simple laboratory investigations that give an excellent guide as to status of haemostasis and renal function. They are: a) platelet count, b) fibrin degradation products and c) serum creatinine. The platelet count in absolute terms gives no guide to

Table 1. Overall results.

Results: Operative Mortality

Group A	Group B
4 (20%)	1 (5%)

Table 2. Volume of blood and blood-derived clotting factors used in 24 h post-surgery.

Results: a) Units of blood;
         b) Units of fresh frozen plasma;
         c) Units of platelets

Group A	Group B
a) 9 (6—25)	4 (2—8)
b) 6 (3—9)	3 (0—6)
c) 12 (6—18)	6 (6)

Table 3. Levels of platelets, fibrin degradation products and creatinine, 24 h after surgery.

Results: a) Platelet count; 10^9/l;
      b) Fibrin degradation products; micrograms/litre
      c) Creatinine; micromoles/litre

Group A	Group B
a) 109 (50—190)	74 (63—140)
b) 24 (16—38)	16 (12—21)
c) 214 (90—440)	120 (94—230)

platelet **activity**, but combined with an estimation of fibrin degradation products alerts clinicians to excessive fibrinolysis and possibly disseminated intra-vascular coagulopathy. The creatinine level is possibly the most sensitive monitor of impending renal complications.

Table 3 sets out these values, at 24 h post-surgery in the two groups of patients.

The platelet count in Group A is significantly higher than in Group B, because of a greater volume of platelet concentrate transfused to these patients. Certainly the higher level of fibrin degradation products in Group A accords with their clinical condition at this time; they were still bleeding enough to cause surgical concern. Experience has shown that further surgery is of no help unless tamponade or sudden excessive haemorrhage occurs.

The difference in creatinine levels between the two groups accords with the clinical picture that patients in Group A, some still bleeding and with a low cardiac output, showed the first signs of renal complications of prolonged blood transfusion and incipient circulatory failure. This was not the case with patients in Group B.

Conclusion

Limited data has been presented indicating that aprotinin may be of considerable help in securing haemostasis in a group of surgical patients whose postoperative recovery may be delayed. The complications of extensive transfusion of blood and blood products may thereby be avoided.

References

1. Bidstrup BP, Royston D, Sapsford RN, Taylor KM (1989) Reduction in blood loss and blood use after cardiopulmonary bypass with high-dose aprotinin. J Thorac Cardiovasc Surgery 97: 364—373
2. Somerville J, Ross DN (1972) Long-term results of complete correction with homograft reconstruction in pulmonary outflow tract atresia. Br Heart J 34: 29—36

Authors' address:
D. N. Ross, J. C. Simpson
National Heart Hospital
Westmoreland Street
London WIM 8 BA
U.K.

The Edinburgh Experience — Low-dose Trasylol

D. H. T. Scott and J. Au

Department of Cardiothoracic Surgery, Royal Infirmary of Edinburgh, Scotland

At the beginning of 1988, preservative-free Trasylol was not available for our patients in Edinburgh. We were able to use a preparation which contained as a preservative benzyl alcohol 9 mg/ml. Concerned about its toxic effects, we consulted the literature and came up with a dosage scheme of 1 mega KIU given over 30 min prior to initiating bypass, and 1.5 mega KIU administered over the first 1.5 h of bypass. This produces a total dose of aproximately half the amount used in the series of Royston et al. [1], Van Oeveren et al. [2] and Bidstrup et al. [3]. The drug was administered to a variety of patients who presented for cardiopulmonary bypass and we are reporting the results of those patients who had repeat cardiopulmonary bypass procedures performed through median sternotomies. As a control group, we have used consecutive patients having repeat cardiopulmonary bypass procedures through median sternotomies in 1987. Patients with a major surgical cause of bleeding confirmed at re-operation were excluded from the analysis. There were 27 patients in the Trasylol group and 24 in the control group. There were no differences in respect of age, sex, bypass time or type of operation. These details are summarised in Table 1.

We measured the amount of blood lost into the mediastinal drain after operation. The mean blood loss in the Trasylol group was 948 mls compared to 1429 mls in the control group. Figure 1 demonstrates the wide range of the volume of drain losses. The difference between the two groups was not significant using the Wilcoxon rank sum test.

The amount of blood administered to each patient throughout their entire hospital stay was obtained from the records of the blood bank. One donation of either red cell concentrate or whole blood was counted as one unit. A mean of 8.3 units were given to the Trasylol group and 9.8 units were given to the control group. These

Table 1. Comparison of treatment and control groups.

	Trasylol	Control
N	27	24
Male	10	13
Mean age	54.2 years	53.6 years
Mean CPB time	119 minutes	109 minutes
Operations		
Coronary artery bypass graft	3	7
Mitral prosthetic replacement	8	6
Aortic prosthetic replacement	9	6
Aortic and mitral valve replacement	4	4
CABG and valve	2	1
Paraprosthetic leak	1	0

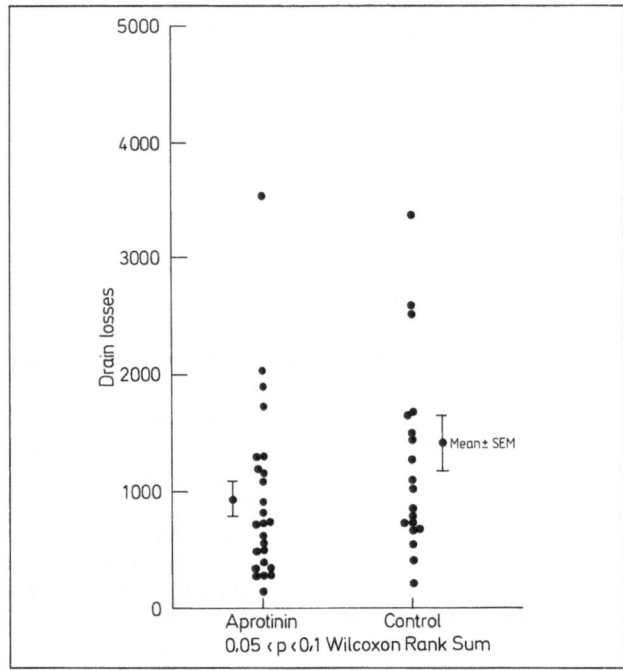

Fig. 1. Comparison of mediastinal drain losses in treated and control patients.

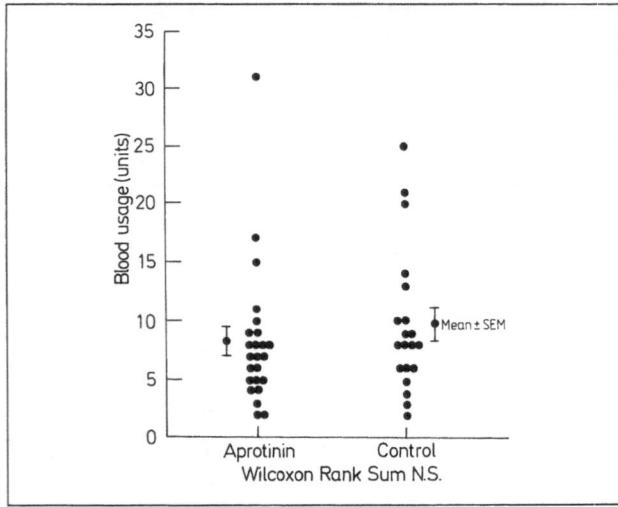

Fig. 2. Comparison of blood use in treated and control patients.

were not statistically different using the Wilcoxon rank sum test. The distribution is shown in Fig. 2.

An average of 4.9 units of platelets were administered in the Trasylol group compared to 5 units in the control. The equivalent figures for fresh frozen plasma were 2.8 and 2.9 units respectively.

Four out of 27 patients in the Trasylol group developed renal failure, as did one patient out of 24 in the control group. There was one death in each group. Neither of these figures is of statistical significance.

Discussion

The mediastinal blood loss of 1429 mls in our control group is directly comparable to the 1509 mls lost by the control patients in Royston's [1] series. The losses in our treated group were considerably higher, 948 mls compared to 246 mls, and it is logical to conclude that this was due to the administration of half the amount of trasylol in our patients. The overall blood use in our series is very much higher, although the difference between our two groups is of the same order of magnitude as the difference in mediastinal blood loss. Our policy was to maintain a patient's haemoglobin around 12 g/dl, and this may have had some influence on the amount of blood administered to our patients. We do not attempt to save blood at all costs, and it is certainly Fox's [4] belief that surgeons tend only to publish blood-loss figures when these are lower than the norm. The losses in the Edinburgh patients compare well with the United Kingdom averages reported by Russell et al. [5].

Conclusions

Trasylol at a dose of 2.5×10^6 KIU tended to reduce post-operative drain losses, but the effect did not reach statistical significance, and it did not materially affect the amount of blood administered to our patients.

References

1. Royston D, Bidstrup BP, Taylor KM, Sapsford RN (1987) Effect of aprotinin on need for blood transfusion after repeat open-heart surgery. Lancet 2: 1289—1291
2. Van Oeveren W, Jansen NJG, Bidstrup BP, Royston D, Westaby S, Neuhof H, Wildevuur CRH (1987) Effects of aprotinin on haemostatic mechanisms during cardiopulmonary bypass. Ann Thorac Surg 44: 640—645
3. Bidstrup BP, Royston D, Taylor KM, Sapsford RN (1988) Effect of aprotinin on need for blood transfusion in patients with septic endocarditis having open-heart surgery. Lancet 1: 366—367
4. Fox MA (1989) "Homologous blood use in Cardiac Surgery" in Blood Use in Cardiac Surgery. Berlin
5. Russel GN, Peterson S, Harper SJ, Fox MA (1988) Homologous Blood use and Conservation techniques for Cardiac Surgery in the United Kingdom. Br Med J 297: 1390—1391

Author's address:
Dr. David H. T. Scott
Department of Cardiothoracic Surgery, Royal Infirmary of Edinburgh, Lauriston Place, Edinburgh, EH3 9YW, Scotland

Reduction of Blood Use by Aprotinin
After Heart-Transplantation

M. Havel, H. Teufelsbauer, W. Zwölfer, A. Laczkovics and E. Wolner

Second Department of Surgery, University of Vienna, Austria

Introduction

Our study comprised a group of 20 patients who underwent orthotopic heart transplantation at the Second Department of Surgery of the Vienna University Clinic Medical School between January and July 1989. All patients were male, with an indication of cardiomyopathy in every case.

Aprotinin dose regimen

Those patients who were allocated to receive aprotinin according to a randomized list, were administered 280 mg aprotinin via a central venous catheter after anesthesia was initiated, yet prior to surgery. Infusion was carried out over a period of 20 min. In addition, 280 mg aprotinin were added to the primary filling of the heart-lung machine.

The patients in the control group received a corresponding volume of normal saline solution.

Measurements

The volumes of blood administered were determined immediately postoperatively, as well as 24 and 48 h after the patients' transfer to the intensive care unit.

Postoperative bleeding was measured 24 and 48 h after surgery.

Statistical analysis

Medians, 0.25 and 0.75 quartiles of postoperative bleeding volumes, and the necessary amounts of blood replacement were calculated for patients with and without aprotinin treatment. Since a normal distribution of these parameters could not be assumed without reservation, the Mann-Whitney U-Test was used to obtain p-values for proving significant differences between both groups.

266

Table 1. Blood loss in ml (median 0.25—0.75 quantile range).

	Aprotinin group		Control group
24 h post-operative	510 (385—780)	$p < 0.01$	820 (665—1025)
48 h post-operative	690 (480—970)	$p < 0.03$	1000 (820—1260)

Table 2. Blood replacement in ml (median; 0.25—0.75 quantile range).

	Aprotinin group		Control group
48 h post-operative	0 (0—250)	$p < 0.04$	500 (0—1000)

Results

There was no difference in the patients of either group with regard to sex, age, height, weight, and extracorporeal circulation time.

Postoperative bleeding in the aprotinin group was significantly lower at 24 and 48 h, respectively, than in the placebo group (Table 1). None of the patients in either group received extra blood during surgery. Corresponding to the increased postoperative bleeding tendency in the group not treated with aprotinin, an increased amount of blood substitution was required; 48 h after completion of surgery, this group required significantly more blood (Table 2).

Discussion

Cytomegalovirus infection, as well as others, are a severe complication in immunosuppressed patients after organ transplantation [1]. Serologically, there are signs of CMV infection in almost 100% of the patients after heart transplantation [2]. Along with the possibility of infection through the donor heart, other sources of infection must be taken into consideration. Thus, a correlation between the number of blood transfusions and the risk of CMV infection can be made [3].

Therefore, it is obviously of most importance to avoid blood transfusions in transplanted and immunosuppressed patients. Our randomized examination of 20 patients after orthotopic heart transplantation showed that by administering proteinase-inhibitor aprotinin, not only postoperative blood loss was significantly lower in the treated group, but also the need for blood transfusion. Seventy percent of the patients of the aprotinin group, compared to 30% in the control group needed neither intra- nor postoperative blood transfusions.

References

1. Wreghitt TG, Gray JJ, Chandler C (1986) Prognostic Value of cytomegalovirus IgM antibody in transplant recipients. Lancet 1: 1157—8

2. Dummer JS, White LT, Ho M, Griffith BP, Hardesky RL, Bahnson HT (1985) Morbidity of cytomegalovirus infection in recipients of heart, heart-lung transplants who received cyclosporine. J Infect Dis 152: 1182—91
3. Adler SP (1983) Transfusion-associated cytomegalovirus infection. Rev Infect Dis 5: 977—993

Authors' address:
Dr. M. Havel
Allgemeines Krankenhaus
Spitalgasse 23
A-1090 Vienna

Blood Damage and Activation in Cardiopulmonary Bypass

Ch. R. H. Wildevuur

Department of Cardiopulmonary Surgery, Research Division, University Hospital Groningen, The Netherlands

Three sources of damage and/or activation of blood in cardiopulmonary bypass (CPB) can be distinguished: mechanical damage, material-dependent, and material-independent blood activation.

The contribution to mechanical blood damage of various components of the extracorporeal circuit used for open-heart surgery cannot easily be analyzed in the complex clinical situation, but requires single-variable comparison in animal experiments.

We have analyzed in animals the hematological damage of priming solutions [24], tubing [10], pumps, oxygenators, and cardiotomy suction [4]. All these factors may induce blood damage, but not to the same extent on preference to different blood elements. In regard to the extent of damage, the blood-air contact plays the most important role in the destruction of blood elements.

We demonstrated experimentally that the damage to blood caused by bubble oxygenators can be minimized by using a membrane oxygenator, but that this only makes sense if the effect of blood-air contact in cardiotomy suction is additionally minimized. This can be achieved by means of an electronically controlled suction system that prevents aspiration of air in the suction line [4, 9].

Since the strict standardization of cardiopulmonary bypass conditions obtained in animal experiments cannot easily be achieved in the clinical situation, the presented differences in animal experiments could not always be demonstrated in randomized clinical studies.

However, categorizing the patients according to the main factors influencing blood damage such as bypass time and type of operation renders it possible to make comparison between groups with a difference in only one major variable. Among different types of open-heart operations, coronary artery bypass grafting (CABG) is probably the best standardized type of operation, and this category of patients is, therefore, mostly used for clinical investigations. We could identify, in this type of patient group with similar perfusion times, the same major mechanical source of blood damage: intensive blood-air contact (as was identified in animal experiments, but to a lesser extent). The significant differences in platelet count between bubble (BO) and membrane (MO) oxygenators demonstrated in animal experiments were not seen in patients [5]. Only by more sensitive measurements of platelet function and their release products, were differences found with regard to these types of oxygenators [3].

Beside direct cellular blood damage, the intensive blood-air contact of the bubble oxygenator also causes plasma protein denaturation, particularly of the proteins of the classical pathway of complement. However, measurement of these alterations in plasma proteins requires more sophisticated assays. Making use of these assays, we found an increase in C4a desarg in patients perfused with bubble oxygenators, whereas virtually no increase was seen in patients perfused with membrane oxygenators [23]. At the same time, C2 was consumed in the BO patients, while C2 levels remained unchanged in the MO patients. This is an important observation because the complement factors of the classical pathway play a major role in such host defense mechanisms as opsonizing capacity and serum bactericidical activity. Opsonization of a particle is required to enable a phagocyte to contact the target. It is completed by C3b-binding, which may occur through alternative or classical pathway activation. The classical pathway, mediated by IgG binding to the particle, plays a predominant role in efficient opsonization [22]. The serum bactericidal activity of serum, the capacity of the effector sequence of complement (C5—C9) to lyse gram-negative bacteria, is also thought to be mainly classical pathway-dependent. Intensive blood-air contact may cause IgG aggregates and subsequent activation and consumption of classical complement components. Indeed, opsonizing capacity and serum bactericidical activity were found to be significantly reduced in patients treated with bubblers, but not with membrane oxygenators [17].

The importance of these mechanisms of host defense was further evaluated in dogs undergoing CPB without antibiotic prophylaxis [13]. Bubblers affected these mechanisms, resulting in 50% sepsis post-bypass, which was not observed when membrane oxygenators were used. Currently since membrane oxygenators are preferred in most hospitals, direct, cellular blood damage and plasma denaturation are substantially reduced. However, material-blood activation still occurs, causing a whole-body inflammatory reaction, as defined by Kirklin in 1983 [12]. Back when he defined the whole body inflammatory reaction, this process was more or less characterized by only C3a being measured and correlated clinically with abnormal bleeding and organ dysfunction.

The question now is whether we are able to prevent the material blood activation, which would imply not only preventing complement activation, but also contact activation.

Of great interest recently is the outcome of various studies using pharmacological inhibitors to modify the blood activation process in CPB. Consistent and reproducible improvement of hemostasis in CPB was obtained with the use of a proteinase inhibitor. Our first study [16] showing this remarkable result in hemostasis was a coincidental finding while we searched for the effect of proteinase inhibitors on possible plasmin-induced complement activation in CPB.

The observed "bone dry" operation field and significantly reduced postoperative blood loss and blood requirements indicated an improvement in hemostatic function *during* and *after* cardiopulmonary bypass. The improvement in hemostatic function was even more convincing in situations where patients had a greater bleeding tendency, such as with reoperations and endocarditis [18]. Therefore, the use of the proteinase inhibitor aprotinin in CPB attracted considerable attention [6].

Five independent double-blind randomized clinical studies in Europe all verified the initial results of hemostatic improvements. Interesting was that the more blood activation occurred, e.g., using bubble oxygenators instead of membrane oxygenators, the greater the hemostatic benefit of aprotinin. The important issue of the improved hemostatic function is now the underlying mechanism that will dictate the optimal way of application. One hypothesis is that aprotinin preserved hemostasis by inhibition of plasmin. However, a pathologically increased fibrinolysis is not commonly observed after CPB. Therefore, this plasmin-inhibiting capacity of aprotinin alone cannot explain the hemostatic benefit of aprotinin.

A second hypothesis is that aprotinin inhibits the kallikrein system and, subsequently, the intrinsic clotting system. To obtain the kallikrein-inhibiting capacity a high circulating concentration of aprotinin (minimal 200 KIU/ml) is required. This hypothesis leads to maximizing the plasma concentration during CPB, and even higher doses of aprotinin, as used in the previous studies, are advocated.

The third hypothesis is based on the experience that hemostasis in cardiopulmonary bypass is related to platelet function, which can be affected by blood activation via, for example, plasmin [1]. Evidence for this hypothesis was obtained by the observation that GpIb platelet receptors were affected in the first 5 min of bypass, but were preserved by aprotinin [14]. Additionally, when aprotinin was only given in the prime of the circuit (2×10^6 KIU) the initial effect on platelets was equally prevented, and hemostasis improved to the same degree as when high continuous doses of aprotinin (6×10^6 KIU) were given to maintain appropriate plasma levels for effective kallikrein inhibition during the whole operation [15].

It can be considered crucial to not only determine the effects on hemostasis by aprotinin treatment, but also the side effects on the plasmatic systems of various doses in particular high vs low doses.

The activation of plasmatic systems can be identified by measurement of split products from the kinin, fibrinolytic, clotting, and complement systems (Fig. 1). We

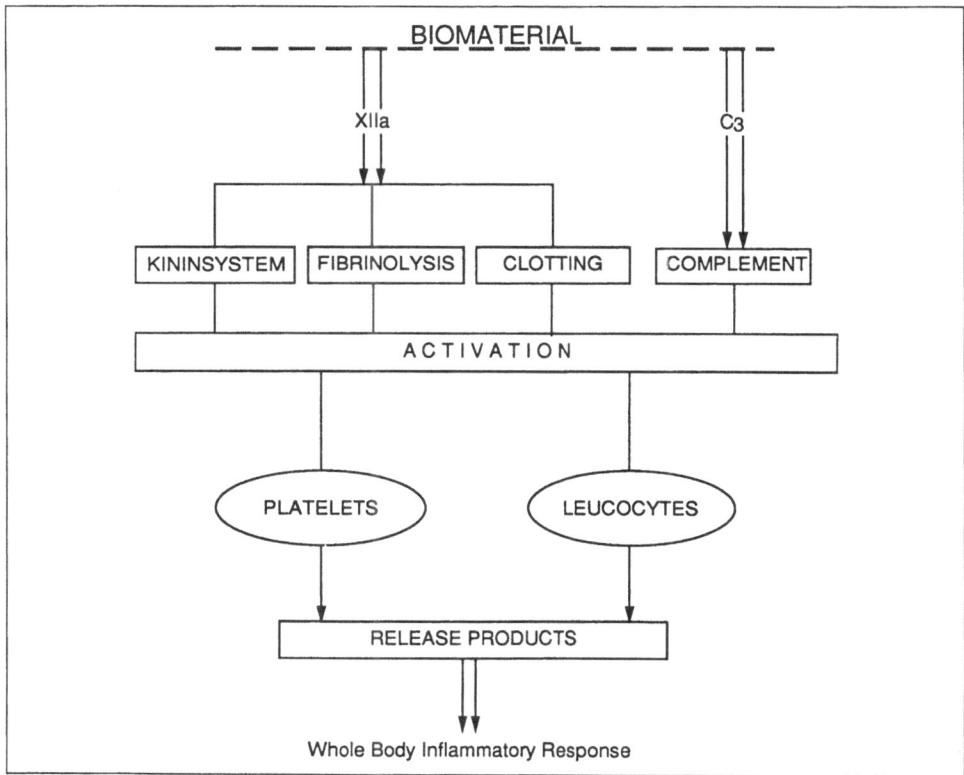

Fig. 1. The activation process of plasmatic systems.

have shown that aprotinin is able to inhibit the kinin, fibrinolytic, and, synergetically with heparin, the clotting system [19]. This latter becomes apparent by the fact that with the routine initial dose of heparin (3 mg/kg body weight) the usual activated clotting time (ACT) of 400—500 s will be increased to 800 s, and no more heparin will be given, if guided by the ACT. Although the high ACT in this respect reflects sufficient inhibition of the *intrinsic* clotting system, it does *not* necessarily reflect inhibition of the *extrinsic* clotting system. The practical consequence of this is that blood in the chest during operation and activated by the extrinsic clotting system and collected in the cardiotomy reservoir might clot when heparin levels are too low.

Interestingly other than aprotinin, plasmin inhibitors like tranexamine acid [7], and also the platelet inhibitor dipyridamol [20], seem to have a similar hemostatic effect in CPB. Furthermore, another protease inhibitor, FUT, is claimed to inhibit (beside the effects on the fibrinolytic and kinin systems) the clotting system, thus it can be used as an anticoagulant [2]. Additionally, FUT also inhibits the classical and alternative pathway of complement, although higher doses seem to be required as for the inhibition of the other systems. Lacking evaluation of the biochemical pathway of inhibition in these studies, little can be predicted of the efficacy and the side effects of those drugs in routine clinical use in various circumstances.

In this regard, not only the assays of the activation of the plasmatic systems are important, but also those of the release factors of the cellular blood components. Aprotinin, for example, specifically reduces the thromboxane release from the platelets, while no effect was seen on the BTG release, nor on any of the release products of the white bloodcells. The observation that BTG-release was not decreased by aprotinin suggests that degranulation of the platelets was not inhibited. As this degranulation is likely induced by ADP-induced activation of platelets or shear force damage, aprotinin appears to protect only against specific platelet agonists.

However, administration of aspirin to improve vein-graft patency will specifically inhibit the arachidonic acid metabolism of platelets and, in addition to the affected platelet adhesive receptors during cardiopulmonary bypass, increases the risk of serious postoperative bleeding. We demonstrated, however, that aprotinin combined with aspirin preserved platelet hemostatic function while platelet aggregatory function remained inhibited. This combination resulted in significantly less bleeding [21] but might still improve vein graft patency.

Specific activation of granulocytes by complement activation during cardiopulmonary bypass could be prevented by corticosteroids which has no effect on complement activation but results in inhibition of LTB4 release, whereas elastase release was virtually unaffected. Most importantly, TNF release from monocytes and macrophages could completely be prevented by corticosteroids [8]. Since TNF release is considered to be caused by endotoxin activation of monocytes, apparently this additional source of blood activation during CPB has to be assumed.

Other than this additional source of blood activation in CPB, still another source of complement activation exists from the heparin-protamine complex after CPB [11]. A safe way of preventing this activation pathway might be not to give protamine to patients who received aprotinin. We already demonstrated that, despite the increased inhibition of the clotting system by aprotinin, hemostasis remained normal *during* operation, which indicates that conversion of heparin *after* operation is no longer needed to restore hemostasis.

272

Although complete pharmacological inhibition of the blood activation processes during CPB might be achieved in the near future, systemic administration of potent drugs always induces unwanted systemic side effects.

Therefore, another promising approach to reduce blood damage and activation during CPB is the use of non-thrombogenic materials or material coatings. In this regard heparin-coated CPB circuits are now under clinical investigation and the preliminary results indicate a decrease in activation of the contact system. Interesting in this regard is that the heparin-coated surfaces resulted in such a change that *no* complement activation occurred after administration of protamine at the end of bypass.

Further evaluation of material coatings with other drugs might elucidate their potentials to completely prevent blood activation in CPB locally and, therefore might eliminate side effects when these drugs are administered systematically. It appears from this survey that by better understanding the blood activation processes in CPB a new break-through in safety of extracorporeal circulation will be introduced in the near future.

Acknowledgement

This survey is based on the work of several coworkers in my group over the years: their contributions are specified in the references.

References

1. Adelman B, Michelson AD, Loscalzo J et al. (1985) Plasmin effect on platelet glycoprotein IB-von Willebrand factor interactions. Blood 65: 32—40
2. Aoyama T, Ino Y, Ozeki M, Oda M, Sato T, Kohiyama Y, Suzuki S, Fujita M (1984) Pharmacological studies of FUT-175, Nafamstat Mesilate I. Inhibition of protease activity in in vitro and in vivo experiments. Jap J Pharmacol 35: 203—227
3. Boonstra PW, van Imhoff GW, Eijsman L, Kootstra GJ, Homan van der Heide JN, Karliczek GF, Wildevuur ChRH (1985). Reduced platelet activation and improved hemostasis after controlled cardiotomy suction during clinical membrane oxygenator perfusions. J Thorac Cardiovasc Surg 89: 900—906
4. Ten Duis HJ, de Jong JCF, van Asseldonk AGM, Smit Sibinga CTh, Wildevuur ChRH (1978). Improved hemocompatibility in open heart surgery. Trans Am Soc Artif Intern Organs 24: 656—660
5. Dungen JJAM van den, Karliczek GF, Brenken U, Homan van der Heide JN, Wildevuur ChRH (1982). Clinical study of blood trauma during perfusion with membrane and bubble oxygenators. J Thorac Cardiovasc Surg 83: 108—116
6. Editorial (1988). Can drugs reduce surgical blood loss? Lancet ii: 155—156
7. Horrow JC, Hlavacek J, Strong MD, Collier W, Brodsky I, Goldman SM, Goel IP (1990). Prophylactic transamic acid decreases bleeding after cardiac operations. J Thorac Cardiovasc Surg 99: 70—74
8. Jansen NJG, Oeveren W van, v. d. Broek L, Oudemans-van Straten HM, Stoutenbeek CP, Chang Njoek Joen M, Roozendaal KJ, Eijsman L, Wildevuur CRH: Inhibition of the reperfusion phenomena in cardiopulmonary bypass by dexamethasone. J Thorac Cardiovasc Surg, in press
9. De Jong JCF, ten Duis HJ, Smit Sibinga CTh, Wildevuur ChRH (1980). Hematologic aspects of cardiotomy suction in cardiac operations. J Thorac Cardiovasc Surg 79: 227—236
10. De Jong JCF, Smit Sibinga CTh, Wildevuur ChRH (1979). Platelet behaviour in extracorporeal circulation. Transfusion 19: 72—755.

11. Kirklin JK, Chenoweth DE, Naftel DC, Blackstone EH, Kirklin JW, Bitran DD, Curd JG, Reves JG, Samuelson PN (1986). Effects of protamine administration after cardiopulmonary bypass on complement, blood elements, and the hemodynamic state. Ann Thorac Surg 41: 193—199

12. Kirklin JK, Westaby S, Blackstone EH, Kirklin JW, Chenoweth DE, Pacifico AD (1983). Complement and the damaging effects of cardiopulmonary bypass. J Thorac Cardiovasc Surg 86: 845—857

13. Oeveren W van, Dankert J, Wildevuur ChRH (1987). Bubble oxygenation and cardiotomy suction impair the host defense during cardiopulmonary bypass: a study in dogs. Ann Thorac Surg 44: 523—528

14. Oeveren W van, Eijsman L, Roozendaal KJ, Wildevuur CRH (1988). Platelet preservation by aprotinin during cardiopulmonary bypass. Lancet ii: 644

15. Oeveren W van, Harder MP, Roozendaal KJ, Eijsman L, Wildevuur CRH (1990) Aprotinin protects against the initial effect of cardiopulmonary bypass. J Thorac Cardiovasc Surg 99: 788—797

16. Oeveren W van, Jansen NJG, Bidstrup BP, Royston D, Westaby S, Neuhof H, Wildevuur CRH (1987). Effects of aprotinin on hemostatic mechanisms in cardiopulmonary bypass. Ann Thorac Surg 44: 640—645

17. Oeveren W van, Kazatchkine MD, Descamps-Latscha B, Maillet F, Fischer E, Carpentier A, Wildevuur CHR (1985). Deleterious effects of cardiopulmonary bypass: a prospective study of bubble versus membrane oxygenation. J Thorac Cardiovasc Surg 89: 888—889

18. Royston D, Bidstrup BP, Taylor KM, Sapsford RN (1987). Effect of aprotinin on need for blood transfusion after repeat open-heart surgery. Lancet i: 1289—1291

19. de Smet AFA, Chang Njoek Joen M, Oeveren W van, Roozendaal KJ, Harder MP, Eijsman L, Wildevuur CRH: Increased anticoagulation during cardiopulmonary bypass by aprotinin. J Thorac Cardiovasc Surg, in press

20. Teoh KH, Christakis GT, Weisel RD, Wong PY, Mee V, Ivanov J, Madonik MM, Levitt DS, Reilly PA, Rosenfeld JM, Glynn MFX (1988). Dipyridamole preserved platelets and reduced blood loss after cardiopulmonary bypass. J Thorac Cardiovasc Surg 96: 332—341

21. Tabuchi N, Oeveren W van, Eijsman L, Roozendaal KJ, Gu Yj, Wildevuur ChRH (1990). Preserved hemostasis during the combined use of aprotinin and aspirin in CABG operations. This Book.

22. Verbrugh HA, Dijk WCvan, Erne M Evan, Peters R, Peterson PK, Verhoef J (1979). Quantitation of the third component of human complement attached to the surface of opsonized bacteria: opsonin-defecient sera and phagocytosis-resistant strains. Infect Immun 26: 808—812

23. Wildevuur CHR, Oeveren Wvan (1987). The membrane artificial lung. Kolff Festschrift; Artificial Organs, Proc int symposium. pp 443—454

24. Woltjes J, de Jong JCF, ten Duis HJ, Wildevuur ChRH (1979). The priming of extracorporeal circuits: the effect on canine blood elements. Transfusion 19: 552—554

Author's address:
MD, PhD. Ch. R. H. Wildevuur
Academisch Ziekenhuis Groningen
Department of Cardiopulmonary Surgery, Research Division
Oostersingel 59
9713 EZ Groningen, The Netherlands

V: Panel Discussion

Changing Concepts of Blood Use in Cardiac Surgery

HETZER:

I welcome you to our panel discussion and I am happy to introduce to you our panelists: Prof. Wolner from Vienna, Prof. Edmunds from Philadelphia, and Dr. Schubel, who is a cardiac surgeon at the Charité University Hospital in East Berlin; also, Dr. Solem from Sweden, Prof. von der Emde from Erlangen, and Dr. Fraedrich from Freiburg, Germany. I would like to divide the discussion in the same manner as the whole symposium was organized, primarily going into practical methods of blood salvage methods. I would like to ask the surgeons what kind of blood loss they presently expect, and what their method of blood transfusion in general is?

Prof. Wolner, what is the average blood loss right now? How many units of blood do you prepare for a regular open-heart case, what kind of blood substitute is this, is it fresh blood, is it a full unit of blood, is it packed cells, fresh frozen plasma, what about platelet concentrates, what number of hemoglobin content do you accept during bypass and after the bypass, and how many patients do you presently expect to be operated without homologous blood transfusion?

WOLNER:

Question No. 1: We have, a mean blood loss of 800 ml in all cases; that is in good agreement with that of other groups. Second question is the blood substitution. We prepare now for every patient 5 units of whole blood. Third question: We give blood in the heart-lung machine when the hematocrit is below 28%, and about the post-operative value, hemoglobin or hematocrit, I must say we have no strict rules. I think that strict rules are senseless, you have to look at the patient since there are a lot of patients who tolerate, let us say 8 g/% hemoglobin, and then you have others who seem to be, from the clinical point of view, also in a worse situation, let us say with 9 g/% or with a hematocrit of about 30%, and so on. So, what is the post-operative transfusion rate and the indication for transfusion? You have to combine laboratory data on the one side and the clinical aspect of the patient on the other side. Last question: How many patients we expect that we can operate without blood. There were in our control group a little bit less than 50%, and in our two studies which we have done with Trasylol there are now over 70%.

EDMUNDS:

We set up blood very differently depending on what the problem is. If it is a problem of valves plus coronaries or a redo or a very elderly patient, 80 years old or even 90 years old, we will set up a little more blood because the incidence of bleeding post-operatively in those patients is greater than it is in a middle-aged or a first-time coronary revascularization, but for most of our patients we would set up two units of blood. Intra-operatively, we use a cell saver and recover the blood, we pack it; we only set up packed cells, we do not set up whole blood; and, post-operatively, usually for those straightforward patients, we will not use retransfusion of shed blood because they just do not bleed much. Now, for the ones who do bleed much, redos, elderly patients patients with very thick ventricles, patients who have a low-cardiac output syndrome, for those patients we will use the outer transfusion device, we will also set up platelet packs, which, in our hospital, come in groups of six. So there were two platelet packs set up in order to have 12 platelet transfusions. We also give additional protamine and FFP post-operatively. We — because of the Federal Food and Drug Administration, which is one of the more repressive regulatory bodies in the United States at the present time — are not able to use any of the new drugs that you have been using — aprotinin, dipyridamole intravenously, etc. So we have no experience with that in the United States.

SCHUBEL:

Some words about the blood loss after the operation. We have in adults on the average 500 to 600 ml. If we have one liter of blood loss after the operation we have to become active and have to take the patient back to the operating room; in reoperations this is another fact. The preperation of the patient; normally we have 5 units of homologous blood prepared. Fresh blood we only use it in children below 15 kg or in patients with reoperations. This year we have introduced Trasylol in our regime and we have seen a reduction of blood loss after the operation, but we have no exact control group. The autologous blood sampling: we are now preparing our center to have the organization and have enough equipment to do this. There are some technical problems and, for us, also some financial considerations.

FRAEDRICH:

For the past 2 years, we have not used blood priming, except for children or patients who are on hemodialysis. We routinely use the cell saver; we retransfuse shed mediastinal blood when there are more than 300 ml within the first 6 h, and with these blood-saving procedures our mean blood is now about 650 ml. We could reduce the blood requirements by about 30% within the last year. We usually transfuse blood when the hemoglobin is below 9%, but dependent on the clinical condition of the patient, of course. Looking at the blood prepared in our blood bank, usually this is five units of packed red cells and three units of fresh frozen plasma, but only half of this will be brought to the operation theatre and the remaining part stays at the blood bank. Even without aprotinin, we are now up to that point to operate on 60% of our elective pts. without any (foreign) blood transfusion. It is also important to point out that we have restricted the use of fresh frozen plasma.

VAN DER EMDE:

Now we have five units of packed cells available for every patient, for a routine patient, and we are not differentiating in secondary operation and primary operation; the average drainage is about 600 cc; the retransfusion rate depends on the nurses and the staff. About 50% will be retransfused or sometimes it is going up to 80%. We are retransfusing up to 1 l, and if it is above this, we think about going back to surgery, because usually then it will be a surgical bleeding and not a coagulation problem. But we set the retransfusion system to run for 12 h, so if it is draining 500 cc or 600 cc, we set it to 50 cc per h, so this goes then automatically for 12 h. The system has also the advantage that if you are in the middle of the night, you can of course postpone going back to surgery, or if you are still in an operation then, you can also postpone it; you have more time and you retransfuse all the time, and then you might retransfuse also 1 or 2 l. We would like to have the hematocrit during extracorporeal circulation above 25%, and in the ICU we keep the hemoglobin at 9 g/%; otherwise we will retransfuse depending on the state of the patient and we will discharge the patient with a hemoglobin of 9 g/%. Sometimes, or regularly, it is above 9%, but if it is below 9%, we will retransfuse. We will not give FFP routinely unless we think it is really a bleeding problem. And we will give additional protamine if the ACT is above 250. We would like to have autologous blood available, predonated, but it is not possible, or it is only exceptional that we have autologous blood available.

SOLEM:

Concerning the bleeding, I can refer to different studies we did. Last year we concluded the desmopressin study including 100 patients; in this study, we had 760 ml of bleeding, and in another smaller group of patients we had 800, and in the data I presented yesterday it was 1 l, so that is our average bleeding at the University Center. The result is, concerning transfusion: We will transfuse at a hematocrit of 28 or 30 or a hemoglobin of 8 in the early post-operative period and between 8 and 9 depending on how the patient is doing. We will transfuse two packed cells and one plasma on average, if we look at the total material of patients. We will order from the blood bank 5 units of packed red cells and 5 plasma and we routinely use retransfusion post-operatively in about 90% of the patients; we do this with the cardiotomy reservoir from the pump and we use an infusion pump. We use a lot of albumin, and no fresh frozen plasma if there is not a special indication. For volume replacement, we use dextrane for the first 24 h. We are very restrictive above platelets and only if the bleeding time is more than 12, 13, 15 min, and sometimes it really is 25 min, then we use platelets. With all this together, we can do about 30% of the surgery without blood.

HETZER:

Thank you. There is quite a uniformity in some aspects, but disparity in several. I think I should give our practice and opinion also. Our average blood loss has been ranging between 500 and 600 cc in the past few years. We still prepare 6 units of packed red cells for every case and for thoracic aneurysm cases we prepare 10 units of packed cells, no fresh blood, and only in hematological indications, post-operatively (but very rarely), and no platelets. We try to aim at a hemoglobin of 8 g/% post-operatively, if the patient is not too old and if the patient does not show symptoms of anaemia but this regime sometimes brings us into frustration, because we then later can see when we need to transfer the patient back to the cardiologist, as a routine 5 or 6 days after the operation, then they are given blood because the cardiologist thinks that 8 g/% is not sufficient. So, I think this has to be taken into account when you look at the whole picture. As I have already mentioned, we can presently count on approximately 60% of the coronary cases to be handled without any blood transfusion; this percentage is not so in the valvular patient group and, of course, not in the pediatric group where we need blood, at least in the infant surgery, to prime the pump. I would like to ask the panel what choice of oxygenators they have at present, whether bleeding coagulation aspects are in any way influenced by the choice of the oxygenator; we now use the membrane oxygenators all the time, but I would like to know whether there is any distinction among the panelists.

FRAEDRICH:

We routinely use membrane oxygenators and we are convinced that this will have an effect on blood saving and contact activation, too, and I think that even in membrane oxygenators there are differences. If you have capillaries, if the blood is going in- or outside of these capillaries and so on, and we are doing investigations focussing on the different effects between different membrane oxygenators.

VON DER EMDE:

We are using membrane oxygenators only in 5% of patients. A couple of years ago, we did a study on the hemoglobin difference using different bubble oxygenators and we could not find any difference concerning the oxygenator, but of course we saw a dependence on the bypass time. Therefore, we are now using the membranes if we expect bypass times above 1 h.

SOLEM:

We use only membranes, too, and we changed to membranes about 1 year ago, and we did not notice any difference concerning the bleeding.

SCHUBEL:

We use, in most cases, the bubble oxygenator, and only for 20% of the patients do we use membrane oxygenators, but I cannot say that in those cases the blood loss is diminished, because these are the cases with longer bypass time.

EDMUNDS:

We now exclusively use a hollowfiber membrane oxygenator but for economic reasons and not for medical reasons. In my opinion, and the data do support this, I do not think that there is any significant difference between the bubble and the membrane oxygenators with respect to coagulation and platelets in the first 2 h. Beyond about 2 h or 1.5 h, I think the membrane oxygenator does have an advantage because bubble oxygenators continue to denature proteins. I think you are going into the actual loss of coagulation factor proteins as you go into the longer bypasses and the membrane oxygenator with a stable surface does not continue this process that much.

WOLNER:

We use, in most of the cases, the bubble oxygenator, and only for the difficult cases, the old patients, do we use the membrane oxygenator, but I must say that this is partially an individual decision from surgeon to surgeon, in accordance with the perfusionist.

HETZER:

I would like to move onto the next part, which comprises the non-pharmacological methods to reduce blood use. I would like to ask the panelists again for their opinion towards blood predonation, the use of the cell saver, whether they use controlled suction for the cell saver, and what is their policy of blood retranfusion, and also what is their policy of using fibrin glue and other topical hemostatics. To be fair, I would like to give our policy briefly.

My colleague, Prof. Schmucker, has shown our system of blood predonation which is not quite complete, because about half of our patients come from all areas of West Germany, where there is a service capable of collecting blood from patients not available everywhere. In Berlin itself, we use a commercial company that runs this fairly well, and we do this mostly also for economical reasons, because they do it in a cheaper way than the university blood bank does it. We initially used the cell saver quite frequently, but we have been somewhat concerned about its use, because I have observed that a number of patients and a higher proportion than other patients — tended to have high fever immediately after the operation; I had my bacteriologist run some studies on the cell saver and he has found out that when you have continuous suction on the cell saver then you probably run a large amount of bacteria by sucking air through the cell saver, and from this experience we have reduced the use of the cell saver only for cases where we expect a higher blood loss, such as multiple re-operation or thoracic aneurysm cases. I would like to have the opinion of the panelists on that. We would essentially use blood retransfusion for 6 h after the operation, but not in patients who have been operated on in a septic state, and we would start when there is more than 200 cc in the cardiotomy reservoir. We use the fibrin glue in a limited way, usually not more than maybe 1 ml a case, and it is a rare instance in which we use more.

WOLNER:
First question: We have no experience, or I would say only in 10 or 20 cases with predonation, but that is one of the things that I have learned here from this symposium, that we have to look more at the autologous blood donation. What we are doing is, immediately after the start of the extracorporeal circulation, we take, depending on each case, 500 cc to 1 l blood, which we can retransfuse immediately after the operation. We use the cell saver for suction, but we only let it work if we have a special amount; I think, if it is more than 300 ml, then we start using it. There are some studies on bacterial contamination and I think we should do bacteriological studies periodically when using the cell saver.
   Concerning fibrin glue, as Dr. Hetzer mentioned before, we were the first to use it in cardiac surgery. It seems that this has now become a routine, but a very restricted routine in our unit since it is very expensive.

EDMUNDS:
In our unit we have over half of patients with postinfarction angina or unstable angina, and for those patients you have to operate on within 12 to 36 h; they are not elective cases, so the autologous blood will never probably have a very big use in our unit or in some other units in the U.S. I think this is the third or fourth study over the last 20 years in which I have participated, and I have never been a co-investigator; none of the studies has shown anything. This really does not show any improvement in bleeding postoperatively, but it seems to show a compelling need to do this study every 1—5 years. We use the cell saver and we use it a lot. I am not too worried about bacterial contamination, although I think the potential is there. You have a whole lot bigger contamination area with the surgical wound. We do use laminar flow in the operating rooms, cardiac operating rooms, in an effort to decrease the infection from the field. The dilution of the cell saver is such that I think unless the bacteria really stick to the red cells you will not get a very big load. You get some load, but not a very big load. And the same is true for the pump itself. Auto-transfusion, postoperatively, there is probably a little more chance of just changing over from the cell saving and hanging up the bag of contamination there. The most important, as far as we are concerned about infection, is the central lines as we call them, and the intravenous tubes for infusing drugs, and so on. And we try to get those out very quickly, postoperatively.

SCHUBEL:
As I said before, we are preparing for the predonation of blood, but I can say the same as Prof. Wolner said, most of our patients live a long distance from our center and they are only 3 days preoperatively in our unit and thus it is difficult to perform such a predonation regime. We have no cell saver, but we use the cardiotomy blood from the heart lung machine, but there are different opinions between the surgeons and anaesthesiologists and we think sometimes there is more blood loss after the operation if we use the blood from the cardiotomy reservoir. We use the drainage blood only in cases with more blood loss than 1 l and re-do's. The last point, fibrin glue. We only use it in cases of aneurysmectomy.

SOLEM:
Concerning predonation: It is very rare in our institution for two reasons: geography, some of the patients will travel 500 km to come to our center and, secondly, is that the blood bank people are

280

not very enthusiastic about it; they have all kinds of excuses not to do it and they have restrictions concerning the diagnosis. They are not allowed to have aortic stenosis, they are not allowed to have severe angina, etc., etc., so it is actually very rare. When the patients come to the clinic 2 days prior to surgery, we do plasmapheresis on them and collect 1 l of plasma, store it for 2 days, and then administer it after surgery. And that is interesting, because we have practically eliminated the use of plasma in these patients. But it is cumbersome and I do not think it will be very popular because it takes 1 h or 2 to do it. Cell saver, we use it for cases where we believe we will have bleeding: redo's, and aneurysms; we are going to put up a sterile suction reservoir, cardiotomy reservoir in all patients, so we can connect the cell saver if we have bleeding post-operatively. I described the earlier use in 90% of the cases and, yes, we do use fibrin glue when we need it.

VON DER EMDE:

Again, concerning pre-donation: We would like to have it more and we think if the surgeon convinces the patients, they will all predonate. But if the cardiologist or the transfusionist talks to them then they will find only a few agreeable ones. And the contamination of the shed blood: I think if you are using a closed system there cannot be any contamination if it is connected in the operating room for the first time. We do use the fibrin glue only congenital heart defects, and nearly never in adult cases.

FRAEDRICH:

I just mentioned our policy, but looking at predonation, I think we all should emphasize this problem. It is an organization problem, but it has to be solved; it is a very important point. Viewing cell saver and fibrin glue, I think that a lot of us use it, but one has to be aware of the costs that are coming with these two systems. And looking at the contamination, we did a study on 30 patients in which we took blood cultures at consecutive points, beginning with the introduction of the anesthesia, heart lung machine, cell saver, in the retransfusion reservoir, after retransfusing a patient, and so on, until the next morning. We found a contamination in 30% of the probes from the devices and in 12% of the probes from the patients, respectively. But only in 3 of these 30 patients we found more than one of the cultures contaminated. So, we are convinced that this system is not in danger of high contamination.

HETZER:

I would like to add a comment on the predonation system. I believe that in West Germany, we probably will have an area-covering system in the near future, where all patients that are scheduled for cardiac surgery in advance can have blood predonated. In Berlin, this is very easy, as you can imagine because the area is limited and, of course, we have to exclude a number of patients as my colleague Schmucker has shown you. Still, I believe that this is a good way to save homologous blood transfusion and in an increasing way it is demanded by the patients themselves because they are more and more aware of the potential dangers of homologous transfusions, and I have been asked several times, and in an increasing number, by the patients themselves whether they can donate their own blood before, and thus avoid transfused blood. Now, relative to the infection via the cell saver, I would like to add that, of course, we have also a laminar flow, but the bacteriologist found out that the higher amount of cultures he found — was mostly related to the number of people in the hall, irrespective of the technical set-ups of the hall.

EDMUNDS:

Yes, this is correct, but the dean requires the students to be in these areas and other people to be there. One thing that has not come up, and I have to ask may co-panelists and perhaps the audience: What about the idea of frozen blood, particularly for a pre-donation. I know that the United States has services, we are interested in and we did have it for quite a while, but I have not heard about it recently, and maybe someone could say why that does not work. I understand that the blood can be preserved for 6 to 12 months.

HETZER:

I believe, Dr. Dietrich in his summary mentioned this. Could you repeat your statement according to that?

DIETRICH:
We use the high glycerol rapid freezing technique, and we are storing the red cells in liquid nitrogen for about 3 months, so we start collection of blood if the patient comes to the waiting list and then we draw the blood. Normally, we take out 2 units of blood and put it in the deep freezer and 1 unit is stored in the liquid phase; it works quite well. The quality of the red cells is not as good as in the normal unit, but it works and the advantage of this is, we are not depending on the time of operation. We have a lot of time between two donations, so the hematocrit can recover in the patient and we are not forced to withdraw some patients from the donation program because of a drop of hemoglobin. So, we are very satisfied with that method and it is not as expensive as it is said to be, so our costs are about 200 DM for a frozen unit of red cells, plasma, fresh frozen plasma; this is the same you pay for a homologous unit.

EMUNDS:
Do you know how long it is safe to store frozen blood?

DIETRICH:
Well, 10 years, or something like that.

HETZER:
I would like to ask the panelists to make a very brief statement on their policy towards Jehovah's Witnesses. I know that is very different from one unit to the other. Some surgeons completely reject Jehovah's Witnesses from open-heart surgery. Others are quite liberal.
I would like to ask whether you operate on Jehovah's Witnesses and what methods or procedures you discuss with the patients beforehand, before you begin operation. Our policy is that we will not operate on an adult patient unless he accepts the cell saver and blood retransfusion of shed blood.

EDMUNDS:
For infants in the United States sometimes a judge will supercede the parents' wishes and rule that when the infant grows to legal age he can decide whether to accept this religious faith that he has inherited.

WOLNER:
Our experience with this group of patients is very limited since these patients in Austria go to Graz. That is the reason why they have had altogether 70 cases there. We have had only a few, and in these few cases our policy is the same as you have mentioned before. The Austrian law is that, in children, even though you have told the parents you will not transfuse blood, when you are in a situation where you have to do it, you can do it.

SCHUBEL:
We have not had many patients who were Jehovah's Witnesses. We have had in the last 10 years, I think, 5 to 6 cases. Very important is the discussion between the patient and the doctor before the operation, and I think there are two different groups. One accepts extracorporeal circulation as being a part of the body, others are strictly against that management and in such cases we do not accept to operate on them. In children there is a special consideration if there is a very dangerous situation, we do transfuse blood and our law is such that we will not be prosecuted.

SOLEM:
In Sweden, we have the situation where Jehovah's Witnesses decided that autotransfusion is okay as long as the line is connected to the patient. So, Jehovah's Witnesses will accept our auto-transfusion, therefore, we operate on adult Jehovah's Witnesses; we actually have had patients who have moved from other areas in Sweden to our referral area to be operated in our clinic as some clinics will not operate on them. We accept their belief, if necessary that they are allowed to die without getting blood. Fortunately, that has not happened in our clinic. However, it happened in a general surgical department where I cooperated as an auto-transfusionist and this man was 40 years old; the surgeons called his wife and explained that the man was going to die if he did not get blood and the

wife refused to compromise and he died. I think one should think about the personnel. You must talk with them, with the anaesthesiologist and nurses, so that everybody knows that this situation can come up because otherwise you get into moral problems with the personnel around you. For children, we never operate without permission to give blood.

VON DER EMDE:
In general, we accept Jehovah's Witnesses and we did quite a lot in the past. If we think that we have to transfuse, for instance, if there is a double valve replacement with a double bypass and the patient refuses blood transfusion, we would not accept him for surgery. We also did some children, no transpositions and no Fallot's, but if we promise the parents or the patients not to give any homologous blood we would be strict on this, but on this closed-loop system of retransfusion, I think this is everywhere accepted by Jehovah's Witnesses.

HETZER:
I think the problem is the priming of the heart lung machine in infants and as I mentioned before, we have operated several children, but in each instance, I had a prior court decision to have the court overtake the right to decide during the time of operation.

VON DER EMDE:
Yes, but the parents have to give permission for the operation, otherwise, they would withdraw.

HETZER:
Certainly, my experience has been that in general. I remember only one case where the mother finally took her child with a transposition to Dublin and the child was operated there, obviously with the promise of the surgeon not to have a transfusion, and the child died. In all the other cases, I could feel some sort of relief on the side of the parents when the decision was taken away from them.

FRAEDRICH:
Prof. Schlosser presented our modalities yesterday. But I think there are two things that have to be mentioned. First you have to mention the increased risk on the consent form for adults, and, secondly, what Dr. Solem said, the entire team must be prepared to operate on these patients, this is quite important.

HETZER:
We come to the final and I guess, the most important point: pharmacological methods to reduce blood loss. The question to the surgeons is: Do you use any pharmacological methods? Do you use aprotinin, routinely, or if not, in which cases? What is your impression? Do you foresee increased use of it in the future?

FRAEDRICH:
I think it is the primary method in patients undergoing reoperations, in patients at high risk of bleeding, let's say on aspirin or anti-coagulation therapy, and we do it in patients who refuse any blood donation. I think before administering it routinely in every open-heart surgical patient, one has to definitely find out the dosage, the concentration we need. One cannot forget all the other blood-saving methods that can be used, especially predonation of blood. And I think one has to be aware of some side-effects. One has to look at renal function and, especially in re-operation, when in a first operation aprotinin has been administered, one has to routinely perform a skin test or antibody test.

VON DER EMDE:
We do not use it routinely, but we used aprotinin in individual cases, but no longer in coronary cases, because we had probably two cases where the bypasses closed. In one case, a redo first performed in another hospital, I did not know why it happened that three bypasses closed off, and so the patient came to our hospital and we put four new bypasses in, quite good coronary vessels, 2 millimeters in diameter and good run-off, and everything was routine. But he closed all four bypasses.

So, this patient had aprotinin before and had it in our hospital also and, therefore, we were a little bit irritated that it might have something to do with aprotinin. But in all other redo cases we use it; we found that in the redo cases, mostly the valve cases, it reduces the blood drainage to half.

SOLEM:
That is our experience; we did a prospective pilot study on aprotinin and we found that it reduced the bleeding to half. We have quite an excessive experience with the DDABP or desmopressin. I myself completed the study of 100 elective coronary bypass cases where we did give DDABP prophylactically to see if it reduced the bleeding and it actually did not. It did not have any effect on the bleeding. However, we could measure a 50% increase of the factor VIII after giving DDABP, and we could also measure an increase in the von Willebrand factor, but it did not influence the bleeding.

HETZER:
As I mentioned before, I was a bit skeptical, because I have been confronted with aprotinin, as was everybody else, for several indications, but finally, I found myself convinced by the experience with patients that were on aspirin before, and re-operations, and also patients who were operated in a septic state, and although we have not been using aprotinin for all routine cases, I do believe that eventually we will come to that.

SCHUBEL:
We do not use Trasylol routinely, but we use it in re-operations and in some risk patients. My impression is that, in most cases, the blood loss is lower, but in some cases we have seen a little more hemolysis and I cannot definitely say that is an effect of Trasylol, but that is my impression.

EDMUNDS:
We, of course, do not use it at all because we are not allowed to. With respect to aprotinin, I think that it has some effect after myocardial revascularization. If it has any effect on the patency of grafts that is going to seriously impede introduction in the United States. Now, as far as the mechanism of action, I think it appears to potentiate the effect of heparin. It seems to inhibit fibrinolysis and I am very persuaded by the Freiburg data that it has an effect on the platelets. This is 6PIb, substantiated by von Oeveren and Wildevuur's work demonstrating the preservation of the 6PIP receptor. So, there is some partial effect on platelets in addition to the inhibition of fibrinolysis. Now, I think the dosis schedule is probably crazy. I am not at all convinced that you have to give it pre-operatively at all. I suspect you have to give it in the prime because the Edinburgh surgeons did not, and they found no effect. And I think you certainly have to give it during bypass because of its half-life. But I am not at all sure that you need to give it in the beginning. The reason that you give it in the beginning is that most of the inner reaction between blood and a foreign surface occurs with the first contact. I am not sure that there is good data that this was going on with aprotinin in bypass systems. And also, you are giving massive doses of it, but maybe this is necessary to inhibit the kallikrein effect. The Freiburg data again show that it really has a relatively low effect on neutrophils.

WOLNER:
There are a lot of pharmacological methods other than aprotinin to control bleeding. The first is that we inform our patients that they should stop aspirin 1 or 2 weeks before operation. I would say that it seems that a high percentage of our patients come on aspirin to operation and we could prevent bleeding in these patients if they would stop aspirin. So, at first this is a question of information. I think that anaesthesia, particularly the pharmacological control of blood pressure, is also very important for bleeding, especially in old patients. The patients who bleed more before going on bypass, usually tend to bleed more after extracorporeal circulation. Concerning Trasylol, we have done some preliminary studies, one of which is very interesting in transplant patients. These transplant patients are usually on coumarin or aspirin when being transferred as an emergency case for transplantation. We have compared 10 patients with and 10 patients without aprotinin and we have seen in the group with Trasylol that we could reduce blood transfusion in 7 of 10 cases. That means there was a drastic drop in blood transfusion.

284

Recently, we started a controlled study with different dosages. It seems that this is also a question; should we take a higher or a lower dosage? We have now a study protocol with a placebo group and two different groups with two different dosage and application protocols, and we shall see what the results of this study will be.

HETZER:

No question, the dosage of aprotinin, the time of application, and the mode of application is still controversial, as we have seen. To come back to the aspirin patients: A large number of patients, who have not followed the advice to stop aspirin beforehand come with aspirin. In the past it was our policy to let them wait a week or two. Now, we have started to operate on those with aprotinin and this aspect really was convincing for me, because we did not have this type of bleeding that we had experienced, at least in some of the aspirin patients in the past.

Ladies and Gentleman, our time is over. I think we should stop at this point. I would like to thank first the panelists, the surgeons. I would like to thank all the speakers, all the experts who have come here and have contributed to a very concise, interesting, and stimulating symposium, and I would also thank the audience. I would like to thank the Bayer Company for sponsoring and organizing this symposium, in particular Dr. Schumann, and I would like to thank Dr. Royston and again my co-worker Dr. Friedel, who have done most of the work. I am sure we will meet again at some necessary future meetings on this same topic; many questions remain to be answered, and I think we are probably in the middle of a process which makes everybody, especially the surgeons, but also the anesthesiologists and the perfusionists more aware of the need to look at blood loss, and to look at how to handle blood loss, and I think we have been quite successful in that.
Thank you.

H. O. Vetter; R. Hetzer; H. Schmutzler (Eds.)

Ischemic Mitral Incompetence

1991. XII, 212 pp. Cloth DM 74,–
ISBN 3-7985-0799-6

Ischemic Mitral Incompetence provides a review of the current knowledge of mitral valve insufficiency. Diagnostic techniques and indications for surgical interventions, particularly coronary bypass operation, valve reconstruction and mitral replacement are presented by leading international scientists. This volume offers a practical overview of the pathophysiological changes in coronary heart disease leading to ischemic mitral incompetence.

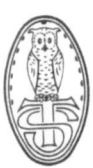

Steinkopff Dr. D. Steinkopff Verlag
Saalbaustr. 12, 6100 Darmstadt/FRG